BARRON'S

ADULT CCRN® EXAM

WITH 3 PRACTICE TESTS

SECOND EDITION

Pat Juarez, MS, RN

ABOUT THE AUTHOR

Pat Juarez, MS, RN, has critical care nursing experience as a clinical nurse specialist (CNS), staff nurse, and educator, and she held the CCRN credential for over 40 years. As the clinical development specialist for critical care, Pat developed and provided oversight for the critical care nursing curriculum for a large health care system for over 10 years. She currently teaches a CCRN certification review course on a consulting basis.

ACKNOWLEDGMENTS

To critical care nurses, I remain in awe of your knowledge, skills, and caring after all these years. The learning and caring are an unending journey.

Published by Kaplan, Inc., d/b/a Barron's Educational Series
750 Third Avenue
New York, NY 10017
www.barronseduc.com

ISBN: 978-1-4380-1234-6

10 9 8 7 6 5 4 3 2 1

Kaplan, Inc., d/b/a Barron's Educational Series print books are available at special quantity discounts to use for sales promotions, employee premiums, or educational purposes. For more information or to purchase books, please call the Simon & Schuster special sales department at 866-506-1949.

CONTENTS

1 Introduction 1

2 Overview of the Adult CCRN Exam 3

3 Pretest 13

   Answers and Explanations 18

4 Cardiovascular Concepts 21

   Cardiovascular Practice Questions 53

5 Respiratory Concepts 63

   Respiratory Practice Questions 102

6 Multisystem Concepts 111

   Multisystem Practice Questions 143

7 Hemodynamics Concepts 151

   Hemodynamics Practice Questions 159

8 Neurological Concepts 165

   Neurological Practice Questions 195

9 Gastrointestinal Concepts 201

   Gastrointestinal Practice Questions 216

10 Renal/Genitourinary Concepts 219

   Renal/Genitourinary Practice Questions 231

11 Endocrine Concepts 235

   Endocrine Practice Questions 243

12 Hematology/Immunology Concepts 247

   Hematology/Immunology Practice Questions 257

13 Behavioral/Psychosocial Concepts 259

   Behavioral/Psychosocial Practice Questions 272

14 Integumentary Concepts 275

   Integumentary Practice Questions 280

15 Musculoskeletal Concepts..283

    Musculoskeletal Practice Questions.....................................288

16 Professional Caring and Ethical Practice Concepts 291

    Professional Caring and Ethical Practice
Practice Questions 296

PRACTICE TESTS

17 Practice Test 1..311

    Answers and Explanations...338

18 Practice Test 2..357

    Answers and Explanations...381

19 References...397

Introduction

1

The art of being wise is knowing what to overlook.

—William James

The purpose of this book is to identify the key concepts you need to master in order to successfully pass the Adult CCRN® exam. This exam is developed and administered by the AACN Certification Corporation, a certification organization for the American Association of Critical-Care Nurses (AACN®). Certification is a process by which a nongovernmental agency validates, based upon predetermined standards, a nurse's qualifications and knowledge for practicing in a defined functional or clinical area of nursing. Achieving certification in your specialty nursing practice is a major professional achievement.

This book is a succinct review. It is not designed to or intended to provide a comprehensive critical care nursing curriculum review, nor does it provide detailed information about every aspect of the test blueprint. You do not need to spend your time studying material that is not covered on the exam. You should spend time understanding and studying the concepts included in the test blueprint. Nurses who have successfully passed this test have reported that self-testing and retesting by using practice questions is one of the best strategies for test preparation. This book and an online practice test provide more than 650 practice questions for you to answer as you study.

This edition reflects all of the latest updates to the official test blueprint, with added content in several chapters and the deletion of content that is no longer tested. It includes the addition of Integumentary Concepts and Musculoskeletal Concepts, brand-new practice questions and answer explanations, and much more. The percentage of topics within the test questions (for the two practice tests at the end of this book as well as the online practice test) has been updated to reflect the percentage of topics from the latest test blueprint.

For detailed information on the qualifications needed to take the Adult CCRN exam and to register for the exam online, go to the official AACN website: *www.aacn.org*.

> **NOTE**
>
> **To access the online practice test, refer to the card at the beginning of this book.**

> Throughout this book, you will see certain subjects or sections marked with a star icon (★). Pay special attention to these concepts, as they are very likely to appear on the Adult CCRN exam!

Overview of the Adult CCRN Exam

2

A journey of a thousand miles begins with a single step.

—Lao Tzu

Congratulations on taking the first step in your certification journey by acquiring *Barron's Adult CCRN Exam*. This chapter will provide you with an overview of this exam as well as strategies that have worked for others who have successfully completed their certification journey by passing the Adult CCRN exam. Although everyone learns at a different pace, one thing's for sure—you will not pass this test if you do not study or if you rely solely on your clinical experience.

BENEFITS OF CERTIFICATION

Before you learn more about the Adult CCRN exam and begin your review, you may be asking yourself the following questions: What are the benefits of critical care certification? Why bother to undertake this professional challenge? Research has demonstrated that certification has the following benefits:

- It validates specialized knowledge.
- It indicates a level of competence.
- It enhances professional credibility.
- It provides access to higher job levels and higher salaries.
- It promotes recognition of nurses by other professionals and patients.
- It improves nurses' confidence and personal satisfaction.
- It increases nurse retention and, in some facilities, garners financial benefits.

The value of certification to patients and their families is that:

- Certified nurses make decisions with more confidence.
- Certification has been linked to better patient safety.
- Certification has been linked to increased patient satisfaction.

More simply expressed…

When you know better, you do better.

—Maya Angelou

EXAM FORMAT

Here are some important facts about the Adult CCRN exam that you should be familiar with:

- This exam is a computerized test that consists of 150 multiple-choice questions, of which only 125 questions will be scored.
  - Note that 25 of the questions on your exam will be in the process of validation by the AACN for future tests, but you will not know which questions are scored versus which ones are in the validation process.
- You will have 3 hours to complete the exam. It is rare that test-takers do not have enough time to complete this test. However, pace yourself and remain aware of the time.
- This test is designed to measure your command of the common body of knowledge needed to function effectively in an acute/critical care setting.
- The test blueprint is based on studies of the acute/critical care nursing practice, as completed by the AACN.
- The **AACN Synergy Model for Patient Care** serves as the organizing framework for the exam. Although no questions refer directly to the Synergy Model, you must understand it, especially to prepare for the 30 questions (20% of the exam) that cover professional caring and ethical practice.
- The Adult CCRN exam is taken to receive or renew one's Adult CCRN, CCRN-E, or CCRN-K credentials.

EXAM BLUEPRINT

The latest Adult CCRN exam blueprint is broken down by test topics as shown in Table 2-1:

Table 2-1. Adult CCRN Exam Blueprint

Section	Number of Questions	% of Test
Clinical Judgment	**120**	**80%**
Cardiovascular*	26	17%
Respiratory	22	15%
Multisystem	21	14%
Neurological**	15	10%
Gastrointestinal**	9	6%
Renal/Genitourinary**	7	5%
Endocrine**	7	5%
Hematology/Immunology**	3–4	2%
Behavioral/Psychosocial**	3–4	2%
Integumentary**	3–4	2%
Musculoskeletal**	3–4	2%

(continued)

Table 2-1. Adult CCRN Exam Blueprint (continued)

Section	Number of Questions	% of Test
Professional Caring and Ethical Practice	30	20%
Advocacy/Moral Agency**	4–5	3%
Caring Practices**	6	4%
Collaboration**	6	4%
Systems Thinking**	3	2%
Response to Diversity**	1–2	1%
Clinical Inquiry**	6	4%
Facilitation of Learning **	3	2%

*Hemodynamics is a part of the Cardiovascular section on the Adult CCRN exam blueprint. However, since Respiratory Concepts and Multisystem Concepts also include hemodynamics, this book separates Hemodynamics into its own chapter.
**The number of questions and percentages in this category may vary slightly from test to test. (For a more detailed breakdown of the specific topics covered within each section of this blueprint, go to *www.aacn.org*.)

QUESTION TYPES

The questions on this exam are all multiple-choice. In order to answer them, you will need to memorize many facts. However, most of the questions will require you to go a step further and apply or evaluate the facts. For instance, you will be expected to know normal hemodynamic parameters. The questions on hemodynamics, though, will test your ability to apply a plan of care for abnormal values. The overall question topic types include:

- Knowledge/Comprehension Questions (~ 36%)
  - These questions require the ability to memorize previously learned information and to demonstrate an understanding of that information.
- Application/Analysis Questions (~ 39%)
  - These questions require the ability to use information appropriately and to recognize commonalities, differences, and interrelationships.
- Synthesis/Evaluation Questions (~ 25%)
  - These questions require the ability to put parts together to form a new conclusion and to judge the value of information.

Note that all phases of the nursing process are included on this exam, with intervention serving as the phase that makes up the greatest percentage of exam material:

- Assessment: ~ 32%
- Planning: ~ 15%
- Intervention: ~ 40%
- Evaluation: ~ 13%

HOW TO APPLY FOR THE EXAM

Understanding the process for applying for this exam is important when creating your study plan. Once you get approval to take the exam, you have **90 days** to schedule and take the exam at an approved testing site. Consider the time of year and the overall personal commitments in your life before developing your plan for studying. For example, if you are getting married on July 1, you probably should not plan on taking the certification exam on June 21! In order to apply to take the exam, you must do the following:

- Go to *www.aacn.org* and have the following available: your RN license, a credit card, and the name, address, phone number, and email address of an RN coworker or supervisor who can verify your eligibility. You will need to enter your member/customer number or email address and password to sign in.
  - Initial exam candidates who are not already in AACN's database must register to create a new customer account.
  - Candidates who are not current AACN members will be given the opportunity to purchase membership and pay member pricing upon certification.
- You will need to provide your current mailing address and email address in order to receive an email confirmation of your registration and to facilitate AACN communication with you in case AACN has questions regarding your registration.
  - Approval to register for the exam will arrive via email several days after you complete the online application.
  - The approval number you receive will be good for 90 days. The clock starts ticking immediately!
- You will use the AACN approval number to go online and schedule the date and time of the exam at an approved testing site.
- You can choose either a morning time or an afternoon time. Choose the time when you tend to be most alert.
- As of the date of this publication, the Adult CCRN exam fee is **$344**, but that fee is reduced to **$239** for AACN members. Membership costs $78 per year.

EXAM RESULTS

After you complete the exam, you will get a printout of the results, with a notification about whether you passed, the number of correct answers that you achieved, what the passing score was for that exam, and a description of each test content area (e.g., Cardiovascular, Respiratory, etc.) with the corresponding % score you achieved for each area. This printout will allow you to see which content areas you did the best on and which areas you may need to brush up on.

During the minutes while you are waiting for your scores, you might be nervous. When you pass, though, the feeling is exhilarating!

PASSING SCORE

- In order to pass this exam, you need to correctly answer approximately 88 out of the 125 questions that are scored (which is approximately 70% of the 125 questions that counted).
- A passing score is evaluated in total, NOT by each category from the blueprint. For example, you can get all 3 behavioral/psychosocial questions wrong and still pass the test if you do well on the other topics.

Familiarizing yourself with the exam blueprint will help guide your study time. For instance, you will probably see only 3 or 4 hematology/immunology questions on your exam, so you should not spend 30 hours studying hematology/immunology. On the other hand, there are

26 cardiovascular questions. Therefore, you should definitely plan on more study time for that topic. Clinical judgment accounts for 80% of this test, while professional caring and ethical practice accounts for 20%.

Keep in mind that the Adult CCRN exam is NOT an easy test. The pass rate has been about the same for years. The latest available test statistics as of December 31, 2018 are shown below.

Table 2-2. Test Statistics from December 31, 2018

Candidates Tested (2018)	First-Time Pass Rate	Total Certificants
15,609	77.3%	78,635

This data should not scare you, but, instead, serve as a reality check. You need to STUDY. However, you only need to study the material covered on the test, not the entire core curriculum for critical care! As T. Boone Pickens said:

A fool with a plan can outsmart a genius with no plan.

Smart critical care nurses without a good study plan have failed this test. So ask yourself, how do you, as an adult learner, learn best? Most nurses would rather study on their own according to a schedule based on the exam blueprint. However, others do better by participating in a study group. Even if you attend an instructor-led course, you cannot walk out of a course and successfully pass the test without studying what was covered in the class.

Strategies for Achieving a Passing Score

The following strategies are recommended for achieving a passing score on the Adult CCRN exam:

- Before studying, take the brief pretest in this book. The pretest questions are primarily knowledge-based questions that provide you with a baseline snapshot of where you are before you begin your review.
- Review the exam blueprint, and determine how much time you will spend studying each topic (e.g., 26 hours devoted to cardiovascular concepts, 3 hours devoted to hematology/immunology concepts, etc.).
- Plan your study time by the number of hours, not by the number of days or weeks. The phrase "weeks of study" is rather vague. Instead, determine how many hours per day/days of the week you are capable of studying.
- You MUST include practice questions when studying.
- Review each chapter of the book, and then attempt the practice questions at the end of each chapter.
- **IMPORTANT:** As you complete the practice questions, answer them without looking back into the chapter review material. You need to test your knowledge, not your ability to look up information. After you score yourself, go back into the review material and review any topics that you are still not confident about.
- For any practice questions that you answered incorrectly, review those topics again within the chapter. Make sure you understand where you went wrong when you first answered the question. Then, take a second attempt at the end-of-chapter practice questions until you get at least 80% of them correct. As you try a second time and improve your score, you will build the confidence that you need to succeed!

- After completing each chapter of this book and working through all of the end-of-chapter practice questions until you can answer at least 80% of each set correctly, take Practice Test 1. Once you've completed the test, review the questions you answered incorrectly and retake the test until you score at least 80%.
- At least 1 or 2 weeks before you are scheduled to take your exam, proceed to Practice Test 2 and follow the same steps that you did for Practice Test 1. By now, your confidence should be increasing.
- The week before your test date, answer 100–150 questions in one sitting at least once; this would be a good time to work through the online exam. This is your mental training. You would not attempt to complete a marathon without training first. Similarly, you should not attempt to sit and answer 150 test questions without practicing at least 100 questions in one sitting. If you don't do this, you may find your attention wavering during the actual exam.
- Do not plan on cramming the night before. This usually results in decreased self-confidence and increased anxiety.
- Remember: Your clinical experience will be an advantage. However, you should not rely totally on your unit practice patterns, which may sometimes vary from correct answers as determined by the AACN.

RECERTIFICATION

The Adult CCRN certification period is 3 years. When it is time for you to renew your Adult CCRN credential, there are specific requirements that you must meet, including:

- Maintaining a current RN or APRN licensure
- Completing 432 hours of direct care of acute/critically ill patients over the 3-year period, with 144 of those hours within 12 months of the renewal date
- Completing the required Continuing Education Recognition Points (CERPs) or retaking and passing the Adult CCRN exam

Note that renewal by CERPs requires 100 CERPs in various categories. For additional information regarding how to renew your CCRN credential, visit *www.aacn.org*.

TEST-TAKING PEARLS OF WISDOM

- Get plenty of rest the night before the test…no alcohol, sedating medications, or overtime shifts! You need to be on your game.
- Plan on taking a watch, a sweater, and glasses (if you need them) to the testing site.
- Eat a healthy meal before the test, including protein and carbs. Avoid eating sugar.
- Remember to bring two forms of ID, and make sure that one of them is a photo ID.
- Plan to arrive early to the testing site, at least 15 minutes before the scheduled time.
- Be aware that prior to beginning the exam, while sitting in front of the computer, you will need to have your picture taken, which will appear on your exam results.
- Control your anxiety:
  - Some anxiety increases performance, but panic does not.
  - Adequate preparation decreases anxiety.
  - Use deep breathing/progressive muscle relaxation.
  - Visualize yourself receiving your passing score.
  - No negative self-talk!

- Approach the exam calmly and confidently:
  - Read each question thoroughly.
  - Look for key words, such as *except, least, most, never, always, initially, first, last, early, late, indicated, contraindicated, priority,* and *best.*
  - After you read the question stem, answer the question without looking at the answer choices. Then, look at the answer choices. If your answer is there, it is most likely right, BUT still go ahead and read all of the options. A different choice may be better than your answer.
  - Do not assume information that is not given.
  - Do not leave any questions blank.
  - If you don't know the answer to a particular question, don't dwell on it after reading the question over a couple of times. Go on to the next question. Come back to the difficult question later since the answer may become more apparent to you.
- Be aware that you will be given one blank sheet of paper and a pen at the testing site to make notations. You will also be able to go back and forth among the questions.
- When it comes to guessing:
  - Use this only as a last resort.
  - First, eliminate any choices that you can.
  - If you still do not know the answer, look for the option that is different from the others.
  - If the content has nothing to do with what you have studied, you can rationalize that perhaps this is one of the 25 questions that will not be counted!
- When it comes to changing your answer:
  - If you tend to answer questions incorrectly because you do not read the question thoroughly and/or you misread the question, change your answer.
  - If you tend to answer questions incorrectly even though you do read them thoroughly, don't change your initial answer—your first selection is most likely correct.
- If any questions ask you what to do first in a situation, look at the choices and see if any of them address the ABCs (airway, breathing, and circulation). Let that guide you. When in doubt, fall back on your ABCs!

ANSWER SHEET
Pretest

1. Ⓐ Ⓑ Ⓒ Ⓓ   6. Ⓐ Ⓑ Ⓒ Ⓓ   11. Ⓐ Ⓑ Ⓒ Ⓓ   16. Ⓐ Ⓑ Ⓒ Ⓓ   21. Ⓐ Ⓑ Ⓒ Ⓓ

2. Ⓐ Ⓑ Ⓒ Ⓓ   7. Ⓐ Ⓑ Ⓒ Ⓓ   12. Ⓐ Ⓑ Ⓒ Ⓓ   17. Ⓐ Ⓑ Ⓒ Ⓓ   22. Ⓐ Ⓑ Ⓒ Ⓓ

3. Ⓐ Ⓑ Ⓒ Ⓓ   8. Ⓐ Ⓑ Ⓒ Ⓓ   13. Ⓐ Ⓑ Ⓒ Ⓓ   18. Ⓐ Ⓑ Ⓒ Ⓓ   23. Ⓐ Ⓑ Ⓒ Ⓓ

4. Ⓐ Ⓑ Ⓒ Ⓓ   9. Ⓐ Ⓑ Ⓒ Ⓓ   14. Ⓐ Ⓑ Ⓒ Ⓓ   19. Ⓐ Ⓑ Ⓒ Ⓓ   24. Ⓐ Ⓑ Ⓒ Ⓓ

5. Ⓐ Ⓑ Ⓒ Ⓓ   10. Ⓐ Ⓑ Ⓒ Ⓓ   15. Ⓐ Ⓑ Ⓒ Ⓓ   20. Ⓐ Ⓑ Ⓒ Ⓓ   25. Ⓐ Ⓑ Ⓒ Ⓓ

Pretest

3

Directions: The purpose of this pretest is to get a quick baseline assessment of your knowledge and understanding before you begin studying. The questions cover all topics on the Adult CCRN exam. However, most are knowledge-based questions and do not cover application, evaluation, and analysis of knowledge. After you complete all chapters of the book and study each chapter's practice questions, but before you take one of the comprehensive practice tests, revisit this pretest. You should notice an improvement! Read each question, and choose the one best response. The answers and explanations can be found at the end of the pretest.

---

1. Which of the following are symptoms of hypoglycemia?

   (A) tachycardia and trembling
   (B) bradycardia and diaphoresis
   (C) anxiety and flushed, dry skin
   (D) flushed, dry skin and tachycardia

2. Which of the following is TRUE for a patient who has had a right-sided stroke and develops increased intracranial pressure?

   (A) The pupils will change before the level of consciousness does, there will be right-sided paralysis, the eyes will be deviated to the left, and there will be a left pupil change.
   (B) The pupils will change before the level of consciousness does, there will be left-sided paralysis, the eyes will be deviated to the right, and there will be a right pupil change.
   (C) The level of consciousness will change before there will be pupil changes, there will be right-sided paralysis, the eyes will be deviated to the left, and there will be a left pupil change.
   (D) The level of consciousness will change before there will be pupil changes, there will be left-sided paralysis, the eyes will be deviated to the right, and there will be a right pupil change.

3. Which of the following interventions would a nurse consider inappropriate for a patient with increased intracranial pressure?

   (A) maintaining oxygenation and normal $PaCO_2$
   (B) feeding the patient via an NG tube
   (C) administering 5% dextrose in water (D_5W) at 75 mL/hour
   (D) using the log roll maneuver when turning the patient

4. Which of the following is associated with mitral regurgitation?

   (A) systolic murmur, sinus bradycardia
   (B) diastolic murmur, heart failure
   (C) systolic murmur, inferior wall myocardial infarction
   (D) diastolic murmur, complete heart block

5. A nurse knows that research supports a patient having unrestricted access to his or her designated support person (according to the patient's wishes). However, the nurse's unit restricts all patient visitors to set times. The nurse's best response would be to:

   (A) gather the facts and propose a policy change to the manager for the unit.
   (B) tell patients/visitors that the unit's policy is outdated but there is nothing that can be done about it.
   (C) continue to follow the unit policy.
   (D) complain to colleagues about the unit's outdated policy.

6. Nitrate therapy is indicated for the treatment of unstable angina and acute heart failure because it:

   (A) decreases preload and increases myocardial O_2 demand.
   (B) increases preload and increases myocardial O_2 demand.
   (C) increases preload and decreases myocardial O_2 demand.
   (D) decreases preload and decreases myocardial O_2 demand.

7. All of the following support the diagnosis of cardiac tamponade EXCEPT:

   (A) widening pulse pressure.
   (B) equalization of right and left heart pressures.
   (C) pulsus paradoxus.
   (D) an enlarged heart on a chest X-ray (CXR).

8. A patient has just consented to a bedside chest tube insertion and requests that his wife be allowed to be present during the procedure. The nurse should:

   (A) explain to the patient that this is against infection control practices.
   (B) tell the patient he will be able to see his wife as soon as the procedure is completed.
   (C) tell the patient it would be too much for his wife to handle.
   (D) prepare the wife for what to expect and allow her to be present.

9. ECG changes associated with ST-elevation myocardial infarction (STEMI) that affect the lateral wall would include changes in which of the following leads?

   (A) II, III, aVF
   (B) V1, V2, V3
   (C) V2, V3, V4
   (D) V5, V6, I, aVL

10. Which of the following laboratory findings are most specifically indicative of disseminated intravascular coagulation (DIC) as the cause of bleeding?

(A) elevated fibrin split products and D-dimer
(B) prolonged PT, PTT, and bleeding time
(C) decreased platelet count
(D) decreased hemoglobin and hematocrit

11. A 29-year-old female has been in the critical care unit for 2 days after a motor vehicle crash, and she has developed acute tubular necrosis (ATN). She was normotensive upon admission. What would be the most likely cause of her ATN?

(A) hemorrhage
(B) rhabdomyolysis
(C) creatinine release
(D) cardiac dysrhythmias

12. A patient with acute tubular necrosis (intrarenal failure) is differentiated from a patient with decreased renal perfusion (prerenal failure) in that ONLY with decreased renal perfusion (prerenal failure) is:

(A) the urine specific gravity low.
(B) the urine osmolality greatly reduced.
(C) the BUN to creatinine ratio at least 20:1.
(D) the urinary sodium 40 to 100 mEq/L.

13. A patient with a history of heroin and alcohol abuse is admitted for treatment of cellulitis. The patient has flushed, slightly moist skin and is slow to respond to verbal stimuli. The affected arm is edematous and hard to the touch, with yellow exudates noted from puncture wounds on the skin. The patient's vital signs are as follows: temperature is 102°F (38.9°C); B/P is 88/50; heart rate is 120 beats/minute; respiratory rate is 26 breaths/minute. The nurse should anticipate orders for:

(A) antibiotic and crystalloid administration.
(B) antipyretic and dopamine administration.
(C) a CT scan of the head and a drug screen.
(D) colloid administration followed by norepinephrine administration.

14. A patient with a history of hyperlipidemia and alcohol abuse reports left upper quadrant abdominal pain. The patient's vital signs are as follows: temperature is 101°F (38.3°C); B/P is 85/50; heart rate is 110 beats/minute; respiratory rate is 24 breaths/minute. Which of the following lab values should the nurse anticipate?

(A) decreased serum amylase level and increased WBC count
(B) decreased hematocrit (HCT) and increased lipase level
(C) decreased sedimentation rate and elevated calcium level
(D) increased LDH and increased SGOT (AST)

15. A patient is admitted with diabetic ketoacidosis (DKA). The arterial blood gas (ABG) on room air shows:

pH   7.22
$PaCO_2$ 21 mmHg
pO_2 94 mmHg
HCO_3 11 mmol/L

The ABG demonstrates:

(A) compensated metabolic alkalosis.
(B) compensated respiratory acidosis.
(C) partially compensated metabolic acidosis.
(D) uncompensated metabolic acidosis.

16. What is the recommended initial position to improve oxygenation for a patient with unilateral pneumonia?

(A) Trendelenburg position
(B) supine position
(C) side lying on affected side
(D) side lying on unaffected side

17. A patient is admitted with a respiratory infection. The patient has shortness of breath with a frequent productive cough and is expectorating light-green sputum. Vital signs are stable, except for the temperature, which is 39°C, and an increased respiratory rate. The nurse should anticipate which of the following ABG results?

(A) respiratory acidosis
(B) respiratory alkalosis
(C) metabolic acidosis
(D) metabolic alkalosis

18. A patient has been receiving mechanical ventilation for 2 days, but the nurse notices that there is no order for nutrition. The nurse's best response would be to:

(A) insert a feeding tube and begin enteral nutritional therapy.
(B) complain about the physician's practice patterns to her colleagues.
(C) ask the physician for an order for enteral feeding for the patient.
(D) assume it is the physician's responsibility for the nutritional plan of care.

19. A patient with status asthmaticus is admitted. His breath sounds are diminished throughout his lung fields, and his respiratory rate is 38 breaths/minute. After giving the patient an aerosol bronchodilator, the patient now has bilateral wheezes. This indicates that:

(A) the patient is getting better.
(B) the patient has gotten worse.
(C) there is a need for anesthesia to be present STAT.
(D) the patient does not have asthma.

20. In a patient with acute lung injury (ALI), which of the following contributes to the development of atelectasis?

(A) loss of surfactant and interstitial fluid accumulation
(B) increased pulmonary vascular resistance and hypoxemia
(C) increased pulmonary compliance and hypoxemia
(D) mucosal edema and mucus plugging

21. All of the following are features of an acute subarachnoid hemorrhage EXCEPT:

(A) a sudden explosive headache.
(B) nuchal rigidity.
(C) a decreased level of consciousness.
(D) pinpoint pupils.

22. A patient with an inferior wall ST-elevation myocardial infarction (STEMI) also has a right ventricular (RV) infarction. He soon develops right ventricular failure. Which of the following data would be consistent with this patient's condition? Note that PAP = pulmonary artery pressure, PAOP = pulmonary artery occlusion pressure, and CVP = central venous pressure.

(A) PAP 38/22; PAOP 20; CVP 6; ST elevation in II, III, and aVF; crackles bilaterally
(B) PAP 54/28; PAOP 14; CVP 14; ST elevation in V_2–V_6; clear lungs
(C) PAP 28/10; PAOP 10; CVP 18; ST elevation in II, III, and aVF; clear lungs
(D) PAP 23/8; PAOP 19; CVP 20; ST elevation in V_2–V_6; crackles bilaterally

23. Which of the following hemodynamic profiles would best exemplify that seen in septic shock? Note that PAP = pulmonary artery pressure, PAOP = pulmonary artery occlusion pressure, CVP = central venous pressure, and SVR = systemic vascular resistance.

(A) PAP 20/4; PAOP 3; CVP 0; SVR 1,400
(B) PAP 22/6; PAOP 5; CVP 1; SVR 600
(C) PAP 45/22; PAOP 21; CVP 8; SVR 1,800
(D) PAP 55/25; PAOP 15; CVP 10; SVR 1,200

24. Which of the following patients is least likely to return to a normal level of functioning after discharge?

(A) the 70-year-old who was admitted with septic shock and is receiving chemotherapy
(B) the 75-year-old who was admitted for a scheduled coronary artery bypass graft procedure
(C) the 21-year-old trauma patient who was admitted with a pneumothorax and a fractured pelvis
(D) the 65-year-old who was admitted with an acute MI and a history of diabetes

25. Which of the following statements is TRUE?

(A) Delirium is a permanent condition.
(B) A patient who develops delirium has an increased risk of mortality.
(C) Most patients with delirium are agitated.
(D) A patient with dementia cannot develop delirium.

ANSWER KEY
Pretest

1. **A**	6. **D**	11. **B**	16. **D**	21. **D**
2. **D**	7. **A**	12. **C**	17. **B**	22. **C**
3. **C**	8. **D**	13. **A**	18. **C**	23. **B**
4. **C**	9. **D**	14. **B**	19. **A**	24. **A**
5. **A**	10. **A**	15. **C**	20. **A**	25. **B**

ANSWERS AND EXPLANATIONS

1. **(A)** When the blood glucose drops, sympathetic stimulation occurs. (Symptoms are masked for a patient who is receiving beta-adrenergic blocker drugs.) Flushed, dry skin is a sign of hyperglycemia.

2. **(D)** Higher brain centers (cerebral cortex) are the first to be affected by increased intracranial pressure. Therefore, the level of consciousness is the first sign (the one exception to that rule is epidural hematoma). Pupil changes are ipsilateral (same side as the injury) due to compression of cranial nerve III against the transtentorial notch. Motor changes are contralateral (opposite side of the injury) due to motor fiber crossing in the brain stem.

3. **(C)** 5% dextrose in water is a hypotonic solution. When administered, it will cause movement of the D_5W into the brain cells, causing swelling and increased intracranial pressure. The other 3 choices are acceptable interventions for a patient with increased ICP.

4. **(C)** Inferior wall MI may result in ischemia and dysfunction (regurgitation) of the mitral valve. The mitral valve is closed during systole (left ventricular ejection). A murmur is produced when the mitral valve is not fully closed during systole.

5. **(A)** The AACN Synergy Model supports patient advocacy. Unrestricted access to a designated support person (according to the patient's wishes) is an evidence-based practice that is included in the "Family Presence: Visitation in the Adult ICU" AACN Practice Alert. Choice (A) is an effective strategy for change.

6. **(D)** Nitrates cause venodilation, which results in a decrease in venous return to the heart (left ventricular preload reduction). The decrease in preload decreases the work of the left ventricle and the myocardial oxygen demand.

7. **(A)** The pulse pressure **narrows** with cardiac tamponade. The other 3 choices ARE seen with cardiac tamponade.

8. **(D)** The AACN Synergy Model supports caring practices and family presence. An AACN Practice Alert indicates that family presence may improve the patient outcome.

9. **(D)** V5 and V6 represent the lower lateral wall of the left ventricle, and I and aVL represent the high lateral wall of the left ventricle, supplied by the left circumflex artery in most of the population.

10. **(A)** DIC is a clotting problem, with massive coagulation. As clots break down, fibrin split products are produced. Therefore, with DIC, FSPs will be high. In fact, this is the most specific test result for DIC. D-dimer is present due to the presence of clots. While not specific for DIC, it is a good rule-out test.

11. **(B)** The motor vehicle crash most likely resulted in a crush injury with destruction of skeletal muscle cells (rhabdomyolysis). This results in the release of massive amounts of creatinine kinase (CK) that, in turn, may "clog" renal tubules and lead to acute tubular necrosis (ATN). Choice (A) is not correct, as there is no history of bleeding. Choice (C), creatinine release, is too vague, could be minor, and does not cause ATN. Cardiac dysrhythmias, choice (D), are not included in this scenario.

12. **(C)** A BUN with a 10:1 ratio is seen in acute intrarenal failure; the 20:1 ratio is typical of prerenal failure. The other 3 choices are typically seen in acute intrarenal failure because they are evidence of damage to the basement membrane of renal tubules with the inability to concentrate urine or "hold on" to sodium.

13. **(A)** This scenario describes septic shock. The patient emergently needs antibiotics and crystalloid administration. The other 3 choices are not as effective as choice (A) is for septic shock.

14. **(B)** This scenario describes acute pancreatitis, which may be hemorrhagic and could cause the hematocrit to drop. Serum lipase increases with acute pancreatitis.

15. **(C)** The pH is low; there is an acidosis. The low bicarbonate indicates that the acidosis is metabolic. Bicarbonate drops as it is attempting to buffer the excess ketoacids. The low $PaCO_2$ is evidence that the lungs are attempting to compensate with hyperventilation, or "blowing off acid." However, compensation is only partial, not complete. (The pH would need to be normal, 7.35, for full compensation.)

16. **(D)** It is best to place the "good" lung down and have the patient on the side that does not have the problem. This is because more blood perfusion is greater to the "down" side due to gravity. If more blood goes to the "bad" side, hypoxemia may occur.

17. **(B)** The increased respiratory rate generally causes hyperventilation, "blowing off CO_2," resulting in a decrease in the $PaCO_2$ and a rise in the pH. Tachypnea does not guarantee hyperventilation. However, nothing in the history of this scenario indicates acidosis or metabolic alkalosis.

18. **(C)** Early nutritional therapy for a patient who is receiving mechanical ventilation improves the patient outcome. Knowledge of evidence-based practices, however, is not enough. A critical care nurse needs to advocate for the patient using strategies that work. Collaboration (a part of the AACN Synergy Model) with the physician would be most likely to provide the patient with what he needs.

19. **(A)** Diminished or absent breath sounds in a patient with an asthma exacerbation are an ominous sign of a lack of air movement through the airways. The development of wheezing is a sign that the patient is improving, with air now moving, although bronchospasm is still present.

20. **(A)** The pathophysiology of acute lung injury includes damage to the Type II alveolar cells (which results in alveolar collapse) and capillary leak (which results in interstitial fluid accumulation). Both alveolar collapse and interstitial fluid lead to atelectasis. Although mucosal edema and mucus plugging may lead to atelectasis, these problems are not associated with acute lung injury.

21. **(D)** Pinpoint pupils are associated with pontine infarcts. The other 3 choices *are* features of an acute subarachnoid hemorrhage.

22. **(C)** When the right ventricle (RV) fails, the pressure that is proximal to the RV (CVP) increases, whereas pressures that are distal to the RV (pulmonary artery pressure and pulmonary artery occlusion pressure) are normal or even low. This results in clear lungs. ECG changes that are indicative of an inferior wall MI are found in leads II, III, and aVF.

23. **(B)** The pathophysiology of septic shock includes capillary leak, which decreases intravascular volume (low CVP and relative hypovolemia), and massive vasodilatation, which decreases systemic vascular resistance (low SVR).

24. **(A)** The AACN believes that a critical care nurse should assess not only the patient's physiological status but also the patient's resiliency, which has been shown to affect the outcome. In addition to acute problems, extremes of age and chronic conditions also need to be considered.

25. **(B)** Studies have shown that delirium produces long-term effects. They also indicate that the more severe the delirium is, the worse is the long-term outcome. The other 3 choices are NOT true regarding delirium.

Cardiovascular Concepts

4

*I'm a great believer in luck, and I find the harder I work,
the more I have of it.*

—Thomas Jefferson

CARDIOVASCULAR TEST BLUEPRINT

Cardiovascular 17% of total test   **26 questions**

→ Acute coronary syndrome (e.g., NSTEMI, STEMI, and unstable angina)
→ Acute peripheral vascular insufficiency (e.g., arterial/venous occlusion, carotid artery stenosis, endarterectomy, fem-pop bypass)
→ Acute pulmonary edema
→ Aortic aneurysm
→ Aortic dissection
→ Aortic rupture
→ Cardiac surgery (e.g., CABG, valve replacement or repair)
→ Cardiac tamponade
→ Cardiac trauma
→ Cardiac/vascular catheterization
→ Cardiogenic shock
→ Cardiomyopathies (e.g., dilated, hypertrophic, idiopathic, restrictive)
→ Dysrhythmias
→ Heart failure
→ Hypertensive crisis
→ Myocardial conduction system abnormalities (e.g., prolonged QT interval, Wolff-Parkinson-White)
→ Papillary muscle rupture
→ Structural heart defects (e.g., acquired and congenital, including valvular disease)
→ TAVR

CARDIOVASCULAR TESTABLE NURSING ACTIONS

☐ Apply leads for cardiac monitoring

☐ Identify, interpret, and monitor cardiac rhythms

☐ Recognize indications for, and manage, patients requiring:

- ○ 12-lead ECG
- ○ Arterial catheter
- ○ Cardiac catheterization
- ○ Cardioversion
- ○ Central venous pressure monitoring
- ○ Defibrillation
- ○ IABP
- ○ Invasive hemodynamic monitoring*
- ○ Pacing: epicardial, transcutaneous, transvenous
- ○ Pericardiocentesis
- ○ QT interval monitoring
- ○ ST segment monitoring

☐ Manage patients requiring:
- ○ Endovascular stenting
- ○ PCI

*Since hemodynamic monitoring also includes respiratory concepts and multisystem concepts, this book places the chapter on hemodynamic concepts after the chapters on respiratory concepts and multisystem concepts.

> Cardiovascular (CV) questions outnumber all of the other clinical topics included on the Adult CCRN exam, so plan on spending the most time studying CV. The 26-question total for CV includes hemodynamic monitoring; therefore, plan to spend about 26 hours reviewing the CV and Hemodynamics chapters of this book and practicing test questions related to CV and hemodynamics.

CARDIOVASCULAR ASSESSMENT

Select assessment concepts are included on the Adult CCRN exam. These concepts may be covered in assessment questions, or they may be incorporated in the cardiovascular disorder questions.

Normal Heart Sounds in Adults

S1

- "Lub"
- Caused by closure of AV (mitral, tricuspid) valves
- Loudest at the **apex** of the heart (midclavicular, 5th intercostal space)
- Marks the end of diastole, the beginning of **systole**

S2

- "Dub"
- Caused by closure of semilunar (aortic, pulmonic) valves
- Loudest at the **base** of the heart (right sternal border, 2nd intercostal space)
- Marks the end of systole, the beginning of **diastole**
- S2 splits on inspiration; wide, fixed splitting of S2 is caused by right bundle branch block (RBBB)
- S2 is **louder with a pulmonary embolism**

> ➤ Each of the 4 valves has an auscultatory point on the chest wall. You need to know these points (Figure 4-1).
>
> ➤ The base of the heart is the aortic area, where S2 ("dub") is loudest. Anatomically, it is at the 2nd intercostal space (ICS), right sternal border.
>
> ➤ The apex of the heart is the mitral area, where S1 ("lub") is loudest. Anatomically, it is at the 5th ICS, midclavicular.

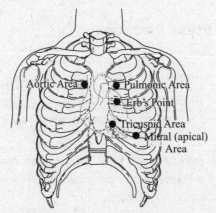

Figure 4-1. Heart auscultatory points on the chest wall and associated valves

Abnormal Heart Sounds in Adults

S3

- Caused by a rapid rush of blood into a dilated ventricle
- Occurs early in diastole, right after S2
- Heard best at the apex with the bell of the stethoscope
- ☆ Associated with heart failure; may occur before crackles
- Ventricular gallop, "Kentucky"
- ☆ S3 is also caused by:
    - Pulmonary hypertension and cor pulmonale
    - Mitral, aortic, or tricuspid insufficiency

TIP

S4 is not heard in the presence of atrial fibrillation . . . why?

No atrial contraction!

S4

- Caused by atrial contraction of blood into a noncompliant ventricle
- Occurs right before S1
- Best heard at the apex with the bell of the stethoscope
- Associated with myocardial ischemia, infarction, hypertension, ventricular hypertrophy, and **aortic stenosis**
- Atrial gallop, "Tennessee"

Pericardial Friction Rub

- Due to pericarditis, associated with pain on deep inspiration
- May be positional

Murmurs

- Valvular disease; see the Valvular Heart Disease section that follows for a detailed discussion of this topic
- Septal defects (atrial or ventricular)

Blood Pressure and Pulse Pressure

- Pulse pressure:

$$\text{Systolic} - \text{Diastolic} = \text{Pulse Pressure}$$

- Normal pulse pressure is 40–60 mmHg (i.e., 120/80).
- Systolic blood pressure is an indirect measurement of the cardiac output and stroke volume.
  - ○ A decrease in systolic pressure with little change or an increase in diastolic pressure is narrowing of pulse pressure; seen most often with severe hypovolemia or a severe drop in cardiac output (CO), i.e., 100/78.
- Diastolic blood pressure is an indirect measurement of the systemic vascular resistance (SVR).
  - ○ A decrease in diastolic pressure that widens pulse pressure may indicate vasodilation, a drop in SVR; often seen in sepsis, septic shock (i.e., 100/38).
- Diastole is normally one-third longer than systole.
- ☆ Coronary arteries are perfused during diastole.

VALVULAR HEART DISEASE

You will most likely see several questions related to valvular heart disease and/or heart sound assessment. Since there are 4 heart valves and each valve may be diseased with either **stenosis** or **insufficiency**, it would be next to impossible to memorize whether each problem is a systolic or diastolic murmur. If you can picture which valves are open and which are closed during each phase of the cardiac cycle (systole and diastole), you will be able to decide what problem is being described in each question. First, let's review some heart sound basics.

- Normal heart sounds, S1 and S2 in adults, are due to valve closure.
- Valves open and close based on the pressure changes in the chamber above the valve and below the valve. When the pressure in the chamber above a valve is higher than that below the valve, the valve opens. When the pressure drops in the chamber above the valve and the pressure is greater below the valve, the valve closes.
- **Systole:** ejection, high pressure
- **Diastole:** filling, low pressure
- Which is longer, systole or diastole? Diastole is one-third longer than systole, needs time for filling.
- When are coronary arteries perfused, during systole or diastole? Diastole!
- Why do the cardiac output and blood pressure drop with extreme tachyarrhythmias? No time for filling, therefore less output.

Causes of Valvular Heart Disease

- Coronary artery disease, ischemia, and acute MI
- Dilated cardiomyopathy
- Degeneration
- Bicuspid aortic valve; genetic
- Rheumatic fever
- Infection
- Connective tissue diseases

Murmurs

- Murmurs of **INSUFFICIENCY** (regurgitation) occur when the valve is **closed**.
  - Acute or chronic
- Murmurs of **STENOSIS** occur when the valve is **open**.
  - Chronic problem, develops over time
  - NOT acute

SYSTOLIC MURMURS (FIGURE 4-2)

Lub . . . shhhb . . . Dub

- Semilunar valves are OPEN during systole.
    - ○ Aortic stenosis
    - ○ Pulmonic stenosis
- AV valves are CLOSED during systole.
    - ○ Mitral insufficiency
        - – Will cause large, giant V-waves on the pulmonary artery, occlusion pressure tracing if the patient has a pulmonary artery catheter
    - ○ Tricuspid insufficiency
- Ventricular septal defect (VSD), which is most common with an acute MI, may result in a systolic murmur. It is heard at the left sternal border, 5th intercostal space (ICS).

DIASTOLIC MURMURS (FIGURE 4-3)

Lub . . . Dub . . . shhhb

- Semilunar valves are CLOSED during diastole.
    - ○ Aortic insufficiency (AI)
    - ○ Pulmonic insufficiency (PI)
- AV valves are OPEN during diastole.
    - ○ Mitral stenosis is associated with atrial fibrillation due to atrial enlargement that occurs over time.
    - ○ Tricuspid stenosis

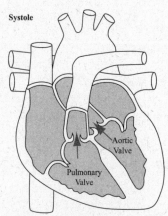

Figure 4-2. Systole, closure
of AV valves, S1
"Lub"
→ The semilunar valves (pulmonic, aortic)
   are OPEN during systole.
→ The AV valves (tricuspid, mitral) are
   CLOSED during systole.

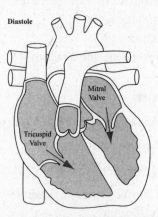

Figure 4-3. Diastole, closure
of semilunar valves, S2
"Dub"
→ The semilunar valves (pulmonic, aortic)
   are CLOSED during diastole.
→ The AV valves (tricuspid, mitral) are
   OPEN during diastole.

- **Mitral insufficiency** occurs when the mitral valve is closed (murmur occurs). When is the mitral valve closed?
  - ➤ Systole!
- **Mitral stenosis** occurs when the mitral valve is open (murmur occurs). When is the mitral valve open?
  - ➤ Diastole!
- **Aortic insufficiency** occurs when the aortic valve is closed. When is the aortic valve closed?
  - ➤ Diastole!
- **Aortic stenosis** occurs when the aortic valve is **open**. When is the aortic valve open?
  - ➤ Systole!

Note: If you can picture what the aortic valve is doing, the pulmonic valve is doing the same (opening or closing). If you can picture what the mitral valve is doing, the tricuspid valve is doing the same (opening or closing).

Does a murmur due to a VSD occur during systole or diastole?

  - ➤ During ejection or systole!

MURMURS ASSOCIATED WITH AN ACUTE MI

- The mitral valve is attached to the left ventricular wall by the papillary muscles and the chordae tendineae. Myocardial ischemia or infarction can affect mitral valve function and lead to acute mitral valve regurgitation.
- Papillary muscle **dysfunction** (Grade I or II), loudest at the apex
- Papillary muscle **rupture** (Grade V or VI), loudest at the apex . . . surgical emergency!
- Ventricular septal defect
  - ○ **Sternal border**, 5th ICS

☆ Several questions on the exam always cover this topic. The questions may describe ECG findings and a clinical picture and then ask about what type of ACS the patient has. Alternatively, the questions may tell you what type of ACS the patient has (e.g., anterior MI) and expect you to know what the typical clinical picture would be for this type of MI. You do not need to have taken a 12-lead ECG class to do well on these types of questions. However, you DO need to understand which leads are associated with which wall of the heart. If you master the following content, you should do well!

Table 4-1. Risk Factors for Coronary Artery Disease

Category	Risk Factors
Non-modifiable risk factors	Age, sex, family history, genetics
Modifiable risk factors	Smoking, atherogenic diet, alcohol intake, physical activity, dyslipidemias, hypertension, obesity, diabetes, metabolic syndrome

Spectrum of Ischemic Heart Disease

- Asymptomatic coronary artery disease (CAD)
- Stable angina, chest pain with activity, predictable, lesions are usually fixed and calcified

Acute Coronary Syndrome

NOTE

Patients may not have chest pain with an MI, especially women and diabetics.

- Due to platelet-mediated thrombosis
- May result in sudden cardiac death
- Types include:

  1. **UNSTABLE ANGINA:** Chest pain at rest, unpredictable, may be relieved with nitroglycerin, troponin negative, ST depression, or T-wave inversion on the ECG
  2. **NON-ST ELEVATION MYOCARDIAL INFARCTION (NSTEMI):** Troponin positive, ST depression, T-wave inversion on the ECG, unrelenting chest pain
  3. **ST ELEVATION MYOCARDIAL INFARCTION (STEMI):** Troponin positive, ST elevation in 2 or more contiguous leads, unrelenting chest pain

☆ **Variant or Prinzmetal's angina**

  ○ A type of unstable angina associated with transient ST segment elevation
  ○ Due to coronary artery spasm with or without atherosclerotic lesions
  ○ Occurs at rest, may be cyclic (same time each day)
  ○ May be precipitated by nicotine, ETOH, cocaine ingestion
  ○ Troponin negative
  ○ Nitroglycerin (NTG) administration results in relief of chest pain, STs return to normal.

Management of Acute Chest Pain

- Stat ECG, done and read within 10 minutes

  ○ Allows categorization to STEMI or NSTEMI/unstable angina
  ○ Allows risk stratification to high, medium, low

ECG Results (3 possibilities)

ST elevation...	ST depression,	No acute change
STEMI	T wave inversion...	
	NSTEMI/UA	

- Aspirin
  - Give **ASAP**; is chewed; improves morbidity/mortality
- ANTICOAGULANT: heparin or enoxaparin
- Antiplatelet agents
  - Clopidogrel (Plavix)
  - Abciximab (Reopro)
  - Eptifibatide (Integrilin)
  - Tirofiban (Aggrastat)
- Beta blocker
  - Unless ACS is due to **cocaine**
  - Use cardioselective such as metoprolol (Lopressor); do not use non-cardioselective such as propranolol (Inderal).
  - Contraindications include hypotension, bradycardia, use of phosphodiesterase-inhibitor drugs such as sildenafil (Viagra).
- Treat pain
  - Nitroglycerin
  - Morphine
- History, risk factor assessment
  - Lab assessment
  - Cardiac biomarkers, lipid profile, CBC, electrolytes, BUN, creatinine, magnesium, PT, PTT
- ☆ **ECG lead changes and location of coronary artery disease**
  - Changes in II, III, aVF → right coronary artery (RCA), inferior LV
  - Changes in V1, V2, V3, V4 → left anterior descending (LAD), anterior LV
  - Changes in V5, V6, I, aVL → circumflex, lateral LV
  - Changes in V5, V6 → low lateral LV
  - Changes in I, aVL → high lateral LV
  - Changes in V1, V2 → RCA, posterior LV
  - Changes in V3R, V4R → RCA, right ventricular (RV) infarct

Differentiation of the Types of Acute MI

⭐ **Inferior MI**

- ○ Associated with right coronary artery (RCA) occlusion
- ○ ST elevation in II, III, and aVF (Figure 4-4)
- ○ Reciprocal changes in lateral wall (I, aVL)
- ○ Associated with AV conduction disturbances: 2nd-degree Type I AV block, 3rd-degree AV block, sick sinus syndrome (SSS), and sinus bradycardia
- ○ Development of systolic murmur: mitral valve regurgitation (MVR) secondary to papillary muscle rupture (posterior papillary muscle tethering distance is significantly greater in an inferior MI than in an anterior MI)
- ○ Tachycardia is associated with an inferior MI → higher mortality.
- ○ Also associated with right ventricular (RV) infarct and posterior MI
- ○ Use beta blockers and NTG with CAUTION.

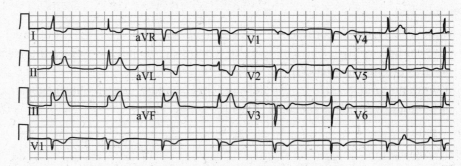

Figure 4-4. Acute inferior wall STEMI

⭐ **Right ventricular (RV) infarct**

- ○ The right coronary artery, which supplies the inferior wall of the left ventricle, also supplies the right ventricle; therefore, about 30% of inferior wall MI patients also have a right ventricular (RV) infarct.
- ○ Size of the infarct will determine symptoms.
- ○ A right-sided ECG (Figure 4-5) may demonstrate the ST changes.
- ○ Signs/symptoms

   - JVD at 45°, high CVP, hypotension, usually clear lungs, bradyarrhythmias
   - ECG with ST elevation in **V4R** (Figure 4-6)

- ○ Treatment

   - Fluids
   - Positive inotropes

- ○ Avoid

   - Preload reducers → nitrates, diuretics
   - Caution with beta blockers, often cannot give initially due to hypotension

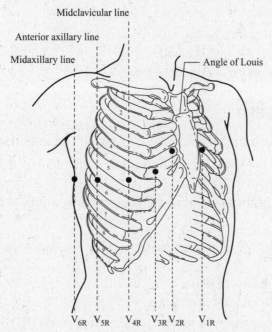

Figure 4-5. Lead placement for right-sided ECG to assess for RV infarct

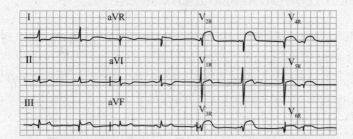

Figure 4-6. Right-sided ECG results with evidence of RV infarct

☆ Anterior MI

○ Associated with left anterior descending (LAD) occlusion

○ ST elevation in V1–V4: precordial leads, V leads (Figure 4-7)

○ Reciprocal changes (ST depression) in inferior wall (II, III, aVF)

○ May develop 2nd-degree Type II AV block or RBBB (the LAD supplies the common bundle of His) → **ominous** sign

○ Development of systolic murmur: possible ventricular septal defect

○ Higher mortality than an inferior MI: **HEART FAILURE**

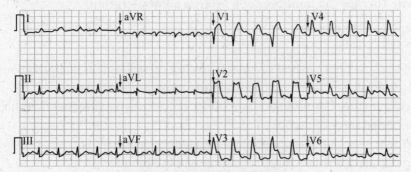

Figure 4-7. Anterior STEMI

- **Lateral MI**
  - ○ ST elevation in V5, V6 (low lateral)
  - ○ ST elevation in I, aVL (high lateral)
  - ○ Generally involves left circumflex artery

Treatment of STEMI

- Determine onset of infarct, if symptoms < 12 hours → **REPERFUSION**
  - ○ Percutaneous coronary intervention (PCI)—standard is door-to-balloon within 90 minutes
  - ○ Fibrinolytic drug therapy—standard is door-to-drug within 30 minutes
- Eligibility criteria
  - ○ ST elevation in 2 or more contiguous leads **or** new onset left bundle branch block (LBBB)
  - ○ Onset of chest pain < 12 hours
  - ○ Chest pain of 30 minutes in duration
  - ○ Chest pain unresponsive to sublingual (SL) nitroglycerin (NTG)

PATIENT CARE FOLLOWING REPERFUSION FOR STEMI

PCI (90 minutes, door-to-balloon inflation in coronary artery at point of lesion)

- Monitor for signs of reocclusion: chest pain, ST elevation → contact physician.
- Monitor for vasovagal reaction during sheath removal → give fluids, atropine.
  - ○ Hypotension < 90 systolic with or without bradycardia, absence of compensatory tachycardia
  - ○ Associated symptoms of pallor, nausea, yawning, diaphoresis
- Monitor for bleeding: sheath site.
  - ○ Immediately apply manual pressure 2 fingerbreadths above the puncture site.
  - ○ Continue manual pressure for a minimum of 20 min (30 min if still on GP IIb/IIIa inhibitors) to achieve hemostasis.
- Monitor for bleeding: retroperitoneal → fluids, blood products.
  - ○ Sudden hypotension
  - ○ Severe low back pain
- Monitor for vascular complications → pulse assessments.

Fibrinolytic Therapy (30 minutes door-to-drug administration)

- Absolute contraindications
  - ○ Any prior intracranial hemorrhage
  - ○ Known structural cerebral vascular lesion (e.g., arteriovenous malformation)
  - ○ Known malignant intracranial neoplasm (primary or metastatic)
  - ○ Ischemic stroke within 3 months EXCEPT acute ischemic stroke within 3 hours
  - ○ Suspected aortic dissection
  - ○ Active bleeding or bleeding diathesis (excluding menses)
  - ○ Significant closed-head or facial trauma within 3 months

☆ **Evidence of reperfusion**

- ○ Chest pain relief: due to fibrinolysis of clot
- ○ Resolution of ST segment deviations: due to return of blood flow
- ○ Marked elevation of troponin/CK-MB: due to myocardial "stunning" when vessel opens
- ○ Reperfusion arrhythmias (VT, VF, accelerated idioventricular rhythm [AIVR]): due to myocardial "stunning" when vessel opens

- ■ Nursing management
  - ○ Assess for major and minor bleeding.
    - – Major bleed, change in LOC, brain bleed
  - ○ Institute bleeding precautions.
  - ○ Assess for reperfusion (see above).
  - ○ Assess for reocclusion as evidenced by recurring chest pain, ST deviation.

Treatment of NSTEMI

- ■ **No** emergent reperfusion
- ■ Same meds as STEMI
- ■ If high risk score **or** continued chest pain, signs of instability, start GP IIb/IIIa inhibitors (Integrilin, Reopro) and prepare for diagnostic cardiac catheterization within 24 hours.

Complications of an Acute MI

ARRHYTHMIAS—MOST COMMON!

- ■ Ventricular tachycardia or ventricular fibrillation
  - ○ Defibrillate VF
  - ○ Drug therapy for stable, sustained VT and to prevent recurrent VF
  - ○ Synchronized cardioversion for unstable, sustained VT

- ■ Bradycardia, heart blocks, sick sinus syndrome (SSS)
- ■ Atrial fibrillation
  - ○ 10% to 15% of all MIs have increased mortality even when returned to NSR.

- ■ Heart failure
- ■ Cardiogenic shock
- ■ Reinfarction
- ■ Thromboembolic events
- ■ Pericarditis
- ■ Ventricular aneurysm
- ■ Ventricular septal defect
- ■ Papillary muscle rupture
- ■ Cardiac wall rupture

Cardiac Catheterization Lab Procedures

- Diagnostic cardiac catheterization
- Percutaneous Coronary Interventions (PCI)
    - Intracoronary stenting: most common PCI procedure
    - Balloon angioplasty without stent (PTCA): seldom used, high reocclusion rates
- Percutaneous balloon valvotomy
- Pacemaker implantation
- Electrophysiology (EP) studies
    - Implantable cardioverter defibrillator (ICD)
    - Cardiac ablation therapy

GOAL OF PCI WITH STENT

- Restoration of blood flow distal to a coronary artery lesion with partial or total occlusion

COMPLICATIONS OF PCI

- In-hospital death is rare, ~ 1.8%.
- In-hospital MI ~ 0.4%
- Coronary artery perforation
- Distal coronary artery embolization
- Intramural hematoma
- Failure of stent deployment
- ☆ **Stent thrombosis is most likely to be on the exam.**
    - Most incidents occur acutely (within 24 hours of stent placement) or subacutely (within the first 30 days).
- Stroke or TIA: greater risk if with aortic stenosis
- Arrhythmias
- Renal failure
- ☆ **Retroperitoneal bleed is most likely to be on the exam.**

PATIENT CARE DURING SHEATH REMOVAL

- Record baseline peripheral pulses and vitals.
- Provide comfort (i.e., morphine 2–4 mg IV) before removal.
- Monitor B/P q 5–10 min during sheath removal.
- Monitor for **vasovagal response** (hypotension < 90 systolic with or without bradycardia, absence of compensatory tachycardia and associated symptoms of pallor, nausea, yawning, diaphoresis).
- Vasovagal management
    - Hold nitrates
    - Atropine 0.5 mg IV (even in absence of bradycardia if other signs occur)
    - IV bolus of 250 mL 0.9 NS if patient is not immediately responsive to atropine
    - Assess for anxiety/pain as contributing factors.

- Achieve hemostasis.
  - Manual pressure for 20 to 30 minutes
  - Mechanical clamp compression using FemoStop or C-clamp
  - Closure device

MANAGE COMPLICATIONS OF PCI

- Monitor for signs of coronary artery reocclusion: chest pain, ST elevation → contact physician.
- Monitor for vasovagal reaction during sheath removal → give fluids, atropine.
- Monitor for bleeding: sheath site.
  - Immediately apply manual pressure 2 fingerbreadths above the puncture site.
  - Continue manual pressure for a minimum of 20 min (30 min if still on GP IIb/IIIa inhibitors) to achieve hemostasis.
- Monitor for bleeding: retroperitoneal → fluids, blood products.
  - Sudden hypotension
  - Severe low back pain
- Monitor for vascular complications: pulse assessments.
- Monitor for hematoma at sheath insertion site: assess sheath insertion site for swelling.

HYPERTENSIVE CRISIS/EMERGENCY

One question may focus on this topic. The question will usually be related to how the topic differs from hypertensive urgency or what drugs are used for treatment.

- Hypertensive **emergency or CRISIS** is elevated B/P with evidence of end organ damage (brain, heart, kidney, retina) that can be related to acute hypertension → needs critical care admission.
- Hypertensive **urgency** is elevated B/P without evidence of acute end organ damage → usually no need for critical care admission.
- Treatment of hypertensive crisis or emergency → emergent lowering of B/P needed.
  - **Nitroprusside (Nipride)**
    - Preload **and** afterload reducer
    - Assess for cyanide toxicity secondary to drug metabolite (Thiocyanate): mental status change (restlessness, lethargy), tachycardia, seizure, a need for ↑ in dose, unexplained metabolic acidosis, especially in those with renal impairment or when a drug is used > 24 hrs.
  - **Labetalol (Normodyne, Trandate)**
    - Intermittent IV doses preferred to a continuous infusion, due to the possibility of continuing the drug beyond the maximum dose of 300 mg.
    - Duration of effect persists 4–6 hrs after IV dose is discontinued.
- Greatest risk is STROKE.

One question about this topic may appear on the exam. That question generally covers **acute** issues that are related to peripheral arterial disease (PAD) or acute symptomatic carotid artery disease.

Peripheral Arterial Disease (PAD)

- Signs and symptoms (the 6 "Ps")
  - **P**ain (activity, rest)
  - **P**allor
  - **P**ulse absent or diminished
  - **P**aresthesia
  - **P**aralysis
  - **P**oikilothermia: loss of hair on toes or lower legs; glossy, thin, cool, dry skin (chronic sign of PAD)
  - Additionally, cool to touch, minimal edema
- Ankle-Brachial Index (ABI)
  - Test to assess for PAD
  - Used to assess the adequacy of lower extremity perfusion
  - Normal is > 0.90
    - Divide the ankle pressure by the brachial pressure on the same side
  - **You only need to remember what a normal ABI is for the exam.**
- Additional diagnostic testing
  - Doppler ultrasound
  - Arteriography
- Patient care management for PAD
  - Embolectomy, bypass graft, angioplasty
- ☆ Bed in reverse Trendelenburg
- ☆ **Do NOT elevate the affected extremity**—will decrease perfusion
- Medications
  - Thrombolytics (tPA)
  - Anticoagulants (heparin)
  - Antiplatelet agents (ASA, clopidogrel)
  - Vasodilators

Acute Symptomatic Carotid Artery Disease

- Signs and symptoms
  - Transient ischemic attack (TIA)
  - Monocular visual disturbances
  - Aphasia
  - Stroke

- Diagnostic testing may include one of the following:
  - Angiography (gold standard): risk of stroke during exam
  - Carotid duplex ultrasound
  - Computed tomography angiography (CTA)
  - Magnetic resonance angiography (MRA)
- Treatment
  - Carotid endarterectomy (CEA)
  - Carotid stenting
  - Aspirin
  - Statin therapy
- Post-procedure monitoring
  - Frequent neurological and motor checks
  - Close blood pressure and heart rate monitoring: patient may experience labile B/P and/or bradyarrhythmia with hypertension, hypotension, or bradycardia.
  - Monitor for bleeding.
  - Patient may develop hypoperfusion syndrome with the signs and symptoms of a headache ipsilateral to the revascularized carotid artery, focal motor seizures, and/or an intracerebral hemorrhage.

ARRHYTHMIA INTERPRETATION, ARRHYTHMIA EMERGENCIES, AND PACEMAKER THERAPY

Test candidates are expected to have mastered arrhythmia interpretation and have an understanding of ACLS principles, so look these over. An exam question may describe the arrhythmia **or** provide an arrhythmia strip for interpretation, but the question will usually be related to patient management.

☆ For exam questions that include the development of an arrhythmia, pay close attention to the patient's clinical response to the arrhythmia. Is the patient stable or unstable? If the clinical description is NOT provided, consider this fact and do NOT assume the patient response!

Conduction Abnormalities

- **Wolff-Parkinson-White (WPW) syndrome** is a genetic conduction abnormality in which an abnormal conduction pathway exists that allows a reentrant tachycardia pathway to bypass the normal AV node conduction pathway, resulting in supraventricular tachycardia. WPW is primarily seen in those younger than 30-years-old.

  - When in sinus rhythm, the ECG demonstrates a short PR interval and the presence of a delta wave (seen as a slow rise of the initial upstroke of the QRS).
  - WPW results in a supraventricular tachycardia (SVT) when the abnormal pathway takes over, but it may also present as **pre-excited atrial fibrillation** (irregular rhythm, rates of 150 beats/minute or greater, and a wide QRS).
  - The signs and symptoms during the SVT include palpitations, dizziness, chest pain, shortness of breath, and syncope.
  - Treatment of WPW

    - Radiofrequency ablation to eliminate the reentrant pathway
    - If unstable SVT is present, perform synchronized cardioversion **or** administer adenosine.
    - If pre-excited atrial fibrillation (AF) is present, administer beta blockers, amiodarone, or procainamide IV.
      - Do NOT give adenosine, digoxin, or calcium channel blockers for pre-excited AF; these agents may enhance antegrade conduction through the abnormal pathway by increasing the refractory period in the AV node, **resulting in ventricular fibrillation**.

- ☆ **Prolongation of the QT interval** (causes, treatment) is often addressed on the Adult CCRN exam. QT prolongation may lead to torsades de pointes. Causes of QT prolongation include:

  - Drugs—amiodarone, quinidine, haloperidol, procainamide
  - Electrolyte problems—hypokalemia, hypocalcemia, hypomagnesemia

- Treatment for torsades VT—magnesium

Pacemaker Therapy

For pacemaker therapy, which includes some knowledge of implantable cardioverter-defibrillator (ICD) devices, review the following information.

PACEMAKER CODE

A = atria   V = ventricle   D = dual (both)

- First initial = chamber **paced**; this was "invented" first
- Second initial = chamber **sensed**; this function came along second
- Third initial = response to sensing; last to be developed

  - I = inhibits (pacer detects intrinsic cardiac activity and withholds its pacing stimuli) . . . demand
  - D = inhibits **and** triggers (pacer detects intrinsic cardiac activity and fires a pacing stimulus in response)
  - O = none

On the Adult CCRN exam, you may see a question that asks how a "VVI" or a "DDD" pacemaker works. If you remember the code, you should be able to figure out the answer.

Sample questions:

    a. Which pacemaker paces both the atria and the ventricles, senses both the atria and the ventricles, and can inhibit and trigger in response to sensing?

    b. Which pacemaker paces the ventricle, senses the ventricle, and inhibits pacing in response to sensing?

Answers: a. DDD   b. VVI

Review the 3 basic pacer malfunctions:

1. Failure to pace (no spike at all when expected)
2. Failure to capture (spikes without a QRS for ventricular pacing)
3. Failure to sense (pacing in native beats)

IMPLANTABLE CARDIOVERTER-DEFIBRILLATOR (ICD)

ICDs can provide "tiered" therapy:

- Programmed to **shock** (defibrillate or synchronized cardioversion)
- Programmed to **burst pace** (sense tachyarrhythmia, provide a series of beats faster than the tachyarrhythmia, and then suddenly stop [with the hope of the recovery of the SA node])
- Programmed to provide pacing for **bradyarrhythmias**

If the ICD does not correct the sudden death arrhythmia, shock as usual; do not place shocking pads directly over the ICD.

- The patient will require special education related to the device and emotional support, since many patients experience a FEAR of being shocked.

HEART FAILURE

Heart failure (HF) is a broad topic. For the exam, if you focus on the following, you will be ready!

    Heart failure may be acute, chronic, acute exacerbation of chronic HF, systolic or diastolic HF, or right-sided or left-sided HF. The most extreme HF occurs when all compensatory mechanisms have failed, and the result is cardiogenic shock. An understanding of these concepts and the management of each, as well as an understanding of heart failure classifications, is needed in order to successfully answer the Adult CCRN exam questions on this topic.

- **Heart failure** is a clinical syndrome that is characterized by signs and symptoms associated with high intracardiac pressures and decreased cardiac output.
- **Acute decompensated heart failure** is the abrupt onset of symptoms that are severe enough to merit hospitalization.

    ○ ~75% of patients with acute decompensated HF have a history of chronic heart failure.

- Heart failure with **systolic dysfunction** (left ventricular systolic dysfunction—LVSD): ejection fraction (EF) is 40% or less, problem with ejection
- Heart failure with **diastolic dysfunction**: EF is > 50%, problem with filling, ejection is OK

TIP

When studying, compare and contrast systolic and diastolic heart failure and differentiate the clinical signs of left-sided and right-sided heart failure.

What Is BNP?

- B-type natriuretic peptide (BNP) is released by the ventricle when the ventricle is under wall stress in attempts to dilate and decrease ventricular pressure.
- BNP is high with heart failure, and BNP is an indicator of a ventricle (left or right) under stress.

Pathophysiology of Acute Decompensated Systolic Dysfunction

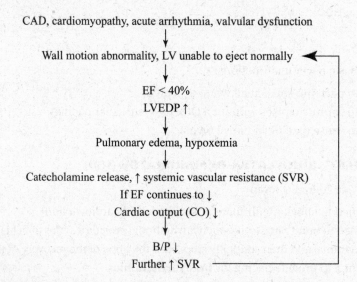

In the figure above: CAD = coronary artery disease; LV = left ventricle; EF = ejection fraction; LVEDP = left ventricular end-diastolic pressure

- When systolic dysfunction is prolonged and becomes chronic, compensatory **hormones** lead to ventricular remodeling over time.
- Drugs are used to decrease neurohormonal effects.

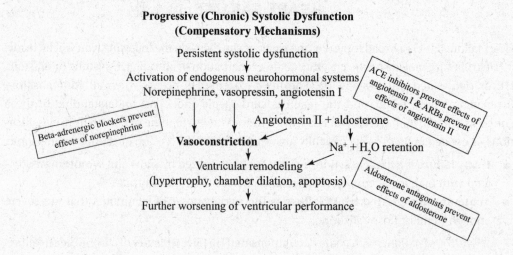

Pathophysiology of HF with Diastolic Dysfunction

Chronic hypertension, valvular disease,
restrictive or hypertrophic cardiomyopathy

↓

Stiff LV due to inability of myofibrils to relax
Impaired LV filling (empties OK, EF normal)
↑ LVEDP

↓

Pulmonary edema

☆ Table 4-2. Summary of the Differences Between Systolic and Diastolic Heart Failure

	Systolic	Diastolic
Primary problem	Ejection problem, dilated chamber • Can fill OK	Filling problem, hypertrophied chamber or septum • Can eject OK
Signs	Dilated left ventricle PMI shifted to left Valvular insufficiency (dilation causes mitral valve insufficiency) EF ≤ 40% Pulmonary edema due to poor ventricular emptying S3 heart sound B/P is normal or low (usually) BNP is elevated	Normal ventricular size Thick ventricular walls and/or thick septum Normal contractile function Normal EF Pulmonary edema due to high ventricular pressure S4 heart sound with hypertension B/P is often high BNP is elevated
Treatment	Beta blockers ACEI/ARB Diuretics Dilators Aldosterone antagonists Positive inotropes	Beta blockers ACEI/ARB Calcium channel blockers Diuretics (low dose) Aldosterone antagonists
Contraindicated	Negative inotropes (calcium channel blockers and, in acute phase, beta blockers)	Positive inotropes Dehydration further worsens filling Tachyarrhythmias decrease filling time and worsen symptoms
Cardiomyopathy Types	Cardiomyopathies that result in systolic HF: • Dilated ○ May result in mitral insufficiency as the left ventricular wall enlarges	Cardiomyopathies that result in diastolic HF: • Idiopathic hypertrophic subaortic stenosis (IHSS) • Hypertrophic cardiomyopathy (HCM) • Restrictive

☆ Chest X-Ray Findings: Systolic vs. Diastolic HF

- Systolic HF may be evidenced by a large, dilated heart **or** by a normal heart size on the chest film.

  ○ An enlarged heart is often associated with a shift of the point of maximal impulse (PMI) from midclavicular to the **left** (Figure 4-8).

- Diastolic HF generally is evidenced by a normal heart size on the chest film. However, on the 12-lead ECG, there **may** be a left ventricular hypertrophy pattern, especially when the patient has a history of uncontrolled hypertension.

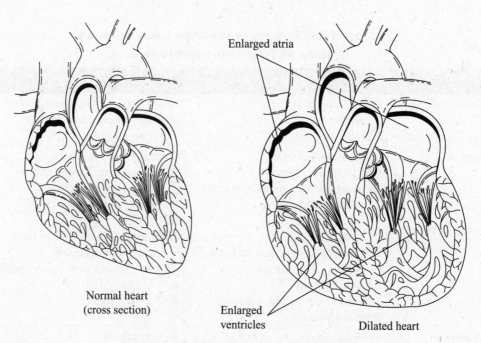

Normal heart
(cross section)

Enlarged atria

Enlarged ventricles

Dilated heart

Figure 4-8. Normal and enlarged heart size

Heart failure may also be categorized according to which ventricle is failing, the right or the left (Tables 4-3 and 4-4). The etiologies and treatment are different. The Adult CCRN exam may present a case scenario with background information, signs and symptoms, and a description of whether the HF is right-sided or left-sided. Then, you will be asked to identify the correct treatment.

Table 4-3. Causes of Right-Sided and Left-Sided Heart Failure

Right-Sided	Left-Sided
Acute RV infarct	Coronary artery disease, ischemia
Pulmonary embolism (massive)	Myocardial infarction
Septal defects	Cardiomyopathy
Pulmonary stenosis/insufficiency	Fluid overload
COPD	Chronic, uncontrolled hypertension
Pulmonary hypertension	Aortic stenosis/insufficiency
Left ventricular failure	Mitral stenosis/insufficiency
	Cardiac tamponade

Table 4-4. Signs and Symptoms of Right-Sided and Left-Sided Heart Failure

Right-Sided	Left-Sided
Hepatomegaly	Orthopnea, dyspnea, tachypnea
Splenomegaly	Hypoxemia
Dependent edema	Tachycardia
Venous distention	Crackles
Elevated CVP/JVD	Cough with pink, frothy sputum
Tricuspid insufficiency	Elevated PA diastolic/PAOP
Abdominal pain	Diaphoresis
	Anxiety, confusion

Heart Failure Classifications

The Adult CCRN exam may include a question related to heart failure classifications. There are two types of classifications: the American Heart Association (AHA) stages of heart failure (which are classified according to heart failure progression and recommended therapy for each stage) and the New York Heart Association (NYHA) four functional classes (which are based on the patient's symptoms and do not include suggested treatment).

- The main cause of death from heart failure is the development of **sudden death arrhythmia**. Select patients with NYHA Class II to IV may be candidates for an implantable cardioverter-defibrillator (ICD).

AMERICAN HEART ASSOCIATION (AHA) STAGES OF HEART FAILURE

- **Stage A**—High risk; no evidence of dysfunction
- **Stage B**—Heart disorder or structural defect; no symptoms
- **Stage C**—Heart disorder or structural defect, with symptoms (past or present)
- **Stage D**—End-stage cardiac disease, with symptoms despite maximal therapy (inotropic or mechanical support)

NYHA HEART FAILURE CLASSES

- **Class I**—Ordinary activity does not cause symptoms, although **EXTRAORDINARY ACTIVITY** results in heart failure symptoms.
- **Class II**—Comfortable at rest, but **ORDINARY ACTIVITY** results in heart failure symptoms.
- **Class III**—Comfortable at rest, but **MINIMAL ACTIVITY** causes heart failure symptoms.
- **Class IV**—Symptoms of heart failure occur **AT REST**; there is a severe limitation of physical activity.

CARDIOMYOPATHY

If the Adult CCRN exam includes a question on cardiomyopathy, it will most likely be on either **dilated** or **hypertrophic** cardiomyopathy (Table 4-5).

Table 4-5. Differences Between Dilated and Hypertrophic Cardiomyopathy

Dilated	Hypertrophic
SYSTOLIC dysfunction, problem ejecting Classical signs • Thinning, dilation, enlargement of LV chamber • Mitral valve regurgitation (MVR) common due to ventricular dilation Symptoms are similar to that of **SYSTOLIC** heart failure. Treatment • Similar to that for systolic heart failure • Heart failure may progress through stages, classes • May need a ventricular assist device (VAD), heart transplant	**DIASTOLIC** dysfunction, problem filling Classical sign • Increased thickening of the heart muscle and septum inwardly at the expense of the LV chamber Symptoms are similar to that of **DIASTOLIC** heart failure. • Fatigue • Dyspnea • Chest pain • Palpitations • S3, S4 heart sounds • Presyncope or syncope Treatment similar to that for diastolic heart failure. **Increased risk of sudden cardiac death!**

CARDIOGENIC SHOCK

When compensatory mechanisms fail to maintain the cardiac output, the most extreme end on the continuum of heart failure occurs—cardiogenic shock (Table 4-6). Cardiogenic shock has several causes. Most commonly, it is due to an extreme drop in stroke volume secondary to systolic dysfunction, which results in:

- Elevated left ventricular preload (PAOP) with associated pulmonary symptoms
- Elevated left ventricular afterload (SVR) due to vasoconstrictive compensatory mechanisms
- A resultant drop in cardiac output to the point where perfusion to organs is no longer adequate

Table 4-6. Clinical Presentation of Cardiogenic Shock

Compensatory Stage	Progressive Stage
Tachycardia	Hypotension
Tachypnea	Worsening tachycardia, tachypnea, oliguria
Crackles, mild hypoxemia	Metabolic acidosis
ABG with respiratory alkalosis or early metabolic acidosis	Worsening crackles and hypoxemia
Anxiety, irritability	Skin is clammy, mottled
Neck vein distention	Worsening anxiety or lethargy
S3 heart sounds (S4 heart sounds if there is also an acute MI)	• At any time, chest pain or arrhythmias may occur
Cool skin	
Urine output is down	
Narrow pulse pressure	
B/P is maintained or lower than baseline	

Etiologies of Cardiogenic Shock

- Acute MI
- Chronic heart failure
- Cardiomyopathy
- Dysrhythmias
- Cardiac tamponade
- Papillary muscle rupture
  - Obliterates the mitral valve
  - Life-threatening emergency
  - Requires immediate surgical intervention

Treatment of Cardiogenic Shock

- Identify the cause
- Manage arrhythmias (brady, tachy) that may be contributing to a decrease in cardiac output
- Reperfusion if there is STEMI (percutaneous coronary intervention or fibrinolytic therapy)
- Emergent surgery if cardiogenic shock is due to a mechanical problem—ruptured papillary muscle, VSD
- Mechanical support
- See Table 4-7

Table 4-7. Treatment of Cardiogenic Shock

Enhance Effectiveness of Pump	Decrease Demand on Pump
Positive inotropic support • Norepinephrine (Levophed) • Dopamine 4–10 mcg/kg/min • Dobutamine, milrinone (Primacor) AVOID negative inotropic agents! Vasodilators • May be used in conjunction with intra-aortic balloon pump (IABP) therapy and positive inotropic agents if the patient is in the progressive stage with hypotension	Preload reduction (or optimization) Afterload reduction Optimize oxygenation Mechanical ventilation Treat pain IABP for short term support Ventricular assist device (VAD) may be used for longer periods of time than IABP

Mechanical Circulatory Support

■ There are several types of mechanical circulatory support devices available, but intra-aortic balloon pump (IABP) therapy is specifically listed on the test blueprint. You will not be tested on the details of this therapy. However, you need to know that it is used in the management of left ventricular heart failure, cardiogenic shock, and cardiomyopathies, and it is also used for patients who are awaiting a heart transplant.

☆ **Benefits of IABP Therapy**

  ○ You will likely have at least 1 question on this.

  ○ Just remember, the balloon does 2 things: it INFLATES and it DEFLATES (Figure 4-9 and Figure 4-10).

Benefits of INFLATION

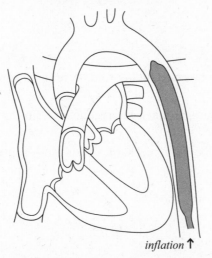

inflation ↑

Figure 4-9. Balloon inflation—increases coronary artery perfusion

→ Inflates at dicrotic notch of the arterial waveform, beginning of diastole

Benefits of DEFLATION

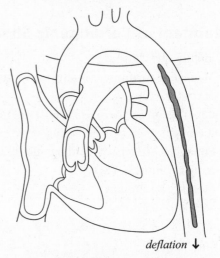

deflation ↓

Figure 4-10. Balloon deflation—decreases afterload

→ Deflates right before systole begins; determined by a set TRIGGER for deflation, R-wave of ECG or upstroke of the arterial pressure wave

Cardiopulmonary Bypass

- Aortic cross-clamping is done, and the heart is stopped during surgery.
- Most common cannulation sites:
  - Aorta
  - Right atrium
- The longer the bypass time, the more bleeding there is and the more complications there may be postoperatively.

Coronary Artery Bypass Graft (CABG) Procedure

- Priming with isotonic crystalloids (hemodilution); enhances oxygenation by improving blood flow
- Hypothermia (28°C–36°C) is induced.
- Anticoagulation with large heparin doses
- Rapid circulatory arrest is achieved during diastole with the infusion of a potassium cardioplegic agent; the cardioplegic agent is reinfused at regular intervals; note that either a warm or a cold cardioplegic agent may be used.

Post-Op Assessment for Complications Related to CABG

- Hemodynamic abnormalities
- Arrhythmias
- ☆ Tamponade
- ☆ Pericarditis
- Electrolyte abnormalities
- Hematologic abnormalities, bleeding
- Pulmonary problems (pneumonia, atelectasis, difficulty weaning from mechanical ventilation)
- Pain, anxiety
- Renal failure
- Endocrine problems (issues with glycemic control)
- Gastrointestinal problems (nausea, vomiting, ileus)
- Infections

☆ **Post-Op Chest Tube Management**
- Maintain patency.
  - Do not allow dependent loops.
  - Milking or stripping chest tubes is not routinely indicated.
    - If clots appear, gently milk the chest tubes.

> **NOTE**
>
> The exam questions related to heart surgery generally focus on complications and nursing care postoperatively.

- Mediastinal chest tubes remove serosanguinous fluid from the operative site, whereas pleural chest tubes remove air, blood, or serous fluid from the pleural space.
- Keep chest tubes lower than patient's chest.
- Do not clamp the system unless you are changing the drainage system or there is a system disconnect. When the tube is clamped, the connection to the negative chamber is lost.
- A chest tube output > 100 mL for 2 consecutive hours generally requires intervention.
    - Maintain hemodynamic stability.
    - Correct the volume status.
    - Administer blood products.

Valve Surgery

Table 4-8. Advantages and Disadvantages of Mechanical and Biological Valves

Mechanical Valve	Biological Valve
Advantages: • Relatively easy to insert • Very reliable • Lasts longer than biological valve Disadvantages: • High risk of thrombosis • Permanent anticoagulation therapy	Advantages: • Only short-term anticoagulation is required (but the patient will need long-term antiplatelet [ASA] therapy) Disadvantages: • Wears down, especially in high-pressure systems

Nursing Considerations Post-Valve Repair or Replacement

- Avoid a drop in preload. Most patients who have had valvular stenosis or chronic regurgitation have had elevated end-diastolic volumes. Sudden preload normalization may result in hypotension.
- Anticoagulation will be needed for mechanical valve replacement; biological valve replacement will require antiplatelet therapy (aspirin).
- Anticipate **conduction disturbances** since the mitral, tricuspid, and aortic valves are anatomically close to conduction pathways. Temporary or permanent pacing may be needed.

Transcatheter Aortic Valve Replacement (TAVR)

- TAVR, which was approved in 2011, is a procedure that involves placement of a collapsible prosthetic valve (either bovine or porcine) over the diseased valve (either a native valve or a previously placed artificial valve).
- Access to the aorta is usually achieved percutaneously or through a small incision, avoiding cross-clamping of the aorta and cardiopulmonary bypass.
- Most TAVR procedures are done via the femoral artery and are performed in a cardiac catheterization laboratory that is modified to accommodate TAVR procedures.
- Ideal candidates for TAVR are those with severe aortic valve disease that is classified as **high-risk** for open surgery.

- Those who are at an intermediate risk for open surgery may qualify for either TAVR or open surgical replacement, depending upon a decision from the interdisciplinary heart valve team based on an evaluation of the patient.
- Patients who are considered extreme high-risk/inoperable or low-risk for open procedure are NOT candidates for TAVR.
- **Note:** There are studies looking at TAVR for a patient who is classified as **low-risk** for an open procedure for aortic valve replacement, but as of the date of this publication, a low-risk patient is not considered an ideal candidate for this procedure.

- Complications: vascular complications associated with femoral access (similar to post-PCI, including hematomas, retroperitoneal bleeding, and arterial occlusion); heart block; stroke; acute kidney injury; and paravalvular regurgitation (associated with a mismatch of the prosthetic valve and the native valve annulus)
- Dual antiplatelet therapy will be required, including aspirin (75–100 mg/day) for life and clopidogrel (75 mg/day) for 3 to 6 months post-procedure.

CARDIAC TAMPONADE

- Etiologies: surgical-related cause (post-op cardiac surgery), medical-related cause (pericarditis, pericardial effusion), trauma
- Signs and symptoms
  - Restlessness and agitation
  - Hypotension
  - ↑ JVD
  - Equalization of CVP, pulmonary artery diastolic pressure, and PAOP
  - Muffled heart sounds
  - Enlarging cardiac silhouette and mediastinum on a chest radiograph
- ☆ Narrowed pulse pressure (i.e., 82/68)
- ☆ Pulsus paradoxus: an excessive drop (greater than 12 mmHg) in the SBP during inspiration, which is the result of cardiac muscle restriction caused by the tamponade with inspiration; the intrathoracic pressure increases, and the venous return decreases

  – Best seen on an arterial waveform as respiratory variation (Figure 4-11).

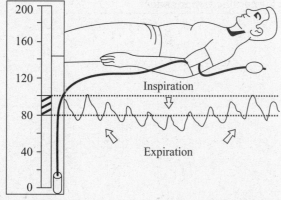

Figure 4-11. Pulsus paradoxus as seen on an arterial waveform

Which valve is most at risk for a rupture due to trauma?

- **Aortic valve** because it is most anterior in the chest
- A myocardial contusion has signs and symptoms that are similar to that for pericarditis, but there are important differences between these two conditions, as outlined in Table 4-9.

Table 4-9. Pericarditis vs. Myocardial Contusion

	☆ Medical—Pericarditis	☆ Trauma—Myocardial Contusion
Etiology	Trauma (rare) Viral After an MI Post-op cardiac surgery Radiation Idiopathic Dressler's syndrome—immune response after an MI, surgery, or traumatic injury	Trauma • Worse outcome than pericarditis • Broken vessels bleed into heart, similar to an MI • Cardiac dysrhythmias • Death can occur within the first 48 hours
Signs and symptoms	Chest pain Pain worsens with inspiration Dyspnea Low-grade temp ↑ Sed rate ST elevation in all the leads Cardiac tamponade Post-MI, Dressler's syndrome, may last months	Signs of trauma Chest pain Pain worsens with inspiration Dyspnea Low-grade temperature ST elevation in the **area of injury**
Treatment	Symptom relief Analgesics Anti-inflammatory agents NSAIDs Steroid Antibiotics Monitor for worsening symptoms Monitor for constrictive pericarditis Monitor for cardiac tamponade	Monitor for arrhythmias Analgesics as needed

An aneurysm is a localized, blood-filled outpouching in the wall of an artery. The larger it becomes, the more likely it is to rupture. The Adult CCRN exam may contain a question about abdominal aortic or thoracic aortic aneurysms.

Etiology of Aneurysms

- Arteriosclerosis
- Hypertension
- Smoking
- Obesity
- Bacterial infections
- Congenital anomalies
- Trauma
- Marfan syndrome

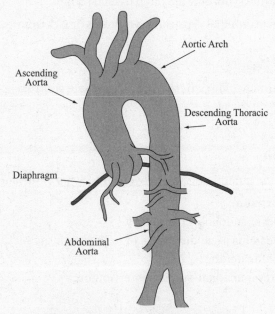

Aortic Arch

Ascending Aorta

Descending Thoracic Aorta

Diaphragm

Abdominal Aorta

Figure 4-12. Types and locations of cardiovascular-related aneurysms

Abdominal Aortic Aneurysms (75% of all CV-related aneurysms)

- Asymptomatic if small
- Pulsations in abdominal area
- Abdominal or low back pain
- Nausea, vomiting
- Shock

Thoracic Aortic Aneurysms (25% of all CV-related aneurysms)

- Sudden tearing, ripping pain in chest that radiates to the shoulders, neck, and back
- Cough
- Hoarseness
- Dysphagia
- Dyspnea
- Dizziness, difficulty walking and speaking
- Widening of mediastinum on a chest X-ray

Treatment of Aneurysms

- Aneurysms that are < 5 cm in diameter and produce no symptoms
  - Monitor regularly.
    - Ultrasound or CT scan
  - Treat hypertension: drug class of choice is beta blockers, which may slow growth.
  - People with Marfan syndrome are often treated sooner.
- Thoracic aortic aneurysm that is causing symptoms or is > 6 cm
  - Surgical repair
  - Dissection: SURGERY
  - Aggressive treatment of hypertension and heart rate control
    - Labetalol drip

Aortic Dissection

Blood passes through the inner lining and between the layers of the aorta.

- The tear is spiral in nature.
- A dissection can occur suddenly or gradually.
- A dissection occurs in the ascending aorta or in the aortic arch.
- A dissection is life-threatening.
- A dissection requires immediate surgical intervention.

Now that you have reviewed the key cardiovascular concepts, go to the Cardiovascular Practice Questions. Answer the questions, and then check your answers. Continue to review the information until you answer 80% of the practice questions correctly.

CARDIOVASCULAR PRACTICE QUESTIONS

1. A 59-year-old male is admitted with complaints of chest pain and dyspnea. ST elevation and T-wave inversion were seen on the ECG in V2, V3, and V4. IV thrombolytic therapy was started in the Emergency Department. Indications of successful reperfusion would include all of the following EXCEPT:

   (A) pain cessation.
   (B) a decrease in CK or troponin.
   (C) reversal of ST segment elevation with a return to baseline.
   (D) short runs of ventricular tachycardia.

2. Which of the following medication orders should the nurse question for the patient described in question 1?

   (A) metoprolol (Lopressor)
   (B) aspirin
   (C) propranolol (Inderal)
   (D) heparin

3. If heart block develops while caring for the patient described in question 1, which of the following types would it most likely be?

   (A) sinoatrial block
   (B) second-degree, Type I
   (C) second-degree, Type II
   (D) third-degree, complete

4. Appropriate drug therapy for dilated cardiomyopathy is aimed toward:

   (A) decreasing contractility and decreasing both preload and afterload.
   (B) decreasing contractility and increasing both preload and afterload.
   (C) increasing contractility and increasing both preload and afterload.
   (D) increasing contractility and decreasing both preload and afterload.

5. An 18-year-old is admitted with a history of a syncopal episode at the mall, and he has a history of an eating disorder. The nurse notes a prolonged QT on the 12-lead ECG and anticipates that a reduction in an electrolyte is the cause. Which of the following is LEAST likely to cause this patient's problem?

   (A) sodium
   (B) magnesium
   (C) potassium
   (D) calcium

6. On the third day after admission for an acute MI, a 67-year-old male complains of chest pain and develops a fever. The pain is worse with deep inspiration and is relieved when he leans forward. There are nonspecific ST changes in the precordial leads of the ECG. The nurse anticipates that this patient will most likely need treatment for:

(A) a thoracic aneurysm.
(B) Dressler's syndrome.
(C) reinfarction.
(D) pleuritis.

7. A patient is admitted to the CCU after PCI with a stent. A femoral sheath is in place, and the site is dry with no hematoma. He suddenly complains of severe back pain. His neck veins are flat, the head of the bed is at 30 degrees, and his heart sounds are normal. His vital signs are as follows: B/P is 78/48, heart rate is 124 beats/minute, and respiratory rate is 26 breaths/minute. What should the nurse suspect?

(A) cardiac tamponade
(B) retroperitoneal bleeding
(C) coronary artery dissection
(D) acute closure of the stented coronary artery

8. A patient admitted with an NSTEMI develops acute shortness of breath, a recurrence of chest pain, and a loud systolic murmur at the apex of the heart. Which of the following has most likely occurred?

(A) The patient has developed acute mitral valve regurgitation.
(B) The patient has developed acute reinfarction.
(C) The patient has developed acute mitral valve stenosis.
(D) The patient has developed an acute ventricular septal defect.

9. A patient has just returned from the OR after insertion of a VVI pacemaker. In order to assess the functioning of this pacemaker accurately, the nurse needs to understand that:

(A) both the atrium and ventricle are paced and sensed and may either inhibit or pace in response to sensing.
(B) the ventricle is paced, ventricular activity is sensed, and pacing is inhibited in response to ventricular sensing.
(C) both the atrium and ventricle are paced, but only ventricular pacing can be inhibited by a sensed intrinsic ventricular impulse.
(D) the ventricle is paced, in response to a sensed intrinsic atrial impulse or inhibited by a sensed intrinsic ventricular impulse.

10. A patient complains of sudden dyspnea 5 days S/P an acute MI (ST elevation in II, III, and aVF, with ST depression in I and aVL). The patient is anxious, diaphoretic, and hypotensive. An examination reveals the development of a loud holosystolic murmur at the apex that radiates to the axilla. The patient has crackles throughout but no S3 heart sound at the apex. What is the most likely cause of this patient's deterioration?

    (A) right ventricular failure related to a right ventricular MI
    (B) ventricular septal defect
    (C) left ventricular failure due to extension of the MI
    (D) acute mitral regurgitation due to papillary muscle rupture or dysfunction

11. A patient with a diagnosis of cardiogenic shock now requires high dose dopamine (greater than 10 mcg/kg/min) to maintain her blood pressure, and the cardiologist is planning to start IABP therapy. This therapy will benefit the patient because it will:

    (A) increase afterload with balloon inflation and decrease diastolic augmentation with balloon deflation.
    (B) decrease afterload with balloon deflation and increase diastolic augmentation with balloon inflation.
    (C) decrease afterload with balloon inflation and decrease diastolic augmentation with balloon deflation.
    (D) increase afterload with balloon deflation and decrease diastolic augmentation with balloon inflation.

12. Four days after mitral valve replacement, a patient goes into atrial fibrillation with a rapid ventricular response. What should be the nurse's initial action?

    (A) Order a 12-lead ECG.
    (B) Evaluate the patient for clinical signs of hypoperfusion.
    (C) Notify the physician.
    (D) Ask the patient to bear down as if having a bowel movement.

13. A patient's 12-lead ECG shows sinus bradycardia at 44 beats/minute and ST segment elevation in leads II, III, and aVF. Which of the following treatments for bradycardia would best resolve the problem for this patient?

    (A) temporary transvenous pacing
    (B) transcutaneous pacing
    (C) percutaneous coronary intervention
    (D) administration of atropine

14. Which drug would most likely be given to a patient with hypertrophic cardiomyopathy?

    (A) metoprolol
    (B) digoxin
    (C) dopamine
    (D) dobutamine

15. A patient is admitted with ST elevation in V2, V3, and V4. Four days after admission, the patient suddenly developed a holosystolic murmur at the lower left sternal border, chest pain, and hypotension. What complication should the nurse expect?

    (A) papillary muscle rupture
    (B) ventricular septal defect
    (C) acute mitral valve stenosis
    (D) acute reinfarction

16. A postoperative patient on the surgical unit suddenly develops chest pain, extreme weakness, and dyspnea and is found to have ST elevation in II, III, and aVF on the stat ECG. Her B/P is 92/62, her heart rate is 58 beats/minute, her respiratory rate is 28 breaths/minute, her lungs are clear, and a heart sound assessment reveals an S4 with no murmurs. In addition to preparing the patient for PCI, which of the following interventions would the nurse anticipate?

    (A) a nitroglycerin drip and the administration of aspirin
    (B) the administration of furosemide (Lasix) and atropine
    (C) transcutaneous pacing and the administration of morphine
    (D) aggressive fluid administration and a right-sided ECG

17. A 52-year-old male presents with complaints of blurred vision and shortness of breath. His B/P is 232/136, his heart rate is 102 beats/minute, his respiratory rate is 28 breaths/minute, he has crackles in the lower lung fields bilaterally, and there are S3 and S4 heart sounds upon auscultation. Which of the following would be indicated for this patient?

    (A) a nitroprusside drip and admission to the critical care unit
    (B) the administration of digoxin and furosemide
    (C) a labetalol drip and admission to a medical unit
    (D) the administration of lisinopril and a calcium channel blocker

18. An 80-year-old female presents with a chief complaint of acute shortness of breath. A clinical exam reveals that her B/P is 180/102, her heart rate is 105 beats/minute, her respiratory rate is 32 breaths/minute, she has lung crackles bilaterally, her pulse oximetry is 88%, and there are S4 heart sounds upon auscultation. An ECG revealed sinus tachycardia and a left ventricular hypertrophy pattern; a chest radiograph showed a normal heart size and pulmonary vascular congestion; and an echocardiogram showed an EF of 55%. Which of the following should be avoided in this patient's treatment plan?

    (A) a calcium channel blocker
    (B) digoxin
    (C) low dose diuretics
    (D) oxygen

19. A patient had a left internal carotid artery stent placed, and the latest assessment reveals that the patient is alert and oriented, has a weakened right hand grasp and a right facial droop, has stable vital signs, and has a dry procedure site without bleeding. The RN should contact the physician because this patient is most likely experiencing which of the following?

(A) a right cerebral hemorrhage
(B) hyperperfusion syndrome
(C) acute cerebrovascular insufficiency
(D) hypovolemia

20. Mrs. Jones has an exacerbation of her heart failure, with signs and symptoms of jugular venous distention (JVD), peripheral edema, and abdominal discomfort. These are clinical signs specific to:

(A) acute left ventricular failure.
(B) chronic right ventricular failure.
(C) acute right ventricular failure.
(D) chronic dehydration.

21. A nurse is managing a post-op CABG patient assesses a sudden drop in B/P, distended neck veins, muffled heart sounds, minimal chest tube output, and a systolic pressure that fluctuates with the breathing pattern. This patient most likely needs:

(A) an emergent return to the OR.
(B) clamping of the chest tube.
(C) a transfusion of PRBCs.
(D) high dose dopamine.

22. Physical assessment findings that are indicative of a significant right ventricular (RV) infarction would include:

(A) bibasilar crackles.
(B) flat neck veins with the patient in Semi-Fowler's position.
(C) jugular venous distention.
(D) tachypnea and frothy sputum.

23. What pulse change might a nurse expect in the presence of cardiac tamponade?

(A) pulsus alternans
(B) pulsus paradoxus
(C) pulsus magnus
(D) pulsus bisferiens

24. A patient with mitral regurgitation develops atrial fibrillation with a heart rate of 88 beats/minute and a B/P of 118/75. Which of the following may be indicated?

(A) beta blockers and vasopressors
(B) cardiac glycosides and calcium channel blockers
(C) beta blockers and calcium channel blockers
(D) antiarrhythmics and angiotensin-converting enzyme inhibitors

25. Which of the following are predominant signs of left ventricular systolic dysfunction?

    (A) pedal edema, ascites, hepatomegaly, weight gain, ejection fraction less than 40%
    (B) S4 heart sound, bibasilar crackles, hypertension, ejection fraction greater than 40%
    (C) S3 heart sound, new cough, bibasilar crackles, ejection fraction less than 40%
    (D) hypertension, murmur, chest pain, weight gain, ejection fraction greater than 40%

26. A nurse was preparing a patient with the diagnosis of STEMI for a percutaneous coronary intervention (PCI). The monitor had previously shown a normal sinus rhythm (NSR); the B/P had been 128/78; and chest pain had improved from a "9" to a "2" on a 0–10 scale. The monitor alarm then sounded, and the rhythm below was observed by the nurse:

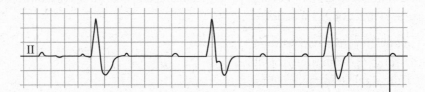

    Based on this information, which of the following statements is TRUE?

    (A) This change is most commonly seen with an acute inferior MI. Assess the patient. If serious signs and symptoms develop, begin transcutaneous pacing (TCP).
    (B) This change is most commonly seen with an acute anterior MI. Assess the patient. If serious signs and symptoms develop, give atropine.
    (C) This change is most commonly seen with an acute inferior MI. Assess the patient. If serious signs and symptoms develop, begin dobutamine.
    (D) This change is most commonly seen with an anterior MI. Assess the patient. If serious signs and symptoms develop, begin transcutaneous pacing (TCP).

27. A 58-year-old patient developed chest pain that he scored as an "8." A rapid assessment included profuse diaphoresis, a B/P of 78/52, a heart rate of 104 beats/minute, a respiratory rate of 20 breaths/minute, clear lungs, and an SpO_2 of 98%. The patient is currently connected to the bedside monitor with a nasal cannula at 2 L/minute in place and intravenous fluids (0.9 NS) being administered at a rate of 10 mL/hour. Which of the following sequences of interventions would be the most appropriate for the nurse to follow at this time?

    (A) Give a chewable aspirin, do an ECG, and then start a fluid bolus.
    (B) Give NTG sublingual, increase the FiO_2, and then give morphine.
    (C) Do an ECG, give NTG sublingual, and then give a chewable aspirin.
    (D) Start a fluid bolus, give a chewable aspirin, and then do an ECG.

28. The location or type of an acute MI is often associated with specific clinical findings. Which of the following statements related to the location of an MI is TRUE?

    (A) An anterior MI is often associated with heart blocks or bradyarrhythmias.
    (B) An inferior MI is often associated with right ventricular wall infarction.
    (C) A lateral MI is most likely to be associated with a posterior MI.
    (D) A posterior MI is most likely to lead to the complication of heart failure.

29. Which of the following statements is accurate regarding heart valves?

   (A) The aortic valve is closed during systole.
   (B) The mitral valve is closed during systole.
   (C) The mitral valve is closed during diastole.
   (D) The aortic valve is open during diastole.

30. The following drugs are all considered positive inotropic drugs that primarily affect the beta-1 receptors in the heart EXCEPT:

   (A) dopamine drip at 12 mcg/kg/min dose.
   (B) dopamine drip at 5 mcg/kg/min dose.
   (C) dobutamine drip at 7 mcg/kg/min dose.
   (D) milrinone at 7 mcg/kg/min dose.

ANSWER KEY

1. **B**	6. **B**	11. **B**	16. **D**	21. **A**	26. **A**
2. **C**	7. **B**	12. **B**	17. **A**	22. **C**	27. **D**
3. **C**	8. **A**	13. **C**	18. **B**	23. **B**	28. **B**
4. **D**	9. **B**	14. **A**	19. **C**	24. **B**	29. **B**
5. **A**	10. **D**	15. **B**	20. **B**	25. **C**	30. **A**

ANSWERS AND EXPLANATIONS

1. **(B)** Coronary artery reperfusion (due to either PCI or fibrinolysis) results in an **elevation** of, NOT a decrease in, creatine kinase (CK) or troponin. The theory is that the return of blood flow distal to the occlusion can result in a "reperfusion injury" of muscle, elevating cardiac biomarkers. The other 3 choices are indicators of successful reperfusion.

2. **(C)** The patient in this scenario is having an acute anterior wall MI. A beta blocker is beneficial for an acute MI, as these agents decrease the work of the heart and increase the threshold for ventricular fibrillation. Although it is a beta-adrenergic blocker like metoprolol, propranolol is NOT a cardioselective beta blocker. It affects beta receptors in heart muscle AND lung tissue. Therefore, it is more likely to cause bronchoconstriction than a cardioselective beta blocker. The other 3 choices (a cardioselective beta blocker, an antiplatelet, and an anticoagulant) are indicated for an acute MI, such as the one that the patient in this scenario is experiencing.

3. **(C)** The patient is having an acute anterior MI, which is generally due to LAD occlusion. The LAD supplies the bundle of His, so an LAD occlusion could result in a second-degree Type II heart block. If symptomatic bradycardia were to occur, the patient may require transcutaneous pacing. The other 3 types of heart blocks are due to SA node or AV node ischemia, which generally occur with an RCA occlusion (inferior wall MI).

4. **(D)** Dilated cardiomyopathy is likely to result in systolic dysfunction, which decreases contractility, causes compensatory arterial constriction, and results in a higher left ventricular preload. To treat this, therapy is aimed at increasing contractility, decreasing afterload (arterial constriction), and decreasing preload that is too high.

5. **(A)** An abnormal level of sodium does NOT cause QT prolongation. In contrast, a low level of magnesium, potassium, or calcium may cause QT prolongation and may result in torsades de pointes ventricular tachycardia and, if self-limiting, a transient syncopal episode.

6. **(B)** The pain described in the scenario is typical of the pain caused by pericarditis. Dressler's syndrome is the pericarditis that may result after an acute MI.

7. **(B)** Retroperitoneal bleeding may cause signs of hypovolemia and hypovolemic shock, as described in this scenario. It may be a complication of a PCI if the femoral artery is the access site during the procedure. Only this problem results in severe back pain; none of the other 3 choices results in back pain.

8. **(A)** The location of the murmur, at the apex of the heart (midclavicular, 5th ICS), is one clue to this answer. In addition, regurgitation occurs when the valve should be closed, and the mitral valve should be closed during systole. Mitral valve stenosis, choice (C), occurs when the mitral valve is open. Additionally, mitral valve stenosis cannot be acute; it develops gradually.

9. **(B)** The first letter indicates chamber paced (ventricle). The second letter indicates chamber sensed (ventricle). The third letter indicates the response to sensing (inhibited in response to sensing).

10. **(D)** The scenario describes a patient having an acute inferior wall MI, which is generally due to occlusion of the RCA. The RCA occlusion may result in papillary muscle dysfunction or rupture of the mitral valve because it supplies the area of the left ventricle where this valve is attached. Although RV infarct could result in RCA occlusion, RV infarct does not result in a holosystolic murmur at the apex of the heart or lung crackles.

11. **(B)** Cardiogenic shock results in a decrease in cardiac output with a resultant drop in coronary artery perfusion and compensatory vasoconstriction. The deflation of the balloon that is placed into the descending aorta is beneficial. Deflation decreases afterload and work of the left ventricle. Inflation of the balloon is beneficial because it "boluses" blood into the coronary arteries, increasing perfusion.

12. **(B)** The patient's response to the arrhythmia will determine whether treatment needs to be emergent and what the treatment will be. Vagal maneuvers (e.g., bearing down) are not known to be effective for atrial fibrillation.

13. **(C)** PCI would address the cause of the problem, not only treat the signs and symptoms, it would also address the cause of the problem. Selection of the other 3 choices presumes that the patient had serious signs and symptoms. Do not read into the questions.

14. **(A)** In hypertrophic cardiomyopathy, there is a problem with filling. A decrease in heart rate provided by a beta blocker such as metoprolol would increase the filling time. Diastolic dysfunction does NOT cause a problem with ejection, and the EF is normal. The other 3 choices may be indicated for systolic dysfunction.

15. **(B)** This scenario describes an acute anterior STEMI, generally caused by an occlusion of the LAD. This type of MI is most likely to result in a VSD. Additionally, the location of the murmur is important. Mitral valve disease–related problems do NOT cause murmurs to be loudest at the left sternal border, whereas a VSD would result in a murmur at this location.

16. **(D)** This scenario describes a patient having an acute inferior STEMI, generally due to RCA occlusion. An RCA occlusion may result in an RV infarct, which this patient has signs of (hypotension with clear lungs). The definitive treatment is emergent PCI. Fluid administration will help increase coronary artery perfusion by correcting hypotension and ensure adequate RV preload. A right-sided ECG may help confirm the RV infarct. Nitroglycerin, diuretics, and morphine may decrease preload, which would worsen the hypotension.

17. **(A)** This patient has signs of organ dysfunction (heart failure) secondary to extreme hypertension. Therefore, he has a hypertensive crisis or emergency. The B/P needs to be emergently decreased. Most often, this treatment is best done in a critical care setting.

18. **(B)** This patient presents with signs of heart failure due to diastolic dysfunction (hypertension, left ventricular hypertrophy, EF > 40%). This patient has a problem with FILLING, not ejection. Digoxin, a positive inotrope, may increase wall stress and worsen filling of the left ventricle.

19. **(C)** Contralateral motor weakness and aphasia may be signs of cerebrovascular insufficiency due to left stent patency issues. A right cerebral hemorrhage (choice (A)) would result in left-sided motor weakness and is not usually associated with post-carotid stent placement. The signs and symptoms of hyperperfusion syndrome (choice (B)) do not include contralateral motor weakness. There were no signs of hypovolemia (choice (D)), such as hypotension or oliguria, described in the question.

20. **(B)** The signs described are those of chronic right-sided heart failure. Acute right ventricular failure may result in JVD, but not peripheral edema or abdominal discomfort (which is due to liver engorgement).

21. **(A)** The signs described in the scenario are those of cardiac tamponade. The treatment for cardiac tamponade for a post-op open heart surgery patient is a return to the OR to drain the pericardial fluid that has accumulated. Development of this problem in other patient populations would necessitate an emergent pericardiocentesis to drain the fluid.

22. **(C)** A right ventricular infarction that is large enough to cause RV failure causes a problem with RV emptying, leading to an elevated right atrial pressure. This causes jugular venous distention. Choices (A) and (D) are signs of left ventricular failure. Choice (B) is a sign of dehydration.

23. **(B)** Pulsus paradoxus is fluctuation of the systolic blood pressure with inspiration and expiration by more than 12 mmHg, best seen when an arterial line is in place. Inspiration increases thoracic pressure. When combined with fluid surrounding the heart in cardiac tamponade, inspiration further decreases venous return to the heart, leading to a drop in systolic pressure by > 12 mmHg during the inspiratory phase of breathing. Pulsus alternans (choice (A)) is characterized by a change in amplitude of the systolic waveform from beat to beat, usually indicative of severe left ventricular failure. Pulsus magnus (choice (C)) is a bounding pulse. Pulsus bisferiens (choice (D)) is a double pulse and is not covered on the Adult CCRN exam.

24. **(B)** This scenario describes the development of atrial fibrillation with a controlled ventricular response and a stable B/P. Even with a normal B/P, the development of atrial fibrillation drops the cardiac output by 20% to 25% due to a loss in "atrial kick" provided by a normal sinus rhythm. A cardiac glycoside (such as digoxin) may be beneficial since it is a weak positive inotrope that may compensate for the loss of atrial kick, and calcium channel blockers will keep the heart rate controlled. Pressors are not needed in this case. The use of both beta blockers and calcium channel blockers would decrease the heart rate too much. ACE inhibitors would offer no benefit in this case.

25. **(C)** An S3 heart sound in an adult is indicative of high left ventricular pressure. A new cough and lung crackles are signs of pulmonary edema secondary to elevated left ventricular end-diastolic pressure (PAOP), although these may be signs of other problems, such as pulmonary fibrosis. The EF is less than 40% in systolic heart failure.

26. **(A)** The patient's clinical status describes a stable B/P, but the development of a bradyarrhythmia specifically a complete heart block with a ventricular rate of 30 beats/minute. This is usually seen with RCA disease, generally associated with an inferior MI. A patient assessment will determine treatment. Transcutaneous pacing would be an appropriate treatment for an unstable patient with this arrhythmia.

27. **(D)** This clinical description may be that of acute coronary syndrome complicated by hypotension. Addressing the hypotension is a priority since this is further decreasing coronary artery perfusion. A fluid bolus would address the hypotension, and no contraindications seem to be present for a fluid bolus since the lungs are clear. Aspirin is indicated for acute chest pain and could be given while preparing to do the ECG, which is needed to help make the diagnosis.

28. **(B)** Since most inferior MIs are due to RCA occlusion and the RCA also supplies blood to the right ventricular muscle wall, an inferior MI is associated with RV infarct.

29. **(B)** During systole (left ventricular ejection), the aortic valve is open, allowing for ejection. The mitral valve is closed at this time. The mitral valve is open during filling (diastole).

30. **(A)** At high doses (> 10 mcg/kg/min), dopamine stimulates alpha receptors in the arteries and causes vasoconstriction. The other 3 drugs/doses affect mainly the beta-1 receptors in the heart, producing a positive inotropic effect.

Respiratory Concepts

5

The difference between a successful person and others is not a lack of strength, not a lack of knowledge, but rather a lack of will.

—Vince Lombardi

RESPIRATORY TEST BLUEPRINT

Respiratory 15% of total test   **22 questions**

→ Acute pulmonary embolus
→ ARDS
→ Acute respiratory failure
→ Acute respiratory infection (e.g., pneumonia)
→ Aspiration
→ Chronic conditions (e.g., COPD, asthma, bronchitis, emphysema)
→ Failure to wean from mechanical ventilation
→ Pleural space abnormalities (e.g., pneumothorax, hemothorax, empyema, pleural effusions)
→ Pulmonary fibrosis
→ Pulmonary hypertension
→ Status asthmaticus
→ Thoracic surgery
→ Thoracic trauma (e.g., fractured rib, lung contusion, tracheal perforation)
→ Transfusion-related acute lung injury (TRALI)*

*This topic is covered in the Hematology/Immunology Concepts chapter of this book.

RESPIRATORY TESTABLE NURSING ACTIONS

☐ Interpret blood gas results
☐ Recognize indications for and manage patients requiring:

   ○ Modes of mechanical ventilation
   ○ Noninvasive positive pressure ventilation (e.g., BiPAP, CPAP, high-flow nasal cannula)
   ○ Oxygen therapy delivery devices
   ○ Prevention of complications related to mechanical ventilation (ventilator bundle)
   ○ Prone positioning

○ Pulmonary therapeutic interventions related to mechanical ventilation: airway clearance, extubation, intubation, weaning

○ Therapeutic gases (e.g., oxygen, nitric oxide, heliox, CO_2)

○ Thoracentesis

○ Tracheostomy

*Note:** Although the test blueprint refers to these topics as respiratory concepts, the terms *respiratory* and *pulmonary* are synonymous and are used interchangeably throughout this book.

Plan on spending approximately 22 hours studying respiratory concepts, since there will be 22 questions related to respiratory topics. The first half of this chapter reviews pulmonary physiological concepts that may appear on the exam. These concepts are the basis of the specific respiratory disorders and treatments that are covered in the second half of this chapter.

PULMONARY ASSESSMENT AND PHYSIOLOGY

Ventilation

- Ventilation is the movement of air in (from the atmosphere) and out (from the body) to maintain appropriate concentrations of O_2 and CO_2.
- Central control (brain stem): primary control

  ○ Senses blood pH, decrease in pH → ventilation is stimulated

  ○ A decrease in pH = acidosis, which results in an increase in the rate and/or depth of breathing

- Peripheral control (PaO_2 "sensors" in aortic arch): secondary control

  ○ Senses PaO_2 of blood, decrease in PaO_2 → ventilation stimulated

  ○ Decrease in PaO_2 = hypoxemia, which results in an increase in the rate and/or depth of breathing

  ○ Chronic $PaCO_2$ retainers rely on mild hypoxemia for ventilator drive. If the PaO_2 is corrected to normal, this may result in a decreased drive to breathe (ventilate).

- What is the clinical indicator of ventilation? How do you know that your patient is ventilating normally?

  ○ You need to know the **$PaCO_2$** (NOT the PaO_2).

- What is minute ventilation?

  ○ Tidal volume (Vt) × respiratory rate (RR)—easily seen on the ventilator of a patient who requires mechanical ventilation

  ○ Normal ventilation is ∼ 4 L/minute.

  ○ An increase in minute ventilation = an increase in **work of breathing**

- What is the primary muscle of ventilation?

  ○ Diaphragm!

  ○ Anything that affects the "health" of the diaphragm (deconditioning, hypoxemia, acidosis, hypophosphatemia) will adversely affect ventilation.

- What is the position for optimal ventilation?
  - Upright sitting position
  - Supine position is NOT good for ventilation; if a patient is in respiratory distress, the worst position for the patient is flat on his or her back!

Dead Space Ventilation

- Volume of air that does not participate in gas exchange
  - Anatomic dead space: ~ 2 mL/kg of Vt
    - We all have this; it is normal.
    - No gas exchange at level of nose down to alveoli
  - Alveolar dead space: pathologic, non-perfused alveoli, PE
  - Physiologic dead space = anatomic dead space + alveolar dead space
- ☆ A **pulmonary embolus** results in increased alveolar dead space! A clot in the pulmonary circulation (a pulmonary embolus): no blood flow past alveoli in that area of the pulmonary circulation (Figure 5-1).

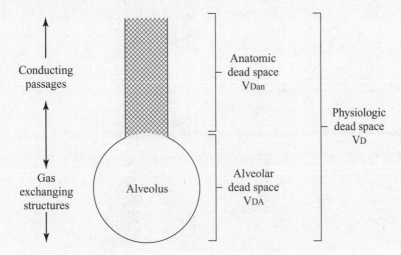

Figure 5-1. Dead space ventilation

Pulmonary Perfusion

The main function of the pulmonary system is gas exchange. For gas exchange to occur normally, there needs to be ventilation. However, movement of air alone is not enough for normal gas exchange. There needs to be perfusion, movement of blood past alveoli.

- Pulmonary perfusion is movement of blood through pulmonary capillaries.
- Any decrease in blood flow past alveoli (e.g., pulmonary embolus, low cardiac output states) will affect the ventilation/perfusion ratio and gas exchange.
- Normal ventilation/perfusion ratio:

$$\frac{4 \text{ L ventilation/min (V)}}{5 \text{ L perfusion/min (Q)}}$$

Ideal lung unit = 0.8 ratio, normal V/Q ratio

Any problem that alters ventilation (V) or perfusion (Q) can result in abnormal gas exchange if compensatory mechanisms are not successful. For example, even though it is not a pulmonary problem, a low cardiac output can result in poor gas exchange.

■ You will not be expected to calculate V/Q ratios for the exam. However, you will need to know that the pulmonary problems (discussed in this chapter) will result in abnormal V/Q ratios, from mild to extreme, depending upon the extent of the problem.

EFFECT OF GRAVITY ON PULMONARY PERFUSION

■ In the upright position, most pulmonary blood is in the lower lung lobes (see A in Figure 5-2). When lying supine, most pulmonary blood is posterior (see B in Figure 5-2). Rarely are ALL lung units perfused, but an example would be vigorous exercise (as in C in Figure 5-2).

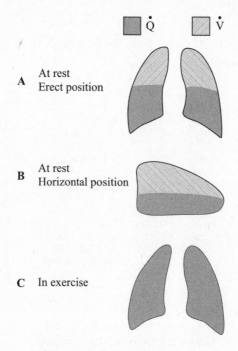

Figure 5-2. Perfused lung units

■ What are the clinical implications?

☆ You want the "good" lung down.

    ○ Large right lung pneumonia: if the patient is turned to the right ("bad" lung), more blood goes to the right, and the patient may become hypoxemic.

    ○ This patient should not be turned to the right side.

V/Q Ratio

☆ Normal V/Q ratio

    ○ When there are no problems with either ventilation or perfusion, the patient will have normal gas exchange on room air (Figure 5-3).

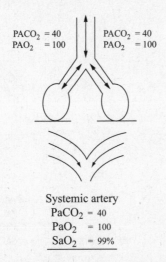

PACO₂ = 40   PACO₂ = 40
PAO₂ = 100   PAO₂ = 100

Systemic artery
$PaCO_2$ = 40
PaO_2 = 100
SaO_2 = 99%

Figure 5-3. Normal V/Q ratio, FiO_2 0.21

■ Abnormal V/Q ratio

○ When there is a problem with ventilation or perfusion, there is a V/Q mismatch.

○ The patient will develop hypoxemia on room air. However, providing oxygen will generally correct the hypoxemia until the etiology can be determined and addressed (Figure 5-4).

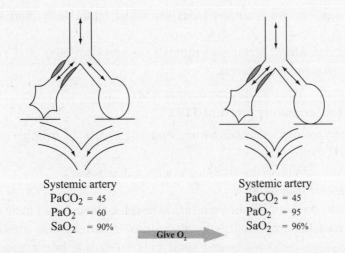

Systemic artery
$PaCO_2$ = 45
PaO_2 = 60
SaO_2 = 90%

Give O₂

Systemic artery
$PaCO_2$ = 45
PaO_2 = 95
SaO_2 = 96%

Figure 5-4. V/Q mismatch (i.e., pneumonia, pulmonary embolism)

○ Treatment of V/Q mismatch

– Give O_2
– Identify and treat the underlying problem

☆ Shunt

○ An extreme V/Q mismatch; even providing 100% FiO_2 will NOT correct the hypoxemia (Figure 5-5).

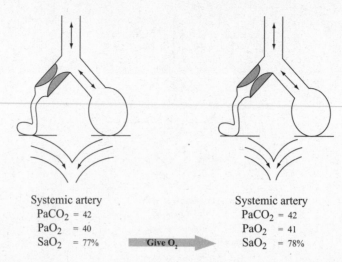

Systemic artery
$PaCO_2$ = 42
PaO_2 = 40
SaO_2 = 77%

Give O_2 →

Systemic artery
$PaCO_2$ = 42
PaO_2 = 41
SaO_2 = 78%

Figure 5-5. Shunt (i.e., acute respiratory distress syndrome (ARDS))

○ A shunt is movement of blood from the right side of the heart to the left side of the heart without getting oxygenated; venous blood moves to the arterial side.

○ Normal physiologic shunt: Thebesian veins of the heart empty into the left atrium. This is why the normal oxygen saturation on room air is 95% to 99%; it cannot be 100% on room air due to this shunt. (With supplemental oxygen, 100% saturation can be achieved.)

○ Anatomic shunt: two examples are a ventricular septal defect and an atrial septal defect.

☆ Pathologic shunt: **ARDS!** Blood goes through the lungs but does NOT get oxygenated, resulting in **refractory hypoxemia.**

○ Treatment of a shunt: administer **oxygen, AND**

○ **Positive end-expiratory pressure (PEEP)**

– Prevents expiratory pressure from returning to zero; by keeping expiratory pressure POSITIVE, it . . .

– ↓ Surface tension of the alveoli, preventing atelectasis

– ↑ Alveolar recruitment

– ↑ Driving pressure, extends time of gas transfer, allows for a ↓ in FiO_2 (Figure 5-6)

– With the addition of PEEP to the airway (provided in cm water pressure, i.e., 10 cm, 15 cm), hypoxemia will be addressed and the FiO_2 may be decreased from 100%.

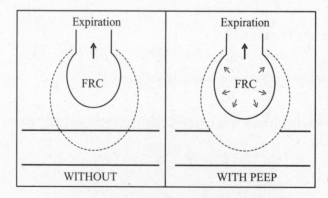

Figure 5-6. Visual representation of PEEP

Assessment of Oxygenation in the Critically Ill

Adequate oxygenation is the delivery of O_2 to meet tissue demands at the **cellular** level. In order to achieve this, each of the following needs to occur:

- Adequate ventilation
- Transfer of O_2 across alveolar-capillary membrane
- Presence of hemoglobin to carry O_2
- Adequate cardiac output to deliver O_2 to the tissue bed
- Release of O_2 from the hemoglobin molecule
- Ability of cells to utilize O_2

At the cellular level, sufficient oxygen is needed for the production of adenosine triphosphate (ATP), which is needed for cell energy and life. See Figure 5-7 to see how oxygen is needed for aerobic metabolism, along with the production of sufficient ATP for cell life. Without sufficient oxygen at the cellular level, lactic acid is produced (LACTIC ACIDOSIS), which is the evidence of anaerobic metabolism, organ failure, and eventual cell death.

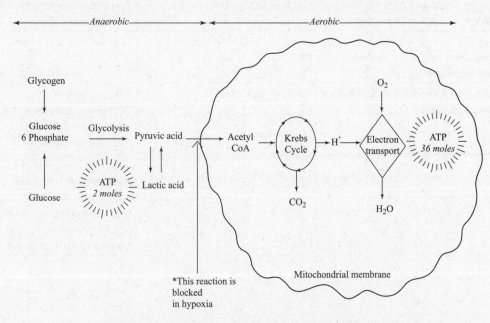

Figure 5-7. Importance of oxygen at the cellular level

It is NOT sufficient to examine only PaO_2 and SaO_2! For example, a patient with sepsis/septic shock may have a normal PaO_2, SaO_2, and hemoglobin; clear lungs; and adequate ventilation and oxygen delivery, yet a lactate level of 10. This is lactic acidosis. Why? Oxygen utilization is affected by sepsis/septic shock and results in anaerobic metabolism at the cellular level. Table 5-1 lists the clinical indicators of oxygenation in the critically ill.

Table 5-1. Indicators of Oxygenation

Parameter	Normal	How It's Calculated/Measured	Clinical Relevance
Arterial oxygen (PaO_2)	80–100 mmHg on room air	Directly measured	Less than 80 mmHg = hypoxemia (classified as mild, moderate, or severe)
Saturation of arterial oxygen (SaO_2)	95–99% on room air	Directly measured	Direct relationship with PaO_2; amount of hemoglobin combined with O_2
Mixed venous oxygen saturation (SvO_2)	60–75%	Direct measurement (pulmonary artery)	Most sensitive indicator of oxygenation at the cellular level
Oxygen content (CaO_2)	15–20 mL/100 mL blood	$CaO_2 = (Hgb \times 1.39 \times SaO_2) + (PaO_2 \times 0.003)$	Severe anemia may result in hypoxia
Oxygen delivery (DO_2)	900–1,100 mL/min	$CaO_2 \times CO \times 10$	Pump problems (heart) will decrease DO_2
Oxygen consumption, utilization (VO_2)	250–350 mL/min	$(SaO_2 - SvO_2) \times Hgb \times 13.9 \times CO$	Low with septic shock
Alveolar-arterial (A-a) gradient	< 10 mmHg	PAO_2 minus PaO_2 $(\% FiO_2 \times 715) - PaCO_2 \div (0.8 - PaO_2)$	Calculates the difference between the alveolar oxygen and the arterial oxygen Indicates whether the gas transfer is normal and, if not, how bad the V/Q mismatch or shunt is; just remember what normal is for the exam

> ☆ **For the exam:**
> ➤ Do not memorize the formulas.
> ➤ Remember that the assessment of oxygenation is more than just examining the PaO_2 or SaO_2.
> ➤ Consider the effects of severe anemia, low cardiac output, and an inability to utilize oxygen even when delivery is adequate (e.g., sepsis).

Most critically ill patients have continuous monitoring of oxygen saturation (SaO_2) that is noninvasively measured with the use of a bedside pulse oximetry (SpO_2). Although the normal SaO_2 on room air is 95% to 99%, the goal for most critically ill patients is to maintain the SpO_2 at 90% or greater, usually with supplemental oxygen. Note from the curve depicted in Figure 5-8 that when the SaO_2 is less than 90%, the PaO_2 is less than 60 mmHg. When the PaO_2 is less than 60 mmHg, cells begin to have difficulty maintaining aerobic metabolism (without compensation, i.e., an increase in heart rate or oxygen delivery).

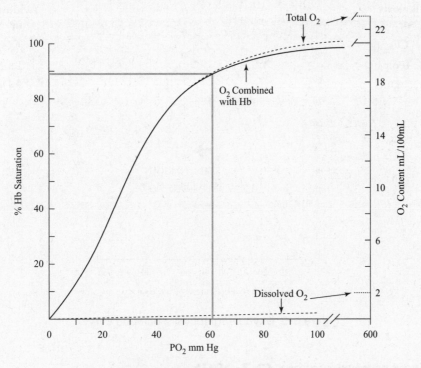

Figure 5-8. PaO$_2$/SaO$_2$ relationship

For the Adult CCRN exam, you will need to understand a high-level concept: the **oxyhemoglobin-dissociation curve**. Certain clinical conditions make hemoglobin "hold on" to oxygen molecules (the curve shifts to the LEFT). Other conditions allow hemoglobin to "release" the oxygen more easily to the tissue (the curve shifts to the RIGHT). See Table 5-2 for conditions that shift the curve to the left and right and Figure 5-9 for an illustration of the oxyhemoglobin-dissociation curve.

**Table 5-2. Clinical Conditions That Cause a Shift
of the Oxyhemoglobin-Dissociation Curve**

Shift to the Left	Shift to the Right
Alkalosis (low H$^+$)	Acidosis (high H$^+$)
Low PaCO$_2$	High PaCO$_2$
Hypothermia	Fever
Low 2,3-DPG	High 2,3-DPG
Remember left is aLkaLosis, coLd, Low Bad for patient; SaO$_2$ is high but O$_2$ is stuck to Hgb	Good for tissues; SaO$_2$ is low but O$_2$ is easily released to the tissues

- Conditions that cause a shift to the left result in a higher SaO$_2$, but the tissues do not get needed O$_2$ as readily.
- Conditions that cause a shift to the right result in a somewhat lower SaO$_2$, but the tissues receive O$_2$ more readily.

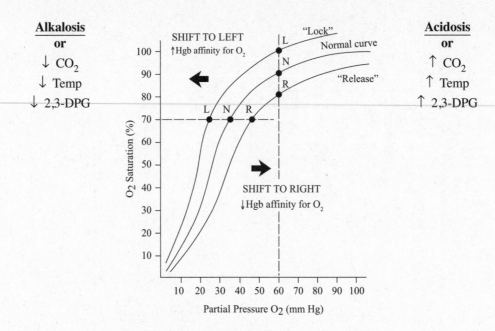

Figure 5-9. Oxyhemoglobin-dissociation curve

2,3-Diphosphoglycerate (2,3-DPG)

- What is 2,3-DPG? It is an organic phosphate, found in RBCs, that has the ability to alter the affinity of Hgb for oxygen.

  - Decreased 2,3-DPG results in hemoglobin holding on to O_2 (Table 5-3).
  - Increased 2,3-DPG results in hemoglobin more readily releasing O_2 (Table 5-3).

Table 5-3. Effect of 2,3-DPG on Hgb Affinity for Oxygen

Decreased 2,3-DPG	Increased 2,3-DPG
Multiple blood transfusions of banked blood	Chronic hypoxemia (e.g., prolonged time spent at high altitudes or chronic HF)
Hypophosphatemia	Anemia
Hypothyroidism	Hyperthyroidism
Result: Less O_2 is available to tissues	Result: More O_2 is available to tissues

Carbon Monoxide Poisoning

- Carbon monoxide (CO) has a greater affinity for hemoglobin than oxygen—approximately 230 times greater (Figure 5-10)!

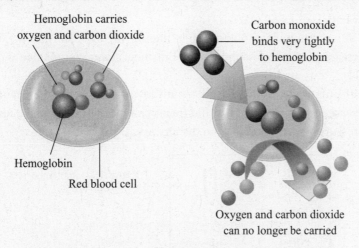

Figure 5-10. Carbon monoxide's effects on hemoglobin

- In the presence of CO, oxygen cannot be carried → tissue hypoxia.
- Do NOT use pulse oximetry to monitor the oxygenation status for a patient with CO poisoning. The pulse oximeter cannot differentiate between CO and O_2. Therefore, an SpO_2 of 95%, in the presence of CO poisoning, only means that the hemoglobin is saturated with a total of 95% molecules.
  - If the CO level of the blood is 40%, the maximum amount of O_2 that can be carried by hemoglobin is 60%.

Carboxyhemoglobin (COHb) levels and associated clinical presentation:

- 0–5% = Normal
- < 15% = Often in smokers, truck drivers
- 15–40% = Headache, some confusion
- 40–60% = Loss of consciousness, Cheyne-Stokes respiration
- 50–70% = Mortality > 50%

☆ Treatment
- 100% FiO_2 until symptoms resolve and carboxyhemoglobin level is < 10%
- Hyperbaric oxygen chamber if available, generally within 30 minutes

Lung Compliance

Think of compliance as the degree of elasticity of tissue. Therefore, a decrease in compliance increases resistance or stiffness.

- **Static compliance:** measurement of the elastic properties of the **lung**

$$\text{Tidal volume} \div \textbf{plateau pressure (minus PEEP)}$$

  - Note that an increase in plateau pressure will decrease compliance.

- **Dynamic compliance:** measurement of the elastic properties of the **airways**

  Tidal volume ÷ **peak inspiratory pressure** (minus PEEP)

  ○ Note that an increase in peak inspiratory pressure will decrease compliance.
- Normal for both is ~ 45–50 mL/cm H_2O.
- Patients with pulmonary problems that mainly involve the airways (i.e., asthma) have a decrease in dynamic compliance, but their static compliance remains normal (Figure 5-11).
- Patients with pulmonary problems that mainly involve the lungs (i.e., pneumonia, ARDS) have a decrease in static compliance, but their dynamic compliance may also decrease as the lung pressures may transmit up to the airways (Figure 5-11).

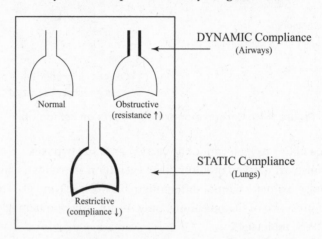

Figure 5-11. Dynamic vs. static compliance

TIP

☆ For the exam, remember that decreased compliance increases the work of breathing.

- Status asthmaticus
  ○ Static compliance (lungs) would be normal.
  ○ Dynamic compliance would be low.
- ARDS
  ○ Static compliance would be low.
  ○ Dynamic compliance would also be low.

ACID-BASE INTERPRETATION

ABGs WILL be tested on the Adult CCRN exam. You need to understand the 4 major acid-base abnormalities as well as states of compensation—uncompensated, partial compensation, and full compensation. Not only will you need to know how to interpret the ABG, but you will also need to know what the clinical implications are for the patient and the treatment, if there are any. How did you do on the ABG question in the pretest of this book? A succinct review of acid-base interpretation is given in Table 5-4. Practice ABGs are also provided later in this section (with answers at the end of this chapter) so that you can practice as needed.

Table 5-4. Normal ABG Parameters

Parameter	Normal Range	Absolute Normal
pH	7.35–7.45	7.40
pCO_2	35–45 mmHg	40 mmHg
HCO_3	22–26 mmol/kg	24 mmol/L
BE	−2 to +2	0
PO_2	80–100 mmHg	
SaO_2	95–99% (on room air)	

The information that follows will focus on acid-base interpretation, not oxygenation, which is covered in other areas of this book.

General Points Related to Acid-Base Balance

- Remember that the pH represents the hydrogen ion (H^+) concentration of the blood.
- Due to the Henderson-Hasselbalch equation, when the H^+ concentration is increased, the pH decreases, and when the H^+ concentration is decreased, the pH increases. There is an inverse relationship between the H^+ and the pH, so don't get confused!
- Think of $PaCO_2$ as an acid. When it increases, there is acidosis. When it decreases, there is alkalosis.
  - The $PaCO_2$ is controlled by the lungs. It is the **respiratory** parameter.
  - The lungs can change the $PaCO_2$ within minutes (rapid change).
- Think of HCO_3 as a base. When it is greater than normal, alkalosis may be present. When it is less than normal, acidosis may be present.
  - The HCO_3 is controlled by the kidneys. It is the **metabolic** parameter.
  - The kidneys alter the HCO_3 over hours to days (slow change).

Table 5-5. Four Primary Acid-Base Disorders and Expected Compensatory Change

Imbalance	pH*	Primary Change	Compensatory Change
Respiratory acidosis	< 7.35	↑ $PaCO_2$	↑ HCO_3
Metabolic acidosis**	< 7.35	↓ HCO_3	↓ $PaCO_2$
Respiratory alkalosis	> 7.45	↓ $PaCO_2$	↓ HCO_3
Metabolic alkalosis	> 7.45	↑ HCO_3	↑ $PaCO_2$

*In the presence of FULL compensation, the pH will enter the normal range.
**Metabolic acidosis may also be evaluated by the anion gap (see below) and the venous CO_2 (which will be lower than normal in the presence of metabolic acidosis).

ANION GAP

The anion gap is the difference between positive and negative anions. In most instances of metabolic acidosis, there is an increase in the anion gap. In several types of metabolic acidosis, though, the anion gap remains normal.

You will NOT need to calculate the anion gap for this exam, but you should know what is normal:

$$(Na^+ + K^+) - (Cl^- + HCO_3{}^-)$$

- Normal is 5–15 mEq/L.
- The anion gap is helpful in determining the cause of and/or response to treatment for metabolic acidosis (Table 5-6). For instance, if a patient with DKA presents with an anion gap of 25 mEq/L, one would expect the anion gap to decrease gradually as the patient responds positively to treatment. Since electrolytes are assessed frequently, the acidosis can be monitored by monitoring the anion gap without getting frequent ABGs.

NOTE

You will not need to know how to calculate the anion gap for this exam.

Table 5-6. Problems Associated with the Anion Gap

Problems Associated with an Increase in the Anion Gap (think "Kussmaul")	Problems Associated with a Normal Anion Gap
Ketoacidosis **U**remia **S**alicylate intoxication **M**ethanol toxicity **A**lcoholic ketosis **U**nmeasured osmoles: ethylene glycol, paraldehyde **L**actic acidosis: shock, hypoxemia	Saline infusion (hyperchloremic acidosis) TPN Diarrhea Acute renal failure, sometimes chronic Note that there are fewer problems associated with a normal anion gap metabolic acidosis than those associated with a high anion gap acidosis.

ACID-BASE COMPENSATION

- Compensation is the body's way of attempting to return the pH to normal (7.35–7.45).
  - Uncompensated
  - Partial compensation
  - Full compensation: **rare** in critically ill, suspect a mixed disorder if present
  - Review Tables 5-7, 5-8, 5-9, and 5-10

Table 5-7. Examples of Compensation for Respiratory Acidosis

Uncompensated	Partial Compensation	Full Compensation
pH 7.30	pH 7.32	pH 7.35
$PaCO_2$ 50	$PaCO_2$ 50	$PaCO_2$ 50
HCO_3 24	HCO_3 29	HCO_3 31

Table 5-8. Examples of Compensation for Respiratory Alkalosis

Uncompensated	Partial Compensation	Full Compensation
pH 7.55	pH 7.50	pH 7.45
$PaCO_2$ 25	$PaCO_2$ 25	$PaCO_2$ 25
HCO_3 22	HCO_3 18	HCO_3 16

Table 5-9. Examples of Compensation for Metabolic Acidosis

Uncompensated	Partial Compensation	Full Compensation
pH 7.30	pH 7.32	pH 7.35
$PaCO_2$ 35	$PaCO_2$ 33	$PaCO_2$ 30
HCO_3 16	HCO_3 16	HCO_3 16

Table 5-10. Examples of Compensation for Metabolic Alkalosis

Uncompensated	Partial Compensation	Full Compensation
pH 7.50	pH 7.47	pH 7.45
$PaCO_2$ 45	$PaCO_2$ 48	$PaCO_2$ 50
HCO_3 32	HCO_3 32	HCO_3 32

COMBINED ACID-BASE DISORDERS—SELDOM SEEN ON THE EXAM

Occurs when 2 single disorders are present simultaneously to produce the **same** abnormality.

- Combined respiratory and metabolic acidosis:

  pH   7.21

  $PaCO_2$ 50

  HCO_3 12

- Combined respiratory and metabolic alkalosis:

  pH   7.59

  $PaCO_2$ 30

  HCO_3 33

MIXED ACID-BASE DISORDERS—SELDOM SEEN ON THE EXAM

- Simple acid-base disorders result from a single process, such as metabolic acidosis.
- In many critically ill patients, multiple acid-base disturbances exist concurrently and result in complex, mixed acid-base disorders.
- For example, a patient with septic shock may present with respiratory alkalosis **and** metabolic acidosis.
- Complex formulas can be applied to determine whether the compensating parameter ($PaCO_2$ or HCO_3) has compensated more than predicted for the primary problem, indicating that a mixed disorder is present. You will not need to know these formulas for this exam.

SYSTEMATIC ASSESSMENT OF ACID-BASE

1. Evaluate the pH → determine whether it is normal, acidotic, or alkalotic.
2. Evaluate respiratory parameters and then renal parameters → determine which, if either, is abnormal.
3. Determine the state of compensation.
4. Evaluate for a mixed disorder.
5. Assess oxygenation (PaO_2, SaO_2).

Practice ABGs

> **Directions:** Interpret each of the following ABGs. Identify the primary problem and the type of compensation. The answers can be found on page 110.

ABG   Interpretation

1. pH 7.48 $PaCO_2$ 32 HCO_3 24

   1. _____

2. pH 7.32 $PaCO_2$ 48 HCO_3 25

   2. _____

3. pH 7.30 $PaCO_2$ 38 HCO_3 18

   3. _____

4. pH 7.28 $PaCO_2$ 60 HCO_3 29

   4. _____

5. pH 7.49 $PaCO_2$ 40 HCO_3 30

   5. _____

6. pH 7.28 $PaCO_2$ 70 HCO_3 33

   6. _____

7. pH 7.50 $PaCO_2$ 49 HCO_3 38

   7. _____

8. pH 7.31 $PaCO_2$ 32 HCO_3 15

   8. _____

9. pH 7.30 $PaCO_2$ 50 HCO_3 25

   9. _____

10. pH 7.48 $PaCO_2$ 40 HCO_3 30

   10. _____

11. pH 7.38 $PaCO_2$ 80 HCO_3 47

   11. _____

RESPIRATORY DISORDERS

About 14 respiratory topics are included in the Adult CCRN test blueprint. However, some topics are more likely to be included on the exam than others. It is highly recommended that you study ARDS, status asthmaticus, pneumonia, and pulmonary embolism in order to do well on the respiratory questions. The physiological concepts that were reviewed previously in this chapter are the foundation for all of the respiratory disorders. Specific respiratory disorders that are likely to be seen on this exam are reviewed in the following sections.

■ Acute respiratory failure is defined as a **rapidly** occurring inability of the lungs to maintain adequate oxygenation of the blood with or without impairment of carbon dioxide (CO_2) elimination. Specifically, the ABG demonstrates:

○ PaO_2 of 60 mmHg or less, with or without an elevation of $PaCO_2$ to 50 mmHg or more with pH < 7.30

■ As seen from the definition, the primary problem may be one of hypoxemia (Type 1) or hypercarbia (Type 2) or both (Type 3). See Table 5-11 for the specific problems that result in each type of acute respiratory failure.

Table 5-11. Types of Acute Respiratory Failure

Type 1 Hypoxemic	Type 2 Hypercapnic	Type 3 Combined
Pneumonia	CNS depression due to drugs (opiates, sedatives)	ARDS
ARDS	↑ ICP	Asthma
Atelectasis	COPD (including asthma)	COPD
Pulmonary edema	Flail chest	
Pulmonary embolism (massive)	ALS	
Interstitial fibrosis	Guillain-Barré syndrome	
Asthma	Multiple sclerosis	
	Myasthenia gravis	
	Spinal cord injury	

■ Clinical signs/symptoms of acute **hypoxemic** respiratory failure

○ Pulmonary: tachypnea, adventitious breath sounds, accessory muscle use

○ Cardiac: tachyarrhythmias (initial), bradyarrhythmias (late), hypertension or hypotension, cyanosis (central, e.g., lips, earlobes)

○ Neurological: anxiety, agitation

■ Clinical signs/symptoms of acute **hypercapnic** respiratory failure

○ Pulmonary: shallow breathing, bradypnea, lungs may be clear or there may be adventitious breath sounds

○ Neurological: progressive decreased level of consciousness (lethargic, obtunded, stuporous, unresponsive)

Prompt identification and treatment may prevent a catastrophic outcome! The etiology of the signs/symptoms may not be the primary focus initially.

Treatment of Acute Respiratory Failure

■ Maintain airway and improve ventilation.

○ Positioning (upright)

○ Suctioning

○ Bronchodilator therapy for wheezing

○ Noninvasive ventilation

○ Intubation, mechanical ventilation if needed

○ Repeat ABGs as needed

- Optimize oxygenation.
  - Adjust FiO_2 to keep $SaO_2 \sim > 0.90$
  - Decrease FiO_2 to 0.50 or less ASAP
  - Do not allow hypoxemia to occur to "prevent O_2 toxicity"
  - Use PEEP/CPAP as needed
  - Use pulse oximetry to monitor response to therapy
- Optimize circulation, cardiac output.
  - Manage hypotension
  - Address cardiac arrhythmias
- Identify the etiology, target treatment accordingly.
- Provide emotional support.

Use of Noninvasive Ventilation for the Management of Acute Respiratory Failure

When used for an appropriate patient, noninvasive ventilation (NIV) has been shown to decrease morbidity and mortality. There are 2 main types of NIV. Generally, though, the exam does not cover the details related to the type of NIV. More importantly, understand those who would NOT benefit from this therapy. Occasionally, a patient may initially be a good candidate for NIV but then, due to a change in condition, the patient should be intubated with an endotracheal tube.

- CPAP—Continuous positive airway pressure
  - Indicated for patients with hypoxemic respiratory failure who have increased work of breathing (e.g., cardiogenic pulmonary edema)
  - Settings include FiO_2 and 1 pressure setting in cm H_2O pressure.
- BiPAP—Bilevel positive airway pressure
  - Indicated for patients with hypoxemic and/or hypercapnic respiratory failure
  - Settings include FiO_2 and 2 pressure settings: the inspiratory positive airway pressure (IPAP) and the expiratory positive airway pressure (EPAP).
  - IPAP assists ventilation and EPAP assists oxygenation.

ADVANTAGES OF NIV

- Buys time for medical treatment to take effect
- Reduces the work of breathing (WOB)
- Decreases preload and afterload
- Improves oxygenation
- Improves ventilation (BiPAP)
- Reduces atelectasis
- Prevents intubation and resultant risks

- ☆ Contraindications for NIV
  - Hemodynamic instability or life-threatening arrhythmias
  - Copious secretions
  - High risk of aspiration
  - Impaired mental status (unable to protect airway)

○ Suspected pneumothorax

○ Inability to cooperate

○ Life-threatening refractory hypoxemia ($PaO_2 < 60$ with FiO_2 1.00)

Use of High-Flow Nasal Cannula (HFNC) Oxygen

HFNC oxygen therapy, which has long been used for pediatric and infant populations, is now used for select adult populations in the treatment of acute respiratory failure and post-extubation.

■ HFNC oxygen delivery systems are able to deliver FiO_2 (up to 100%) of heated and humidified gas at flow rates up to 60 L/minute via a nasal cannula.

■ Advantages of HFNC therapy

○ Able to provide high FiO_2 (up to 100%)

○ Heated and humidified oxygen may improve secretion clearance and decrease airway inflammation

○ Able to meet high inspiratory flow demands of tachypneic patients

○ Seems to promote alveolar recruitment and increase FRC

○ Decreases dead space ventilation

○ More comfortable than CPAP or BiPAP masks, allows access to the mouth without removal of a mask

■ Limitations of HFNC oxygen therapy

○ Unable to deliver higher airway pressures (PEEP or CPAP), and the low levels of airway pressure provided are variable when mouth breathing

○ Provides limited pressure support for a patient with hypercapnic respiratory failure

■ Indications: community-acquired pneumonia; cardiogenic pulmonary edema when NIV is not tolerated; preoxygenation prior to intubation; post-extubation (even in low-risk patients); for a patient who refuses intubation (DNI) but accepts alternate treatment measures

■ HFNC oxygen therapy may also be used in conjunction with NIV post-extubation to prevent re-intubation.

■ Nursing implications

○ Monitor for deteriorating oxygenation/ventilation (the patient may require NIV or intubation and mechanical ventilation)

○ Assess for nasal skin irritation

CHRONIC OBSTRUCTIVE PULMONARY DISEASE (COPD): ACUTE EXACERBATION

■ COPD includes emphysema, asthma, and bronchitis (more details on status asthmaticus are in the next section).

■ In general, with each type of COPD, it is easier for air to enter the pulmonary system than to exit it; inspiration is easier than exhalation.

■ Physiological consequences of COPD include:

○ Dynamic hyperinflation occurs due to too much air in the lungs.

○ Air trapping and auto-PEEP are common.

○ Expiratory flow rates are LOW.

○ An acute exacerbation results in a V/Q mismatch due to a problem with ventilation and an increase in the $PaCO_2$.

○ The patient may have chronic CO_2 retention; if so, the patient will have partial or complete compensation and high HCO_3 on the ABG.

○ COPD may result in right ventricular enlargement (cor pulmonale) and elevated CVP.

■ Signs of an acute exacerbation of COPD include:

○ Worsening dyspnea

○ Increase in sputum purulence

○ Increase in sputum volume

○ Hypercapnia, hypoxemia

■ Management of an acute exacerbation of COPD includes:

○ Titrate FiO_2 to $PaO_2 > 60$ mmHg or $SaO_2 > 90\%$ with care not to overcorrect hypoxemia and decrease respiratory drive

– Must address **severe** hypoxemia; do not withhold oxygen only because hypoventilation may occur . . . cells still need oxygen

○ Bronchodilator therapy

– Inhaled short-acting beta-agonist (SABA), e.g., albuterol

– Inhaled anticholinergic

○ Corticosteroid therapy

○ Antibiotic therapy (when pneumonia is thought to be the trigger)

○ Proceed with mechanical ventilatory support if needed (noninvasive or invasive).

– Multiple studies have shown that noninvasive ventilation (NIV) is beneficial for patients with an acute exacerbation of COPD.

■ Status asthmaticus is airway hyper-reactivity that produces severe airway narrowing that is refractory to aggressive bronchodilator therapy, which may result in respiratory failure. Status asthmaticus can be fatal as evidenced by the pathophysiology diagram in Figure 5-12.

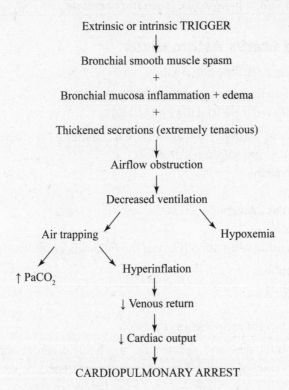

Extrinsic or intrinsic TRIGGER

↓

Bronchial smooth muscle spasm

+

Bronchial mucosa inflammation + edema

+

Thickened secretions (extremely tenacious)

↓

Airflow obstruction

↓

Decreased ventilation

Air trapping   Hypoxemia

↑ PaCO$_2$ Hyperinflation

↓ Venous return

↓ Cardiac output

CARDIOPULMONARY ARREST

Figure 5-12. Pathophysiology of status asthmaticus

Clinical Presentation of Status Asthmaticus

■ Dyspnea, tachypnea
■ Cough, chest tightness
■ Accessory muscle use
■ Wheezing → decreased breath sounds → absent breath sounds . . . ominous sign!
■ V/Q mismatch
■ Chest X-ray may have flattened diaphragm (sign of air trapping).
■ Tachycardia
■ Pulsus paradoxus ≥ 15 mmHg (severe is > 18 mmHg)
■ Anxiety → ↓ LOC
■ May have elevated WBC, eosinophils
■ Peak flow rate < 80% of predicted, < 50% is severe
■ History of previous intubations (higher mortality)
■ Table 5-12 describes ABG changes.

Table 5-12. ABG Progression in Status Asthmaticus (on Room Air)

Stage 1	Normal PaO_2, respiratory alkalosis ($\downarrow PaCO_2$)
Stage 2	Mild hypoxemia, respiratory alkalosis ($\downarrow PaCO_2$)
Stage 3	Worsening hypoxemia, normalization of pH and $PaCO_2$
Stage 4	Severe hypoxemia, respiratory acidosis

Management of Status Asthmaticus

- Measure presenting peak flow rate (PFR).
  - Admit the patient to the hospital if the PFR is 50–70%.
  - Admit the patient to the ICU if the PFR is < 50%.
- Bronchodilator: short-acting beta-2 agonists, e.g., albuterol (Ventolin)
- Anticholinergics, e.g., ipratropium (Atrovent)
- Corticosteroids (systemic)
- O_2, pulse oximetry
- Hydration to prevent thickened secretions
- Avoid sedation agents.
- Intubation, mechanical ventilation if any of the following ominous signs occurs:
  - Respiratory acidosis
  - Severe hypoxemia
  - Silent chest
  - Change in the level of consciousness (LOC)
- If the patient is intubated and sedated on mechanical ventilation, avoid paralytics because paralytics combined with steroids increase incidences of neuropathy.

☆ Ventilator management for status asthmaticus
  - Use low rate to increase exhalation time.
  - Use low tidal volumes to prevent auto-PEEP.
  - Increase inspiration/expiration (I/E) ratio, often greater than 1:3–4, to allow time for optimal exhalation and to prevent auto-PEEP.

PULMONARY EMBOLISM

- A pulmonary embolism (PE) is a partial or complete obstruction of the pulmonary capillary bed by a blood clot or another substance such as fat, air, amniotic fluid, or a foreign material, with a disruption of blood flow to an area of the lung.
  - Massive: > 50% occlusion
  - Submassive: < 50% occlusion
  - 80–90% result from DVT
- Although a pulmonary embolism may be the result of a variety of causes, venous thromboembolism (VTE) is the primary cause. VTE and a fat embolism are the 2 types of embolism that are most likely to be covered on the Adult CCRN exam. Refer to Table 5-13 for the risk factors for VTE and Figure 5-13 for the pathophysiology of PE.

Table 5-13. Risk Factors for Venous Thromboembolism (VTE)

Strong	Moderate	Weak
Fracture (hip or leg)	Arthroscopic knee surgery	Bed rest > 3 days
Hip or knee replacement	Central venous lines	Prolonged sitting
Major trauma	Chemotherapy	Increasing age
Spinal cord injury	HF or respiratory failure	Laparoscopic surgery
	Hormone replacement therapy	Obesity
	Malignancy	Pregnancy, antepartum
	Oral contraceptives	Varicose veins
	Stroke	
	Pregnancy, postpartum	
	Previous VTE	

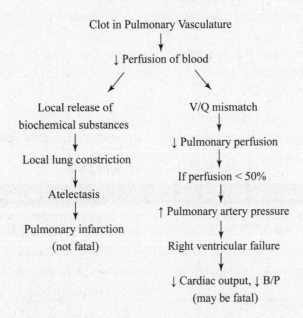

Clot in Pulmonary Vasculature

↓ Perfusion of blood

Local release of biochemical substances

V/Q mismatch

Local lung constriction

↓ Pulmonary perfusion

Atelectasis

If perfusion < 50%

Pulmonary infarction (not fatal)

↑ Pulmonary artery pressure

Right ventricular failure

↓ Cardiac output, ↓ B/P (may be fatal)

Figure 5-13. Pathophysiology of pulmonary embolism

Refer to Table 5-14 for the signs and symptoms of a PE.

Table 5-14. Signs and Symptoms of a PE

Most PEs	Massive PEs
Dyspnea, tachypnea	Hypoxemia
Tachycardia, chest pain	Hypotension
Right-sided S3 or S4 heart sounds	EKG changes—RBBB, right axis deviation on the ECG, tall peaked P-waves in lead II, RV strain pattern, ST elevation in V1 and V2
Anxiety, apprehension	
Cough, hemoptysis, crackles	Cardiopulmonary arrest—PEA
Syncope	
Petechiae (fat emboli)	
Low-grade fever	
Respiratory alkalosis	

Types of PE

- **Venous thromboembolism—DVT**
- **Fat emboli—long bone, pelvic fractures**
- Air emboli—surgery, IV lines
- Catheter embolization
- RA/LA or RV embolus—AFib/flutter (left atrial leading to stroke is more common)
- Amniotic fluid embolism (rare)—amniocentesis, abruptio placenta, or abortion
- Tumor emboli—malignancy causes an increase in thrombin
- Septic emboli—bacterial/viral

Diagnosis of PE

- Pulmonary angiography—gold standard!
- V/Q scan: "high" probability, "low" probability, not definitive
- High-speed CT scan
- D-dimer: good rule-out test; if positive, it means that a clot is present in the body; therefore, if symptoms ARE due to a PE, expect the D-dimer to be positive
- Venous Doppler (helps with source)

TIP

☆ A PE will increase alveolar dead space!

Note: ∼ 2/3 of PEs never get diagnosed!

Table 5-15 lists mechanical and pharmacological agents that are used to **prevent** PEs.

Table 5-15. Prevention of PEs

Mechanical	Pharmacological
Graduated compression stockings (GCS) and/or	Low–molecular-weight heparin (LMWH): enoxaparin (Lovenox) **DAILY**
intermittent pneumatic compression (IPC)	Low-dose unfractionated heparin: **t.i.d.**
Use continuously except while ambulating!	rivaroxaban (Xarelto): **DAILY**
	apixaban (Eliquis): **b.i.d.**

Treatment of PE

- Maintain adequate airway, ventilation, and oxygenation
- Fluids!
- Anticoagulation
    - Heparin (80 units/kg IVP and then 18 units/kg/hr drip)
    - Low–molecular-weight heparin (1 mg/kg q 12 hrs)
    - Coumadin **on the first treatment day** if able
    - The patient may require long-term anticoagulation.

NOTE

You will not need to know drug doses for this exam.

- Fibrinolytic therapy: **for all patients with hemodynamic compromise with a low risk for bleeding**
- Maintain cardiac output (inotropes, fluids)
- Analgesics for a patient who experiences pain

PULMONARY HYPERTENSION

Pulmonary hypertension (PH) is included on the test blueprint. However, you are more likely to see questions that cover status asthmaticus, PE, pneumonia, and ARDS than questions that cover PH. Keep this in mind when studying.

- PH is defined as a MEAN pulmonary artery pressure that is greater than 25 mmHg at rest and a PAOP that is less than 16 mmHg at rest with secondary right heart failure.
  - The normal mean pulmonary artery pressure is ~ 20 mmHg. Since the RV normally pumps into a low-pressure system, the wall of the RV is thin compared to that of the LV. Pulmonary hypertension results in cor pulmonale and right ventricular failure.
- 5 groups of PH, as defined by the World Health Organization (WHO)
  - Group 1—Pulmonary arterial hypertension (PAH); sporadic and hereditary due to localized small pulmonary muscular arterioles (i.e., collagen vascular diseases, drug/toxin induced)
  - Group 2—Pulmonary hypertension (PH) due to left heart disease, such as LVF or valvular (mitral, aortic) disease
  - Group 3—PH due to lung diseases or hypoxemia
  - Group 4—PH due to chronic thromboembolic problems
  - Group 5—PH that has unclear factors or is multifactorial (e.g., sarcoidosis)

Signs and Symptoms of Pulmonary Hypertension

- Exertional dyspnea, lethargy, and fatigue due to an inability to increase cardiac output with activity
- Progression to RV failure, chest pain, syncope with exertion, and peripheral edema
- Passive hepatic congestion may cause anorexia and ABD pain
- Ortner's syndrome—cough, hemoptysis, and hoarseness
- Systolic ejection murmur, increased intensity of pulmonic component of S2 heart sound, diastolic pulmonic regurgitation murmur, right-sided murmurs, and gallops are augmented with inspiration.
- RV hypertrophy, elevated JVD, hepatomegaly, ascites, and pleural effusion

Treatment of Pulmonary Hypertension

- Treat the underlying cause as able.
- Each "group" has specific treatments based on the cause.
- All regimens should consider diuretics, oxygen, anticoagulants, digoxin, and exercise training.
- Use dilators, which include calcium channel blockers or phosphodiesterase-5 inhibitors, e.g., sildenafil (Viagra), tadalafil (Cialis), or treprostinil (Remodulin).
- For patients who are refractory to all medical interventions—lung transplantation (bilateral or heart-lung transplant) or possible atrial septostomy (right-to-left shunt)

Pneumonia is an acute inflammation of the lung parenchyma (caused by an infectious agent) that can lead to alveolar consolidation.

Causative agents include:

1. Bacterial
2. Viral
3. Fungal
4. Parasitic

Pneumonia may also be classified according to where it developed:

- Community-acquired pneumonia (CAP)
    - Outside the hospital
    - Common pathogens: *Streptococcus pneumoniae, Legionella pneumophila, Klebsiella pneumoniae, Haemophilus influenzae, Staphylococcus aureus, Mycoplasma pneumoniae, Pseudomonas aeruginosa*
- Hospital-acquired pneumonia (HAP)
    - Acute care
    - Long-term care
    - Nursing home
- ☆ Ventilator-associated pneumonia (VAP); now referred to as ventilator-associated event (VAE)
    - By definition, develops 48 hours or more after admission to the hospital
    - Common pathogens: *P. aeruginosa, Escherichia coli, K. pneumoniae, Acinetobacter baumannii, Staphylococcus aureus* (especially diabetes and head trauma), MRSA
    - HAP has higher mortality than CAP.

Risk Factors for Pneumonia

Multiple factors will increase the risk, including:

- Age
- Preexisting pulmonary disease
- Smoking
- ↓ level of consciousness (LOC)
- Artificial airways
- Chronic illness
- Malnutrition
- Immunocompromised
- Increased secretions
- Atelectasis
- Immobility
- Depressed cough or gag reflexes
- Concurrent antibiotic therapy
- Aspiration
- Organisms spread from another site (gut, wound) to the lungs.
- Multiple organ dysfunction syndrome (MODS)

Signs and Symptoms of Pneumonia

- Chills, diaphoresis, fever, malaise
- Tachycardia, chest pain
- Confusion (especially for the elderly)
- Productive cough
- Use of accessory muscles
- Dehydration
- Over area of consolidation on the chest:

  - ↑ Tactile fremitus
  - Dull to percussion
  - Bronchial breath sounds or diminished breath sounds
  - Bronchophony (louder/clearer)
  - Egophony ("e" to "a")
  - Whispered pectoriloquy (whisper heard better with a stethoscope)

Diagnosis of Pneumonia

- CXR: consolidation or diffuse patchy infiltrates
- Sputum culture with Gram stain
- Blood cultures
- WBC: high but may be normal or low in immunocompromised or elderly people
- WBC differential: increased bands > 10%
- ABGs: hypoxemia
- Thoracentesis for effusions

Treatment of Pneumonia

- Optimize oxygenation and ventilation.

  - Titrate FiO_2

☆ Positioning—GOOD lung DOWN
  - Bronchial hygiene, chest physiotherapy
  - Noninvasive ventilation or intubation/mechanical ventilation as needed
  - Bronchoscopy (with lavage, if needed)
  - Mobilize, clear secretions

- Identify organism

  - Sputum culture and sensitivity (C&S)
  - Blood cultures

- Antibiotic therapy

  - Empiric therapy: choice of agent is based on the likely causative organism (as determined by a patient assessment and the types of pneumonia seen in the community and in the institution) and whether that organism may be resistant to therapy
  - Timing: first dose within 4 hours if the patient first presents to the Emergency Department (and is later admitted to the hospital); the first antibiotic dose should be given in the Emergency Department; note that if the patient has sepsis, the antibiotic timing differs (see Chapter 6 of this book)
  - Organism-specific therapy: as soon as the results of the C&S are available

- System support
  - Hydration
  - Fever management
  - Glucose control
  - Nutrition
- General preventative measures
  - Smoking cessation
  - Pneumonia vaccine for those who are 65 and older
  - Flu vaccine

Prevention of Hospital-Acquired Pneumonia

- Practice hand hygiene.
- Keep HOB elevated 30 degrees or greater.
- Prevent bacterial translocation from GI tract: use the gut, feed patient.
- Practice oral hygiene!
- Provide education on common institution pathogens and the rates of nosocomial pneumonia.
- Use evidence-based confirmation of feeding tube placement.

  - Confirm with an X-ray prior to using for feeding.
  - Mark the exit site with an indelible marker for future reference.
  - Assess patency every 4 hours.
  - Observe for a change in the length of the external portion of the feeding tube (as determined by movement of the marked portion of the tube).
  - Review routine chest and abdominal X-ray reports to look for notations about tube location.
  - Observe changes in volume of aspirate from feeding tube.
  - If pH strips are available, measure the pH of feeding tube aspirates if feedings are interrupted for more than a few hours.
  - Observe the appearance of feeding tube aspirates if feedings are interrupted for more than a few hours.
  - Obtain an X-ray to confirm tube position if there is doubt about the tube's location.

Prevention of Ventilator-Associated Pneumonia

Prevention involves all of the interventions for preventing hospital-acquired pneumonia, plus:

- Drain accumulated condensate from tubing.
- Prevent backflow of tubing condensate into endotracheal tube (ETT).
- Change ventilator tubing only when it is contaminated.
- Mobilize the patient.
- Utilize aseptic technique for ETT, tracheostomy suctioning.
- Adhere to mouth care protocol, chlorhexidine mouth rinse.
- Brush teeth to remove plaque.
- Keep ETT cuff inflated.
- Perform subglottic suctioning prior to cuff deflation.
- Perform routine oropharyngeal suctioning.

ASPIRATION

Aspiration is the inhalation of toxic substances into the lung, with an injury to the lung that is the result of the chemical, mechanical, and/or bacterial characteristics of the aspirate.

- Oropharyngeal is most common!
- May or may not involve an infection
- May be acute or chronic: micro or massive
- Table 5-16 shows management techniques.

Table 5-16. Emergent Management of Aspiration

Witnessed Aspiration	All Aspirations
Place patient in slight Trendelenburg and turned to the right side to aid drainage Suction mouth and pharyngeal areas Bronchoscopy for large particles	O_2, titrate up as needed Intubation/mechanical ventilation as needed Monitor for the onset of noncardiogenic pulmonary edema (ARDS) or pneumonia Monitor for ↓ B/P

☆ Due to the anatomy of the right mainstem bronchus (shorter, wider, and with less of an angle), most aspirations occur in the RIGHT lung. Although aspirations may occur in both lungs, they seldom are isolated solely to the left lung.

Etiology of Aspirations

- Altered level of consciousness
- Drug or alcohol abuse
- Depressed gag, cough, or swallowing reflexes
- Presence of feeding tubes (all types)
- Improper patient positioning
- Presence of artificial airways
- Ileus or gastric distension
- History of dysphagia, GERD, esophageal strictures, ↓ GI motility
- Increased secretions

Signs and Symptoms of Aspirations

- Acute respiratory distress
- Presence of gastric contents in oropharynx
- Tachycardia
- Hypoxemia
- Crackles
- Copious secretions due to alveolar edema
- Hypotension (massive fluid shifts may occur)

ARDS and ALI are syndromes caused by a variety of acute conditions that trigger an inflammatory response, resulting in an increase in the permeability of the pulmonary capillary membrane, which allows a transudation of proteinaceous fluid into the interstitial and alveolar spaces. They may also be referred to as "noncardiogenic pulmonary edema." Damage to Type II alveolar cells is one of the pathological consequences. Since these are the cells that are responsible for the production of surfactant, massive atelectasis occurs.

ALI is similar to ARDS in that both involve a shunt, which results in hypoxemia. The degree of the shunt is represented by the PaO_2 to FiO_2 ratio, as described in Table 5-17. Note that you will not be expected to differentiate between ALI and ARDS on this exam.

- All of the criteria in Table 5-17 must be present for a diagnosis of ARDS or ALI. The pulmonary edema is not due to heart failure. Hypoxemia is REFRACTORY, meaning that the FiO_2 is increased to the maximum of 100% and hypoxemia is still present.

- Since a shunt is present, PEEP needs to be provided in order to increase alveolar recruitment and treat the refractory hypoxemia.

Table 5-17. Differentiation of ARDS and ALI

ARDS	ALI
Acute onset with precipitating event	Acute onset with precipitating event
Bilateral infiltrates consistent with pulmonary edema	Bilateral infiltrates consistent with pulmonary edema
$PaO_2/FiO_2 \leq 200$ mmHg, regardless of the level of PEEP	PaO_2/FiO_2 between 201 and 300 mmHg, regardless of the level of PEEP
PAOP* ≤ 18 mmHg	PAOP* ≤ 18 mmHg

*PAOP = pulmonary artery occlusive pressure

PaO_2/FiO_2 Examples

- The patient is receiving 50% FiO_2 and PaO_2 is 90:

$$90 \div 0.50 = 180$$

- The patient is receiving 30% FiO_2 and PaO_2 is 110:

$$110 \div 0.30 = 367$$

- The patient is receiving room air and PaO_2 is 62:

$$62 \div 0.21 = 295$$

- The patient is on 100% FiO_2 and PaO_2 is 95:

$$95 \div 1.00 = 95$$

Remember: It is not only the PaO_2/FiO_2 that is considered when diagnosing ALI or ARDS; the other 3 factors also need to be present.

Surfactant

- Phospholipid/lipoprotein produced by Type II alveolar cells
- Stabilizes alveoli, "keeps them open"
- Increases lung compliance
- Eases work of breathing
- Therefore, with ARDS (destruction of Type II alveolar cells):
  - Massive atelectasis, alveolar collapse
  - Decreased compliance
  - Increased work of breathing
  - Decreased functional residual capacity (FRC)

Figure 5-14 and Tables 5-18 and 5-19 show the pathophysiology, etiology, and signs and symptoms of ARDS and ALI.

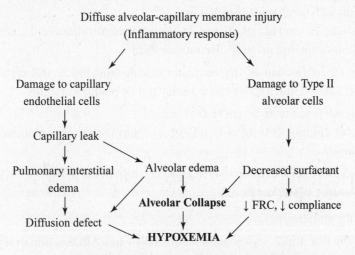

Figure 5-14. Pathophysiology of ARDS/ALI

Table 5-18. Etiology of ARDS/ALI

"Direct" Injury	"Indirect" Injury
Aspiration	Sepsis
Pneumonia	Shock
Pulmonary contusion	Head injury
Fat/air embolism	Non-thoracic trauma
O_2 toxicity	Blood transfusion
Inhalation injury	Pancreatitis
Drowning	Burns
Transthoracic radiation	Heart bypass
	DIC

Table 5-19. Signs and Symptoms of ARDS/ALI

Early	Late
Tachycardia	Tachycardia, episodes of bradycardia
Apprehension, restlessness	Agitation
Mild dyspnea	Extreme dyspnea
Respiratory alkalosis	Respiratory and metabolic acidosis
Few crackles	Crackles, wheezes
Chest X-ray → isolated infiltrate or "ground-glass" appearance	Chest X-ray → whiteout/bilateral infiltrates
PaO_2 on room air ∼ 60 mmHg	PaO_2 on room air ∼ 30 mmHg, refractory hypoxemia despite ↑ FiO_2

Treatment of ARDS/ALI

☆ Pulmonary stabilization strategies

- ○ Intubation with mechanical ventilation
- ○ PEEP, usually 15 cm H_2O or greater; monitor for barotrauma and ↓ cardiac output; treat hypotension, but do NOT discontinue PEEP
    - – Note: Disconnection of the ventilator circuit (and PEEP) will result in alveolar derecruitment and hypoxemia that may not be readily corrected.
- ○ Limit plateau pressure to 30 cm H_2O or less.
- ○ Limit tidal volume (Vt) to 5–6 mL/kg → "permissive hypercapnia" to prevent volutrauma.
    - – A low Vt will cause a rise in the $PaCO_2$ and a drop in the pH; however, patients tend to tolerate a pH as low as 7.2.

- Cardiovascular stabilization
    - ○ Support the B/P (fluids, vasopressors, especially when ARDS is due to septic shock).
    - ○ Monitor for and treat arrhythmias.
- Prone positioning: helps deliver blood flow to underperfused lung units, thereby improving ventilation/perfusion; keeps alveolar lung units open, thus improving gas exchange and preventing further injury
    - ○ Use extreme caution to avoid misplacement or loss of airway.
    - ○ Prevent a pressure injury.
- Monitor acid-base balance.
- DVT and stress ulcer prophylaxis
- Analgesia, sedation
- Nutritional support
- Nitric oxide, prone positioning may provide improvement in oxygenation.
- Coordinate the interdisciplinary team—PT, OT, and dietitian.
- Prevent, identify organ failure.
- Provide emotional support (to the patient and the patient's family).
- Monitor for complications.
- Use steroids? **NO!**

Complications of ARDS/ALI

The mortality from ARDS is still around 30%, although patients do not die from hypoxemia. Instead, they die from multiple organ dysfunction syndrome (MODS) and other complications, as listed below:

- Secondary infections
- Pulmonary embolus
- Ileus
- Skin breakdown
- Malnutrition
- Barotrauma: pneumothorax, subcutaneous emphysema

PNEUMOTHORAX

Pneumothorax (Figures 5-15 and 5-16 and Table 5-20) is included in the Adult CCRN test blueprint. A simple, unilateral pneumothorax is generally not life-threatening, unless it occurs in a patient with end-stage chronic lung disease. A tension pneumothorax, however, may be life-threatening. Therefore, you must know the difference between the two types. The test makers also expect you to have an understanding of chest tube management.

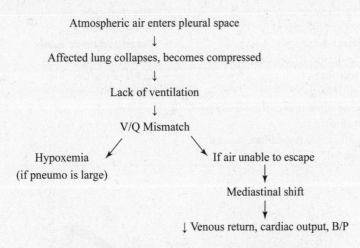

Atmospheric air enters pleural space
↓
Affected lung collapses, becomes compressed
↓
Lack of ventilation
↓
V/Q Mismatch

Hypoxemia
(if pneumo is large)

If air unable to escape
↓
Mediastinal shift
↓
↓ Venous return, cardiac output, B/P

Figure 5-15. Pathophysiology of a pneumothorax

Types of Pneumothorax

- Spontaneous
- Traumatic
    - Open (penetrating chest trauma)
    - Closed (blunt chest trauma)
    - Iatrogenic (due to therapeutic or diagnostic procedures) (Figure 5-16)
- ☆ **Tension**
    - Air is unable to exit → mediastinal shift
    - Life-threatening

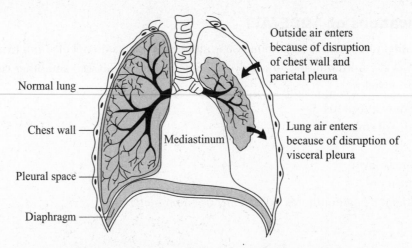

Normal lung

Chest wall

Mediastinum

Pleural space

Diaphragm

Outside air enters
because of disruption
of chest wall and
parietal pleura

Lung air enters
because of disruption of
visceral pleura

Figure 5-16. Pneumothorax (no mediastinal shift)

Table 5-20. Signs and Symptoms of a Pneumothorax

Spontaneous or Traumatic	Tension
Depends upon the size of the pneumothorax and depends upon the underlying lung disease (if any) • Dyspnea, tachypnea • Chest pain (not all cases) • Unequal chest excursion • Tracheal deviation (if present) **toward** the affected side • Hypoxemia (if large) • Decreased or absent breath sounds on the affected side • Mediastinum remains midline, no shift (see Figure 5-17)	Similar to a traumatic pneumothorax, EXCEPT: • Tracheal deviation **away from the** affected side (see Figure 5-18) • Tachycardia • **Distended neck veins** • **Mediastinal shift** • **HYPOTENSION** • Life-threatening!

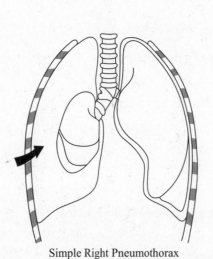

Simple Right Pneumothorax

Figure 5-17. Simple right pneumothorax
(no tension)

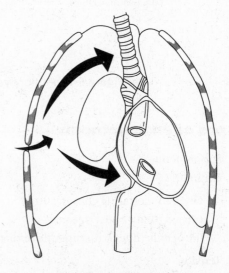

Right Tension Pneumothorax

Figure 5-18. Right tension pneumothorax,
mediastinal shift

HEMOTHORAX

- Usually due to trauma; presents as lung collapse, with blood in the pleural space or in the mediastinal space
  - Dullness to percussion
  - Absent breath sounds on the affected side
  - Tracheal deviation toward the unaffected side

Treatment for a Pneumothorax

- Pneumothorax > 20%
  - Chest tube: reestablish negative pleural pressure
  - Supplemental O_2
  - Treat pain, if needed.
- Pneumothorax < 20%
  - O_2
  - Monitor for lung reexpansion.
  - If there is a pneumothorax plus an underlying lung disease, the patient may need a chest tube.

☆ Chest Tube Assessment and Management

- Close assessment of the patient's respiratory status, which should improve after chest tube insertion
- Pain assessment, treatment
- Entry site—dressing assessment
- Tubing—no dependent loops!
- Drainage collection chamber
  - Keep lower than chest
- Water seal chamber
  - Tidaling with deep inspiration is normal.
  - Air leak
    - Bubbling in water seal chamber is not normal.
    - May be present postoperatively; if there has not been a leak and now there is bubbling, notify the physician.
    - Avoid high airway pressures with chest tubes in place in order to avoid an air leak.
- Suction control chamber: gauge or water level determines the amount of suction, NOT the wall suction source.
- Clamp only when changing the system, with inadvertent disconnection, or with a physician order.
  - Clamping cuts off the negative pressure water seal chamber; expanded lung may recollapse.

Endotracheal Tube Placement

- Confirmation of correct placement is done immediately after intubation.
    - Waveform capnography is most accurate.
    - End-tidal CO_2 detector
    - Auscultation
- Cuff inflation to 20 cm H_2O pressure
- Obtain a chest radiograph for placement confirmation; should be **3–5 cm above the carina**.
- Assess and document tube placement at the level of the teeth or gum line for an ongoing assessment of correct placement.
- If the tube migrates down, it most often migrates to the right lung due to the anatomy of the mainstem bronchi (right is shorter/wider, with less of an angle, than the left).
- Get ABGs within 20 to 30 minutes of intubation to assess acid-base status.
- The endotracheal tube:
    - Is narrow and increases airway resistance, similar to breathing through a straw
    - Is longer than a tracheostomy tube; therefore, it has a greater degree of dead space ventilation than a tracheostomy tube

Ventilator Management

- Ventilator breaths may be delivered at a set volume (most common for adults) or at a set pressure.
- The main focus of the exam is how the ventilator settings may differ depending upon the patient's primary problem (e.g., ARDS or asthma); nontraditional modes of ventilation are not covered on this exam.

VENTILATOR MODES

- Assist-control (AC) mode
    - The patient receives the **set tidal volume** at the set breath rate; the patient also receives the **set tidal volume** for each breath triggered by the patient's spontaneous effort made above the set breath rate.
        - For example, if the AC is set at a rate of 12 breaths/minute, at a tidal volume of 700 mL, and the patient's total rate per minute is 20, the tidal volume of the 8 extra breaths initiated by the patient is 700 mL because the extra breaths are sensed by the machine and the set tidal volume (700 mL) is given.
    - All breaths are machine breaths.
    - Provides full ventilatory support
    - Not used as a weaning mode unless it is being alternated with periods of spontaneous breathing (reducing the AC rate does nothing if the patient is spontaneously breathing)
    - Can result in overventilation and/or hyperinflation of the lungs at higher spontaneous breathing rates

- Synchronized intermittent mandatory ventilation (SIMV) mode
  - The patient receives the set tidal volume at the set breath rate, and all breaths above the set rate are spontaneous breaths at the patient's own tidal volume.
    - For example, if the SIMV is set at a rate of 12 breaths/min, at a tidal volume of 700 mL, and the patient's total rate per minute is 20, the tidal volume of the 8 extra breaths will vary from breath to breath because the breaths that are spontaneously initiated by the patient are at the patient's own tidal volume.
  - All machine breaths are synchronized with the patient's breathing effort.
  - Provides full or partial ventilatory support
  - Reducing the SIMV rate will allow the patient to assume more of the work of breathing.
  - Spontaneous breaths may be pressure supported.

VENTILATOR SETTINGS

Positive End-Expiratory Pressure (PEEP)

- Positive pressure is applied to the airways at the end of exhalation.
- Increases lung volume at the end of exhalation (FRC), creating more surface area for gas exchange; increases alveolar recruitment
- Can be applied to patients via artificial airways, full face mask, nasal mask, and nasal prongs (neonates)
- Think oxygenation!

Continuous Positive Airway Pressure (CPAP)

- CPAP is PEEP applied to a spontaneously breathing patient.
- The patient does not receive machine breaths.
- The patient assumes all of the work of breathing.
- Usually the last step in the weaning process
- All breaths may be pressure supported.
- The patient may experience fatigue if left on CPAP for an extended period of time.

Pressure Support Ventilation (PSV)

- The patient receives an increase in airway pressure during inspiration to augment (boost) the spontaneous tidal volume.
- Patient-triggered mode (if the patient is paralyzed and/or sedated, PSV will not be triggered on)
- Rate, tidal volume, inspiratory flow rate, and inspiratory time are determined by the patient's effort.
- You cannot use PSV with assist-control mode.
- PSV is frequently used during weaning to **reduce the work of breathing** and to overcome imposed work of ETT and ventilator circuit.

Breath Rate

- The breath rate is determined by the $PaCO_2$, generally 12–16 breaths/minute on full ventilator support.

Tidal Volume (Vt)

- The tidal volume (Vt) is determined by the patient's ideal body weight and medical problem.
- Generally, the Vt is 6–8 mL/kg.
- For ARDS, in order to prevent "volutrauma," it is 5–6 mL/kg.

Fraction of Inspired Oxygen (FiO$_2$)

- The fraction of inspired oxygen (FiO$_2$) is generally set at 100% on intubation and is then adjusted down according to the PaO$_2$; the goal is to decrease it to 50% or less as soon as you are able to.

VENTILATOR ALARMS

- Alarms are set for patient safety.

Cause of High-Pressure Limit Alarms

- Agitation
- Coughing
- Secretions
- Aspiration
- Kinked/occluded ETT or ventilator circuit
- Bronchospasm or mucosal edema
- Decreasing lung compliance (ARDS)
- Pneumothorax

Cause of Low-Pressure Limit Alarms

- Ventilator circuit disconnection or leak
- Inadequate tidal volume
- Cuff leak
- Chest tube leak

If You Are Unable to Troubleshoot an Alarm, What Should You Do?

- Disconnect the ventilator from the airway, and ventilate with a bag/valve device.
- A bag/valve device should be at the bedside of every patient who is receiving mechanical ventilation, with the mask available as well, in case there is an issue with the artificial airway.
- As noted in the section on ARDS, disconnecting the ventilator circuit (and PEEP) for a patient who requires high PEEP will result in alveolar derecruitment and hypoxemia, which may not be readily corrected.

☆ Refer to Table 5-21 for the different ventilator setting guidelines used for ARDS and asthma.

Table 5-21. Ventilator Setting Guidelines Used for ARDS and Asthma

ARDS	Asthma
Plateau (static) pressure (< 30 cm) Low tidal volume (5–6 mL/kg) High PEEP (15–20 cm)	Provide short inspiratory time and long expiratory time • Low breath rate • Low Vt • High peak flow rate Monitor for auto-PEEP

WEANING FROM MECHANICAL VENTILATION

Criteria for weaning from mechanical ventilation and initiating a spontaneous breathing trial:

- Original reason for intubation is being resolved.
- Resting minute ventilation (ideally < 10 L/min)
- Spontaneous tidal volume (ideally > 5 mL/kg)
- Negative inspiratory force (NIF) (ideally > –25 cm H_2O)
- Rapid shallow breathing index (respiratory rate/Vt) (ideally < 105 breaths/min/L)
- Vital capacity (ideally above 10 mL/kg body weight)
- ABGs/oxygenation acceptable with FiO_2 50% or less

Criteria for stopping the spontaneous breathing trial:

- Respiratory rate (> 35 breaths/minute)
- Respiratory rate (< 8 breaths/minute)
- SpO_2 (< 88%)
- Respiratory distress
- Mental status change
- Acute cardiac arrhythmia
- Acute hypotension

Now that you have reviewed the key respiratory concepts, go to the Respiratory Practice Questions. Answer the questions, and then check your answers. Continue to review the information until you answer 80% of the practice questions correctly.

RESPIRATORY PRACTICE QUESTIONS

1. Which of the following developments would indicate that a patient, who is receiving noninvasive ventilation, may require intubation with an endotracheal tube?

   (A) a need for an increase in FiO_2 from 0.30 to 0.40
   (B) a dry cough and a fever
   (C) a change in mental status with difficulty to arouse
   (D) positive blood cultures

2. A patient was discharged from the medical unit 7 days ago following an acute ischemic stroke and is now anxious and complaining of severe shortness of breath. The patient demonstrates tachycardia, tachypnea, hypotension, an SpO_2 of 88% on 3 L/nasal cannula, and a temperature of 37.9°C. Breath sounds are present, clear, and equal bilaterally. A chest X-ray is clear. ABGs reveal respiratory alkalosis. Based on this history and assessment, which of the following problems exists and which interventions should the nurse anticipate?

   (A) increased dead space ventilation; fibrinolytic therapy
   (B) decreased dynamic compliance; bronchodilators
   (C) infection; antibiotics
   (D) shunt; PEEP therapy

3. A patient who is receiving mechanical ventilation has a peak inspiratory pressure of 70 cm H_2O and a plateau pressure of 35 cm H_2O. What intervention would be most beneficial for this patient?

   (A) Increase the FiO_2.
   (B) Administer morphine.
   (C) Obtain stat ABGs.
   (D) Administer a bronchodilator.

4. Which of the following is an appropriate intervention for a patient with status asthmaticus who is on a ventilator?

   (A) Decrease the peak flow rate.
   (B) Increase the tidal volume.
   (C) Check for auto-PEEP.
   (D) Increase the breath rate.

5. Which of the following interventions has been demonstrated to decrease ventilator-associated pneumonia?

   (A) Provide sedation.
   (B) Maintain the head of the bed at 20° or greater.
   (C) Adhere to a mouth care protocol.
   (D) Deflate the endotracheal tube cuff prior to suctioning.

6. A 49-year-old male, who weighs 70 kg, is admitted to the ICU with smoke inhalation and ARDS. He is receiving mechanical ventilation with the following ventilator settings: $FiO_2 = 0.80$, assist-control mode = 10 breaths/minute, Vt = 400 mL, and PEEP = 15 cm of pressure. Arterial blood gases are as follows: pH 7.39, $PaCO_2$ 42, PaO_2 96, HCO_3 22, and O_2 sat 98%. Which of the following interventions is appropriate?

    (A) Decrease the FiO_2.
    (B) Increase the tidal volume.
    (C) Decrease the PEEP.
    (D) Do not make any changes.

7. Which of the following statements about lung compliance is TRUE?

    (A) An increase in the peak inspiratory pressure will decrease static compliance.
    (B) A decrease in compliance increases the work of breathing.
    (C) Static compliance is decreased with an asthma exacerbation.
    (D) The plateau pressure is used to calculate dynamic compliance.

8. Each of the following is a clinical feature of ARDS EXCEPT:

    (A) bilateral chest infiltrates on an X-ray.
    (B) PAOP > 18 cm H_2O.
    (C) refractory hypoxemia.
    (D) tachypnea.

9. A patient has mild tachypnea, a productive cough, bronchial breath sounds in the right mid and lower lobes, dullness to percussion over the right lower chest, and an SpO_2 of 92% on 0.40 FiO_2. Which of the following interventions would be appropriate for this patient?

    (A) Contact the physician for an order for a bronchodilator.
    (B) Use noninvasive ventilation.
    (C) Avoid turning the patient to the right side.
    (D) Maintain the patient in a supine position.

10. Drug therapy that is most likely to be prescribed for a patient with status asthmaticus includes which of the following drug categories?

    (A) bronchodilators and anticoagulants
    (B) corticosteroids and diuretics
    (C) antibiotics and expectorants
    (D) bronchodilators and corticosteroids

11. The following interventions may improve oxygenation EXCEPT:

    (A) increasing the FiO_2.
    (B) giving PRBCs.
    (C) giving fluids or pressors to increase a low B/P.
    (D) increasing the ventilator breath rate.

12. While monitoring a patient post-thoracotomy, the nurse suspects that there is hypoventilation. Which characteristic best defines hypoventilation?

    (A) $PaCO_2 > 45$ mmHg

    (B) respiratory rate < 12

    (C) pH < 7.35

    (D) $PaO_2 < 60$ mmHg

13. A patient who was admitted with a carboxyhemoglobin (COHb) level of 45% is lethargic and complains of a headache. The patient is receiving 100% O_2 per a face mask and is noted to have an SpO_2 of 100%. Which of the following is indicated?

    (A) Administer hydrocodone with acetaminophen.

    (B) Continue the FiO_2 of 1.00.

    (C) Decrease the FiO_2.

    (D) Intubate and initiate mechanical ventilation.

For questions 14 and 15

A 38-year-old female is admitted with respiratory failure secondary to viral pneumonitis. She is receiving mechanical ventilation and suddenly becomes restless, tachypneic, tachycardic, and hypotensive. The high-pressure ventilator alarm is continuous, and pulse oximetry (SpO_2) decreases to 0.83. Breath sounds are diminished on the right with tracheal deviation to the left.

14. Based on this information, what condition is likely developing?

    (A) ARDS (acute respiratory distress syndrome)

    (B) hemothorax

    (C) tension pneumothorax

    (D) pulmonary embolism

15. Treatment for the patient described in this scenario would likely include which of the following?

    (A) morphine and furosemide

    (B) addition of PEEP

    (C) vasopressors

    (D) chest tube

For questions 16 and 17

A 63-year-old male is admitted with acute respiratory distress. Symptoms include marked shortness of breath and circumoral cyanosis. He is awake and complains of shortness of breath. He has a history of COPD (chronic obstructive pulmonary disease). Blood gases reveal the following information:

pH	7.22
$PaCO_2$	62
PaO_2	54
SaO_2	81%
HCO_3	25
FiO_2	30%

16. Based on this information, what condition is likely developing?

    (A) congestive heart failure
    (B) ARDS
    (C) acute respiratory failure
    (D) pulmonary emboli

17. What would be the priority treatment indicated at this time?

    (A) Increase the FiO_2.
    (B) Intubate and initiate mechanical ventilation.
    (C) Use postural drainage treatment.
    (D) Administer a bronchodilator.

---

18. Which of the following may be an effect of mechanical ventilation and PEEP (positive end-expiratory pressure)?

    (A) atelectasis
    (B) oxygen toxicity
    (C) ARDS
    (D) reduced cardiac output

19. Which of the following is NOT a clinical finding seen in pneumonia?

    (A) a chest X-ray with an area of consolidation
    (B) hypoxemia refractory to O_2 administration with a need for PEEP
    (C) normal WBCs with increased immature neutrophils (bands)
    (D) bronchial breath sounds, diminished breath sounds, or crackles on auscultation

20. Which of the following would be the earliest sign of hypoventilation?

    (A) respiratory rate of 20 breaths/minute
    (B) anxiety
    (C) decreased level of consciousness
    (D) SpO_2 of 85%

21. A 70 kg patient with ARDS is intubated and mechanically ventilated. The patient is on a continuous vecuronium infusion to maintain a twitch of "1." The peak inspiratory pressure is 55 cm H_2O, and the plateau pressure is 50 cm H_2O. The PaO_2 is 60. The physician orders the following ventilator settings: assist-control mode = 12 breaths/minute, tidal volume 700 mL, FiO_2 1.00, and PEEP 15. The nurse knows that:

    (A) continuous positive airway pressure (CPAP) is an appropriate setting for a patient who is receiving vecuronium.
    (B) a tidal volume of 700 mL is inappropriate for this patient.
    (C) the PEEP should be decreased to 5 cm H_2O pressure to improve oxygenation.
    (D) the plateau pressure is appropriate for this patient.

22. When caring for a postoperative patient with a chest tube, care of the patient needs to include:

(A) loop tubing right above the collection chamber.
(B) placing the collection chamber on the IV pole when turning the patient.
(C) clamping the chest tube during patient transport.
(D) reporting sudden bubbling in the negative pressure chamber.

23. A patient with an acute exacerbation of COPD is minimally responsive, tachypneic, and tachycardic. The ABG results include pH 7.20, $PaCO_2$ 68, and PaO_2 65. The nurse anticipates that the next intervention will be:

(A) initiating noninvasive ventilation.
(B) endotracheal intubation.
(C) beginning low-flow oxygen per a nasal cannula.
(D) administering sodium bicarbonate to correct acidosis.

24. A patient with a known history of asthma is admitted with asthma exacerbation. The critical care nurse needs to be aware of the potential clinical signs that may indicate a need for intubation and initiation of mechanical ventilation. Which of the following would indicate a possible need for intubation?

(A) difficulty to arouse
(B) respiratory alkalosis
(C) bilateral wheezing
(D) SaO_2 92%

25. Which of the following factors would DECREASE the release of oxygen from hemoglobin at the tissue level?

(A) a temperature of 39°C
(B) increased levels of 2,3-DPG
(C) arterial pH of 7.30
(D) a massive transfusion of stored, banked blood

26. A trauma patient with multiple long bone fractures suddenly develops agitation, tachypnea, tachycardia, and mild hypoxemia. Her lungs are clear, and a petechial rash is noted on her upper body. Which of the following is suspected?

(A) acute respiratory distress syndrome
(B) fat embolism
(C) deep vein thrombosis
(D) delirium

27. A patient's arterial blood gas (ABG) is as follows: pH 7.32, $PaCO_2$ 33, and HCO_3 16. Based on this ABG, what might be this patient's problem?

(A) anxiety
(B) shock
(C) drug overdose
(D) electrolyte imbalance

ANSWERS AND EXPLANATIONS

1. **(C)** Noninvasive ventilation is not safe for a patient who is unable to protect his or her airway. A depressed level of consciousness increases the risk of airway obstruction or aspiration. Choice (A) can be provided with NIV. Choices (B) and (D) do not put a patient who is receiving NIV at a greater risk for a poor outcome.

2. **(A)** This scenario describes a patient who is experiencing a pulmonary embolism (PE). Signs of hypotension and hypoxemia indicate that it is a massive PE. The PE increases dead space ventilation due to the drop in pulmonary perfusion. Fibrinolytic therapy (tissue plasminogen activator) is indicated for a massive PE. For any of the other choices to be correct, the patient would have to have abnormal breath sounds.

3. **(D)** This clinical picture is one of asthma. Asthma is an airway problem that results in bronchospasm, which increases airway pressure as evidenced by an elevated inspiratory pressure while the lung pressure itself (the plateau pressure) remains normal. Symptoms would be relieved with a bronchodilator. The other choices would not relieve these symptoms.

4. **(C)** A patient with asthma has difficulty with expiration. Therefore, with each breath air may get trapped, resulting in elevation of the end-expiratory pressure without PEEP being set on the ventilator. This may decrease cardiac output because it decreases venous return. The other interventions would all increase the air trapping.

5. **(C)** Mouth care decreases bacterial colonization in the mouth, which decreases the possibility of microaspiration of bacteria in lower airways. The other 3 choices have NOT been found to decrease incidences of ventilator-associated pneumonia. Sedation should be minimized. The head of the bed should be greater than 30°. The ETT cuff should not be deflated prior to suctioning but, instead, prior to ETT removal. (At that time, the mouth and the subglottic space should be well suctioned.)

6. **(A)** The goal is to get the FiO_2 down to 50% or less ASAP for a patient who requires high FiO_2. This patient's oxygenation status would allow for a decrease in the FiO_2. During acute ARDS, the tidal volume needs to be low to prevent volutrauma, and the PEEP needs to be maintained to limit atelectasis.

7. **(B)** Decreased compliance increases "stiffness" and therefore requires more work to ventilate. Choice (A) is not correct because an increase in the peak inspiratory pressure will decrease dynamic compliance. Choice (C) is not correct because asthma decreases dynamic (airway) compliance, not static (lung) compliance. Choice (D) is not correct because dynamic compliance is calculated using the peak inspiratory pressure.

8. **(B)** If the PAOP is high, the pulmonary edema is most likely cardiac in origin, whereas in ARDS, the pulmonary edema is noncardiogenic in origin. The other 3 choices (bilateral infiltrates, refractory hypoxemia, and tachypnea) are all present in ARDS.

9. **(C)** This clinical scenario is one of right-sided pneumonia. Therefore, the right side is the "bad" side. Due to the effects of gravity on perfusion, the patient generally does better with the "good" lung DOWN. With the "bad" lung down, there is an increased risk of worsening hypoxemia. Choice (A) is not correct because the patient is not wheezing. Therefore, there is no indication for a bronchodilator. Choice (B) is not correct because this condition does not warrant NIV. Choice (D) is not correct because the best position for a patient with a pulmonary problem is sitting upright, not lying flat.

10. **(D)** A patient with asthma needs a bronchodilator (to treat the bronchospasm caused by smooth muscle contraction around the airways) and steroids (to treat the airway inflammation). There is no indication for anticoagulants, diuretics, or antibiotics to treat asthma.

11. **(D)** An increase in the ventilator breath rate will influence the $PaCO_2$ (ventilation), not oxygenation. The other 3 choices will improve oxygenation at the tissue level. An increase in the FiO_2 will provide more oxygen at the alveolar-capillary membrane. A blood transfusion will increase oxygen content by increasing hemoglobin, which is the carrier of oxygen. Increasing a low blood pressure will increase oxygen delivery.

12. **(A)** The best clinical indicator of effective ventilation is the $PaCO_2$. Although a breath rate less than 12 may indicate hypoventilation, it is not as sensitive an indicator as is $PaCO_2$. In addition, the breath rate does not include the other determinant of effective ventilation (depth of ventilation or tidal volume). Although a low pH may indicate hypoventilation, it may also indicate metabolic acidosis. Hypoxemia (PaO_2 less than 80 mmHg on room air) may be present during hyperventilation.

13. **(B)** If the patient has a COHb level of 45%, the best SaO_2 achievable is 55% since saturation of hemoglobin cannot be greater than 100% total. The patient needs 100% FiO_2 until COHb levels have returned to normal and symptoms (alteration in the level of consciousness and headaches) are relieved. Opiates may depress the level of consciousness and mask the patient's response to FiO_2. A decrease in the FiO_2 would decrease the driving forces of oxygen and prolong abnormal COHb levels. Intubation would not help oxygenation since the same FiO_2 can be provided with a face mask. Intubation would be indicated for a ventilation problem, but the patient does not have signs of hypoventilation.

14. **(C)** This clinical scenario describes a pneumothorax. As a result of hypotension and tracheal deviation to the opposite side of the pneumothorax, the pneumothorax is a life-threatening tension pneumothorax with symptoms that are the result of a mediastinal shift. If ARDS was the problem, the patient would have bilateral crackles. If a hemothorax was the problem, there would generally be a history of trauma, not an infection. A mediastinal shift (tracheal deviation to the opposite side and hypotension) is not usually present with a hemothorax. If the problem was a PE, the breath sounds would be equal bilaterally.

15. **(D)** The treatment for a tension pneumothorax is a chest tube (generally after emergent needle decompression). None of the other choices is beneficial for treating a tension pneumothorax.

16. **(C)** Not enough information is provided to select any condition other than acute respiratory failure. Acute respiratory failure is an ABG diagnosis, and this ABG meets the requirements of acute respiratory failure. Do NOT read into the questions.

17. **(A)** This patient has severe hypoxemia that needs to be addressed first in order to prevent all of the associated effects of the severe hypoxemia. Although the patient is not ventilating normally, the elevated $PaCO_2$ is less of a problem, as indicated by the patient's mental status. The level of consciousness is not depressed. There is no indication in the scenario for choices (C) or (D).

18. **(D)** Initiation of mechanical ventilation (even without PEEP) that delivers positive pressure breaths results in a mild increase in the intrathoracic pressure with a resultant decrease in venous return. PEEP increases the intrathoracic pressure even more and causes a decrease in venous return. Mechanical ventilation and/or PEEP do not cause any of the other 3 choices.

19. **(B)** Pneumonia results in a V/Q mismatch, not a shunt. Therefore, the administration of oxygen will correct the hypoxemia. PEEP is not required as it is for a shunt (ARDS). The worse the pneumonia, the greater the FiO_2 requirement will be. The other 3 choices are possible clinical indicators of pneumonia.

20. **(C)** As ventilation decreases, the $PaCO_2$ rises and affects the brain by decreasing the level of consciousness from lethargy to an obtunded state, to a stupor, to a comatose state. Although the patient MAY have hypoventilation with a respiratory rate of 20 breaths/minute, it would not be considered a typical sign. Anxiety and SpO_2 are more likely signs of hypoxemia than early signs of hypoventilation.

21. **(B)** Since the patient has ARDS, low tidal volumes (5–6 mL/kg) are indicated (permissive hypercapnia) in order to prevent volutrauma. Since the patient weighs 70 kg, a Vt of 700 mL is too high. CPAP requires that the patient has a spontaneous breathing effort. Therefore, CPAP is not appropriate for this patient. A patient with ARDS requires high PEEP to prevent atelectasis and hypoxemia. Therefore, a decrease in PEEP would worsen the hypoxemia. The plateau pressure should be kept at 30 cm H_2O or less. Therefore, this patient's plateau pressure is too high, and a decrease in the Vt may help decrease the plateau pressure.

22. **(D)** Sudden bubbling in the negative pressure chamber is an indication of a possible air leak; this should be reported to the physician. All of the other choices should be avoided when caring for a patient with a chest tube. Loops will increase pressure in the system. The collection chamber needs to be kept below the level of the chest at all times. Clamping the chest tube cuts off the negative pressure provided by the negative pressure chamber and could result in lung re-collapse.

23. **(B)** Due to the patient's decreased level of consciousness, the need for improved ventilation is a priority. NIV would address the hypoventilation, but it would not be considered safe for a patient with minimal responsiveness. Providing oxygen alone would not address the main problem (hypoventilation), which in this case is worse than the problem of hypoxemia. This patient has respiratory acidosis and should not be treated with sodium bicarbonate.

24. **(A)** A depressed level of consciousness may be an indication of hypoventilation (respiratory acidosis) and a precursor to respiratory arrest for a patient with asthma exacerbation. Respiratory alkalosis and bilateral wheezing are common early manifestations during an asthma exacerbation. Mild hypoxemia should be treated with an increase in FiO_2 but is not considered ominous unless it is severe.

25. **(D)** Banked blood does not have normal 2,3-DPG. Low levels of 2,3-DPG shift the oxyhemoglobin dissociation curve up to the left, which will decrease hemoglobin's release of oxygen at the tissue level. The remaining 3 choices—a fever, increased levels of 2,3-DPG, and acidosis—all shift the curve to the right, which increases the release of oxygen from hemoglobin.

26. **(B)** This clinical scenario is one of a pulmonary embolism. With the history of long bone fractures and the development of petechiae, a fat embolism is most likely. ARDS does not present with clear lungs. DVT does not always result in a PE. If it did, though, the PE would be due to a blood clot and petechiae would not be present. Delirium may result in agitation but not the other symptoms.

27. **(B)** The low pH indicates acidosis. The low bicarbonate indicates that the acidosis is metabolic, and the low $PaCO_2$ indicates that hyperventilation has started in order to compensate. The only option that causes metabolic acidosis is shock. Anxiety generally causes respiratory alkalosis. An opiate drug overdose results in respiratory acidosis. An electrolyte imbalance (low chloride) causes metabolic alkalosis.

ANSWERS TO PRACTICE ABGs

1. Respiratory alkalosis, no compensation
2. Respiratory acidosis, no compensation
3. Metabolic acidosis, no compensation
4. Respiratory acidosis, partial compensation
5. Metabolic alkalosis, no compensation
6. Respiratory acidosis, partial compensation
7. Metabolic alkalosis, partial compensation
8. Metabolic acidosis, partial compensation
9. Respiratory acidosis, no compensation
10. Metabolic alkalosis, no compensation
11. Mixed disorder: respiratory acidosis and metabolic alkalosis

Multisystem Concepts

6

By failing to prepare, you are preparing to fail.

—Benjamin Franklin

MULTISYSTEM TEST BLUEPRINT

Multisystem 14% of total test   **21 questions**

→ Acid-base imbalance*
→ Bariatric complications**
→ Comorbidity in patients with transplant history
→ End-of-life care
→ Healthcare-associated conditions (e.g., VAE, CAUTI, CLABSI)
→ Hypotension
→ Infectious diseases
   ○ Influenza (e.g., pandemic or epidemic)
   ○ Multi-drug resistant organisms (e.g., MRSA, VRE, CRE)
→ Life-threatening maternal/fetal complications (e.g., eclampsia, HELLP syndrome, post-partum hemorrhage, amniotic embolism)
→ Multiple organ dysfunction syndrome (MODS)
→ Multisystem trauma
→ Pain: acute, chronic
→ Post-intensive care syndrome (PICS)
→ Sepsis
→ Septic shock
→ Shock states
   ○ Distributive (e.g., anaphylactic, neurogenic)
   ○ Hypovolemic
→ Sleep disruption (including sensory overload)
→ Thermoregulation
→ Toxic ingestion/inhalations (e.g., drug/alcohol overdose)
→ Toxin/drug exposure (including allergies)

*This topic is also covered in the Respiratory Concepts chapter of this book.

**This topic is covered in the Gastrointestinal Concepts chapter of this book.

MULTISYSTEM TESTABLE NURSING ACTIONS
☐ Manage continuous temperature monitoring
☐ Provide end-of-life and palliative care
☐ Recognize risk factors and manage malignant hyperthermia
☐ Recognize indications for, and manage, patients undergoing:
○ Continuous sedation
○ Intermittent sedation
○ Neuromuscular blockade agents
○ Procedural sedation—minimal
○ Procedural sedation—moderate
○ Targeted temperature management (previously known as therapeutic hypothermia)

> The number of questions in the multisystem section of the Adult CCRN test blueprint has significantly increased in recent years. There are now 21 multisystem-related questions on this exam (as opposed to only 12 previously). Therefore, plan on studying the content in this chapter for approximately 21 hours.

SHOCK

Overview

- Although blood pressure (hypotension) is generally thought of when discussing shock, shock is actually a **cellular disease** due to either inadequate perfusion (the oxygen demand is greater than the oxygen delivered) or the inability of cells to utilize the delivered oxygen (issues with oxygen utilization/consumption).

- Refer to Figure 6-1 to study the pathophysiology of shock.

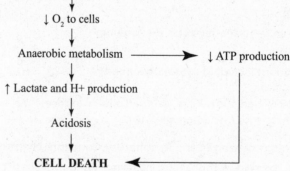

Inadequate tissue perfusion **or** impaired O_2 uptake

↓ O_2 to cells

Anaerobic metabolism ⟶ ↓ ATP production

↑ Lactate and H+ production

Acidosis

CELL DEATH

Figure 6-1. Pathophysiology of shock

- There are 3 stages of all types of shock:
  1. Compensatory
  2. Progressive
  3. Refractory

- The rapidity with which a patient progresses through these stages varies depending upon many factors.
- During the **compensatory stage** of shock (Figures 6-2 and 6-3), the blood pressure (B/P) is maintained as a result of 2 mechanisms: stimulation of the sympathetic nervous system and activation of the renin-angiotensin-aldosterone system (RAAS).

Sympathetic Nervous System Stimulation

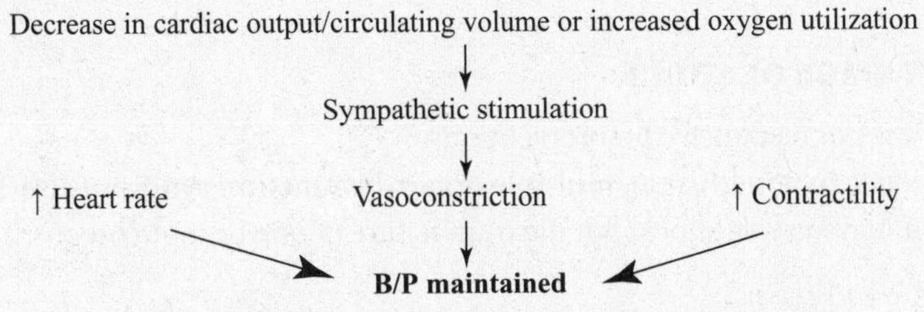

Decrease in cardiac output/circulating volume or increased oxygen utilization

↓

Sympathetic stimulation

↓

↑ Heart rate   Vasoconstriction   ↑ Contractility

B/P maintained

Figure 6-2. Physiology of compensatory stage of shock

Renin-Angiotensin-Aldosterone System (RAAS) Activation

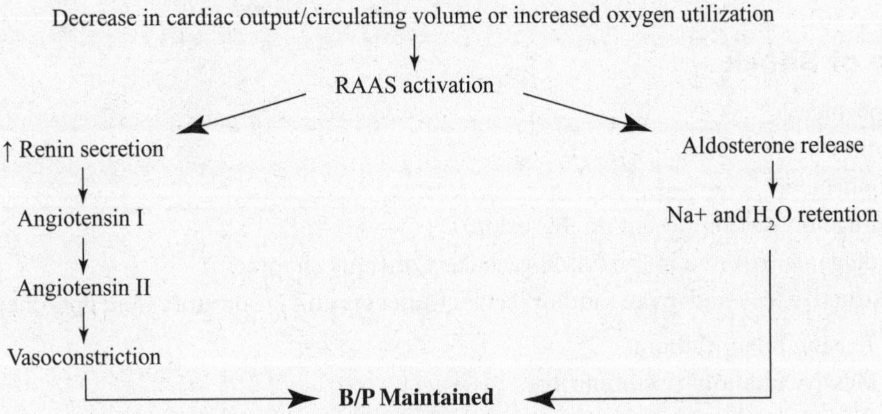

Decrease in cardiac output/circulating volume or increased oxygen utilization

↓

RAAS activation

↑ Renin secretion   Aldosterone release

↓   ↓

Angiotensin I   Na+ and H_2O retention

↓

Angiotensin II

↓

Vasoconstriction

B/P Maintained

Figure 6-3. Compensatory stage of shock due to RAAS

Clinical Signs/Symptoms of the Stages of Shock

COMPENSATORY STAGE OF SHOCK (BLOOD PRESSURE MAINTAINED)

- Tachycardia
- Tachypnea, respiratory alkalosis
- Normal PaO_2
- Oliguria
- Skin is pale, cool (except in early sepsis)
- Restlessness, anxiety
- Complaints of thirst
- **Remember, B/P maintained!**

PROGRESSIVE STAGE OF SHOCK (COMPENSATORY MECHANISMS FAILING)

- **Hypotension**
- Worsening tachycardia, tachypnea, oliguria
- Metabolic acidosis
- Decreased PaO_2
- Clammy, mottled skin
- Further change in LOC
- The patient may complain of nausea.

REFRACTORY STAGE OF SHOCK

- The patient is not responsive to interventions.
- Severe systemic hypoperfusion, **multiple organ dysfunction syndrome (MODS)**
- The patient may survive shock, but die from failure of one or more organs.
  - Pulmonary (ARDS)
  - Kidney (acute tubular necrosis)
  - Heart (failure, ischemia)
  - Hematologic (disseminated intravascular coagulation)
  - Neurological (encephalopathy, stroke)
  - Liver (failure)

Types of Shock

- Hypovolemic
- Septic
- Anaphylactic
- Neurogenic (seldom tested on this exam)
- Cardiogenic (covered in the Cardiovascular Concepts chapter)
- Obstructive (covered in the Cardiovascular Concepts and Respiratory Concepts chapters)
  - Tension pneumothorax
  - Massive pulmonary embolism
  - Cardiac tamponade

HYPOVOLEMIC SHOCK

- Critical reduction in the circulating intravascular volume, leading to inadequate tissue perfusion
- Most common type of shock
  - Internal causes—third-spacing or pooling in the intravascular compartment
  - External causes—hemorrhage, GI or renal losses, burns, excessive diaphoresis
- Hypovolemia effects on pulse pressure:
  - Systolic decreases, diastolic maintains or elevates, NARROW pulse pressure
  - Example:
    - Baseline is 130/80
    - Volume loss → 110/80, 100/80, 90/70

- Hemodynamics
  - ↓ B/P
  - ↓ Pulse pressure
  - ↓ Right atrial pressure (CVP)
  - ↓ Cardiac output, O_2 delivery
  - ↓ Left atrial pressure (PAOP)
  - ↓ SvO_2
  - ↑ Systemic vascular resistance (SVR)

Everything is decreased except SVR.

Treatment of Hypovolemic Shock

- Identify the etiology and correct it, if possible.
- Replace volume appropriately, "Fill up the tank!"
  - Rapid and vigorous volume loading
  - Requires at least 2 large bore IV sites (hemorrhagic); a central line is not necessary but may assist fluid replacement.
  - Use a fluid warmer if > 2,000 mL of fluids are administered in 1 hour (ALL fluids for trauma patients).
- Hemorrhagic vs. nonhemorrhagic
- Fluid resuscitation: goal is to maintain O_2 delivery (DO_2) and O_2 uptake (VO_2) into tissue and sustain aerobic metabolism.
- Fluid resuscitate to clinical targets (e.g., decreased tachycardia, increased urine output)
  - Use isotonic fluid: 0.9 normal saline or lactated Ringer's.
  - Which is better? There are advantages and disadvantages to each (Table 6-1).

Table 6-1. Comparison of Normal Saline and Lactated Ringer's

Normal Saline	Lactated Ringer's
Isotonic crystalloid, effects last approximately 40 minutes, then leaves vascular space	Isotonic crystalloid, effects last approximately 40 minutes, then leaves vascular space
Disadvantage—large volumes may lead to hyperchloremic acidosis	Best mimics extracellular fluid (ECF) minus proteins, recommended resuscitation fluid by the ACS Committee on Trauma
Do not give to those with hypernatremia or renal failure	Has the potential to correct lactic acidosis; yet in severe hypoperfusion, it may promote lactic acidosis due to lactate accumulation
• Has 154 mmols Na^+ and 154 of Cl^-; does **NOT** contain any K^+, Ca^{++}, or lactate	Do not give through a blood product transfusion line or to those who should not receive K^+ or lactate
	• Has 130 mmols of Na^+, 109 Cl^-, 4 K^+, 2.7 Ca^{++}, 28 lactate

- Resuscitation endpoints
  - ○ MAP $\geq$ 65 mmHg
  - ○ CVP $\sim$ 6 mmHg (not well-defined)
  - ○ Urine OP 0.5 mL/kg/hr
  - ○ Heart rate decreased
  - ○ Hgb $>$ 7.0 g/dL and coagulation/platelet abnormalities are corrected.
    - – Hemoglobin and hematocrit measurements are not accurate during active blood loss.

Hemorrhagic Shock

The severity of hemorrhagic shock is categorized into 4 classes (Table 6-2).

Table 6-2. Classification of Hemorrhagic Shock

	Class I	Class II	Class III	Class IV
Blood loss (mL)	Up to 750	750–1,500	1,500–2,000	> 2,000
Blood loss (% blood vol)	Up to 15%	15–30%	30–40%	> 40%
Heart rate	< 100	> 100	> 120	> 140
Blood pressure	Normal	Normal	Decreased*	Decreased
Pulse pressure	Normal or ↓	Decreased	Decreased	Decreased
Capillary refill	Normal	Decreased	Decreased	Decreased
Respiratory rate	14–20	20–30	30–40	> 40
Urine output (mL/hr)	> 30	20–30	5–15	Scant
Mental status	Slightly anxious	Mildly anxious	Anxious, confused	Confused, lethargic

*Note that the blood pressure does not decrease in hemorrhagic shock until Class III, a loss of 1,500–2,000 mL of blood.

- Class I: treat with crystalloids
- Class II: treat with crystalloids
- Class III: treat with crystalloids + blood
- Class IV: treat with crystalloids + blood

Treatment of Hemorrhagic (Hypovolemic) Shock

- STOP the bleeding.
- Blood transfusion
  - ○ Optimal threshold remains controversial.
  - ○ 7.0 g/dL Hgb is fairly well established in the critically ill.
  - ○ Goal may be higher in the presence of:
    - – Active bleeding
    - – Severe hypoxemia
    - – Myocardial ischemia
    - – Lactic acidosis

- Packed red blood cells (PRBCs), unlike whole blood, do not have plasma or platelets; therefore, the patient will need a replacement of the coagulation components of blood with a transfusion of multiple units of PRBCs.
  - Fresh frozen plasma
  - Platelets
  - Cryoprecipitate
- Risks of blood product administration
  - Hemolytic and non-hemolytic reactions
  - Transfusion-mediated immunomodulation
  - Viral infection transmission
  - Transfusion-related acute lung injury (TRALI)
  - Hypothermia—WARM blood products to prevent this
    - Consequences of hypothermia
      - ➤ Impairment of red cell deformability
      - ➤ Platelet dysfunction
      - ➤ Increase in affinity of hemoglobin to hold onto O_2
  - Coagulopathy: monitor coagulation status, provide plasma and platelets
  - Hypocalcemia, hypomagnesemia (citrate in transfused blood binds ionized Ca^{++} and Mg^{++})
  - Banked blood does not have adequate 2,3-DPG. What is the consequence?
    - Shifts the oxyhemoglobin-dissociation curve to the LEFT (see the Respiratory Concepts chapter); increases the affinity of hemoglobin to hold onto O_2.

Massive Transfusion Protocols

- Designed to provide rapid infusion of large quantities of blood products to restore oxygen delivery (DO_2), oxygen utilization (VO_2), and tissue perfusion (blood pressure)
- Indications include traumatic injuries, ruptured abdominal aortic or thoracic aortic aneurysms, liver transplant, OB emergencies.
- Definition: 10 units of RBCs in 24 hours or 5 units in less than 3 hours
- Mortality > 50%
- Need to prevent the **triad of death**:
  - Hypothermia
  - Acidosis
  - Coagulopathy

SEPSIS AND SEPTIC SHOCK

Most acute care settings have developed protocols for the treatment of sepsis and septic shock to provide timely, evidence-based, life-saving treatment for this patient population and to meet the requirements set forth by the Centers for Medicare and Medicaid Services (CMS). Whereas older medical studies stressed the importance of CVP and $ScvO_2$ measurements, more recent medical studies that discuss sepsis and septic shock place less importance on those measurements and instead stress fluid resuscitation, timeliness of obtaining blood cultures and serum lactate level measurements, the administration of antibiotics, and the initiation of vasopressors if necessary.

Overview

- There are at least 1.7 million incidences of sepsis in American adults annually, with ~ 270,000 deaths per year.
- Sepsis is the #1 cause of death in the non-coronary ICUs.
- As per the CDC, 1 in 3 patients who die in a hospital have sepsis.
- Numbers are expected to increase due to high incidences of sepsis in the older adult population.
- The current Adult CCRN test blueprint expects you to understand sepsis and septic shock. Systemic inflammatory response syndrome (SIRS) and severe sepsis are not included in the latest blueprint (most likely due to the changes introduced in the Sepsis-3 definitions, which were published in 2016). Brief descriptions of all of these terms are provided in the following sections, but exam questions will most likely focus on sepsis and septic shock.

Systemic Inflammatory Response Syndrome (SIRS)

- SIRS is a systemic inflammatory response to a wide variety of severe clinical insults, manifested by 2 or more of the following:
  - Temperature $\geq 38°C$ or $< 36°C$
  - Heart rate > 90 bpm
  - Respiratory rate > 20 breaths/minute or $PaCO_2 < 32$ mmHg
  - WBC > 12,000 or < 4,000 **or** bands > 10% (shift to the left)
- A patient **may have SIRS without sepsis** (i.e., traumatic injury, pancreatitis, burns).
- Studies have shown that SIRS is a poor predictor of sepsis, and thus SIRS was eliminated from the Sepsis-3 definitions.

Sepsis

- Sepsis is a life-threatening organ dysfunction that is caused by an abnormal host response to an infection. Initially, the infection may be "suspected," rather than "proven," based on the clinical examination and the patient's history.
- A "suspected" infection is the presence of one or more of the following:
  - Positive culture results from blood, sputum, urine, etc.
  - Receiving antibiotic, antifungal, or another anti-infective therapy
  - Altered mental status in the elderly
  - Possible pneumonia (infiltrate on the chest radiograph)
  - Nursing home patient with an indwelling urinary catheter
  - Pressure ulcers
  - Acute abdomen
  - Infected wounds, especially with a history of diabetes
  - Immunosuppression
- Sepsis = infection + organ dysfunction
- Organ dysfunction may be identified by assessing the patient's qSOFA score or SOFA score.

EXAMPLES OF ORGAN DYSFUNCTION

- Hypotension
- Acute hypoxemia
- Acute drop in urine output (< 0.5 mL/kg)
- Lactate 2 mmol/L or greater
- Abrupt mental status change
- Platelets below 100,000
- Coagulopathy

qSOFA (QUICK SEPSIS RELATED ORGAN FAILURE ASSESSMENT) SCORE

- The qSOFA score is included in the Sepsis-3 definitions, but it is not currently included in the Adult CCRN test blueprint (although it could be added in the future).
- The qSOFA score is a bedside evaluation (without the need for labs) to identify patients with suspected **organ dysfunction**.
- The qSOFA score evaluates 3 criteria, assigning 1 point for each of the following:
  - Systolic B/P ≤ 100 mmHg
  - Respiratory rate ≥ 22 breaths per minute
  - Glasgow coma scale < 15 (altered mentation)
- A qSOFA score of **2 or 3** indicates a high probability for organ dysfunction.

Severe Sepsis

- Severe sepsis (as defined prior to the publication of the Sepsis-3 definitions in 2016) is sepsis **PLUS** markers of organ dysfunction.
- Note that severe sepsis is not included in the Sepsis-3 definitions, and it has been eliminated from the Adult CCRN test blueprint.

NOTE

"Severe sepsis" is included in the Sepsis-2 definitions (from 2001) and is still used by the CMS, but it is not included in the Sepsis-3 definitions (from 2016) or in the current Adult CCRN test blueprint. The Sepsis-3 definition of "sepsis" includes organ dysfunction, whereas the Sepsis-2 definition instead calls it a "systemic response (SIRS positive) to an infection." Due to changing nomenclature and "bundles" of care (1-hour, 3-hour, 6-hour) as defined by various organizations, it is unlikely that "severe sepsis" will be mentioned in an exam question. However, just in case you need a quick refresher on the differences between the Sepsis-2 definitions and the Sepsis-3 definitions and how they define SIRS, sepsis, severe sepsis, and septic shock, refer to Table 6-3.

Table 6-3. Differences Between the Sepsis-2 Definitions and the Sepsis-3 Definitions

Condition	Sepsis-2 Definitions	Sepsis-3 Definitions
SIRS	Systemic response to a wide variety of clinical insults (may or may not be an infection)	SIRS criteria is not assessed
Sepsis	Presence of an infection AND a systemic response (SIRS positive) to an infection	Presence of an infection AND **organ dysfunction**
Severe sepsis	Sepsis PLUS markers of **organ dysfunction**	Severe sepsis is not included in these definitions
Septic shock	Hypotension due to an infection; includes markers of hypoperfusion, which persists despite adequate fluid resuscitation; requires the administration of pressors	Hypotension due to an infection; includes markers of hypoperfusion, which persists despite adequate fluid resuscitation; requires the administration of pressors

Septic Shock

- Of all deaths in hospitals annually, more than 40% are the result of septic shock.
- Clinically identified by an infection, **PLUS**:
  ○ Vasopressor requirement to maintain a MAP of ≥ 65 mmHg, despite adequate fluid resuscitation
  ○ Serum lactate > 2 mmol/L, despite fluid resuscitation

Differentiation of Infection, Sepsis, and Septic Shock

Match the condition in the left-hand column with the clinical signs of patients in the right-hand column, each of which has a documented infection.

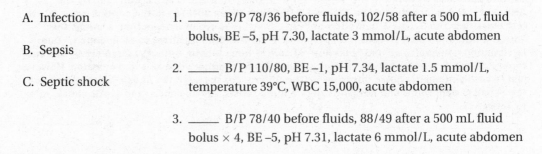

A. Infection

B. Sepsis

C. Septic shock

1. _____ B/P 78/36 before fluids, 102/58 after a 500 mL fluid bolus, BE –5, pH 7.30, lactate 3 mmol/L, acute abdomen

2. _____ B/P 110/80, BE –1, pH 7.34, lactate 1.5 mmol/L, temperature 39°C, WBC 15,000, acute abdomen

3. _____ B/P 78/40 before fluids, 88/49 after a 500 mL fluid bolus × 4, BE –5, pH 7.31, lactate 6 mmol/L, acute abdomen

The answers are located at the end of the "Sepsis and Septic Shock" section on page 124.

Pathophysiology of Sepsis/Septic Shock

- Sepsis/septic shock is a process of malignant intravascular **inflammation**.

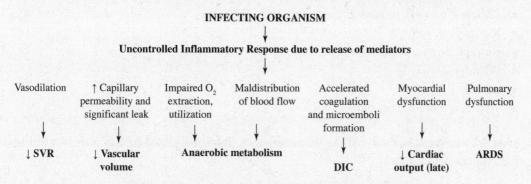

Figure 6-4. Pathophysiology of sepsis/septic shock

- Activation of coagulation, inflammatory cytokines, complement, and kinin cascades with the release of a variety of endogenous mediators
- Causative organisms include:
  - Gram-negative bacteria
  - Gram-positive bacteria
  - Fungi, viruses, *Rickettsia*, parasites

Risk Factors for Sepsis

- Extremes of age
- Chronic health problems
- Invasive procedures and devices
- Surgical wounds
- Genitourinary infections
- Prolonged hospitalizations
- Translocation of GI bacteria (NPO)
- Acquired immunodeficiency syndrome
- Use of cytotoxic and immunosuppressive agents
- Alcoholism
- Malignant neoplasms; bone marrow suppression
- Transplantation procedures
- History of a splenectomy

Signs/Symptoms of Early Septic Shock

- Tachycardia, bounding pulse
- B/P is low, responsive to vasopressors
- Skin is warm, flushed
- Respirations are deep, somewhat fast
- Lactate > 2 mmol/L
- Confusion → mental status change (especially in elderly people)
- Oliguria
- Fever (temperature > 38°C)

Signs/Symptoms of Progressive (Later) Septic Shock

- Hypotension, may not be responsive to pressors
- Tachycardia, pulse is weak and thready
- Lactate 4 mmol/L or greater
- Skin is cool, pale
- Respirations are rapid *or* may be slow
- Lethargy, coma
- Anuria
- Hypothermia (temperature < 36°C)

MYTH

A patient with sepsis or septic shock always has a fever and an elevated WBC.

Table 6-4 shows the hemodynamics of septic shock. Table 6-5 lists the diagnostic test results that indicate septic shock.

Table 6-4. Hemodynamics of Septic Shock*

Early	Progressive (Late)
CO/CI ↑	CO/CI ↓
RA, PA, PAOP ↓	RA, PA, PCWP ↑
SVR ↓	SVR (variable)
SvO$_2$ ↑	SvO$_2$ (variable)
O$_2$ delivery ↑	O$_2$ delivery ↓
O$_2$ consumption ↓	O$_2$ consumption ↓
*Key: ↓ = decrease; ↑ = increase	

Table 6-5. Diagnostic Test Results That Indicate Septic Shock*

Early	Progressive (Late)
ABGs → respiratory alkalosis, mild ↓ PaO$_2$, or may have a combined respiratory alkalosis and metabolic acidosis	ABGs → metabolic acidosis, ↓↓ PaO$_2$
PT, PTT ~ or ↑	PT, PTT ↑↑
Platelets ~ or ↓	Platelets ↓↓
WBC ↑, ~, or ↓	WBC ↓
Bands ↑	Bands ↑↑
Glucose ↑	Glucose ↓
Lactate ↑	BUN, creatinine ↑
Troponin ↑	Liver enzymes ↑
	Lactate ↑
	Troponin ↑
*Key: ↓ = decrease; ↑ = increase; ~ = no change	

- Only 30–50% of patients who present with sepsis/septic shock have positive blood cultures.

MYTH

A patient with sepsis or septic shock always has positive blood cultures.

Treatment for Sepsis/Septic Shock

- Initial fluid challenge should be the administration of 30 mL/kg of crystalloid (2.1 L for a 70 kg or 154 pound person) **as early as possible** to achieve the goals listed below:
  - MAP ≥ 65 mmHg
  - UO ≥ 0.5 mL/kg/hr
  - Decrease in tachycardia

- If hypotension persists despite fluid resuscitation, start:
  - Vasopressor: pressor of choice is norepinephrine.
    - **Norepinephrine (Levophed)** is first-line.
    - **Epinephrine** (drip) is recommended when a second vasopressor agent is needed.
- IF the B/P does not respond to high-dose initial pressor and fluids, the patient may have **catecholamine-refractory septic shock**, whereby alpha receptors in the arterial bed are not responsive to pressors.
  - Start a **vasopressin drip** at 0.03–0.04 units/min, generally not titrated.
    - **NOT** a first-line agent for hypotension
    - Used to enhance the effectiveness of the initial pressor that was used for treating septic shock
  - If vasopressin is not effective, consider extreme metabolic acidosis or corticosteroid insufficiency related to a critical illness; treatment with sodium bicarbonate or steroids may be considered, although neither have demonstrated that they can improve mortality rates.
- Obtain two **blood cultures as early as possible** that are drawn simultaneously from two different sites prior to antibiotic administration.
- Begin broad-spectrum **antibiotic therapy as early as possible** after recognizing sepsis/septic shock and **after** blood cultures are drawn; administer within 3 hours of recognition of sepsis/septic shock (preferably within 1 hour of recognition, if possible).
  - In one study, for every hour that the administration of antibiotics was delayed, there was an approximately 12% decrease in the probability of survival.
- Obtain serum lactate **as early as possible** and remeasure within 2–4 hours if the first lactate is > 2 mmol/L.
- Identify the source of infection ASAP (which may direct antibiotic and/or interventional therapy).
- If the MAP remains below 65 mmHg **OR** the lactate is 4 mmol/L or greater, **reassess the fluid status**.
  - Ask a licensed independent practitioner to complete a focused clinical assessment, **OR**
  - Perform an assessment of 2 of the following: measure the CVP; assess the patient's fluid responsiveness with either a passive leg raise or a fluid challenge; perform/assess a bedside ECHO; measure the $ScvO_2$.
- Inotropic therapy—**dobutamine** is recommended (by itself or in addition to a vasopressor) for patients with cardiac dysfunction, as evidenced by high filling pressures and low cardiac output, or clinical signs of hypoperfusion after successfully restoring the blood pressure with effective volume resuscitation.
- Oxygenation goals for septic shock
  - Maintain SpO_2 95% or greater
  - Goal = $ScvO_2 \geq 70\%$ or $SvO_2 \geq 65\%$ (when CVP and MAP goals are met)
  - If $ScvO_2$ or SvO_2 goals are not achieved:
    - Consider further fluids
    - Dobutamine infusion, max 20 mcg/kg/min
    - Consider a transfusion of PRBCs if the Hgb is 7.0 or less

Summary of Therapeutic Endpoints for Septic Shock

- MAP $\geq$ 65 mmHg
- Decreased lactate/improved base deficit
- Normalization of heart rate
- UO $\geq$ 0.5 mL/kg/hr
- Warm extremities
- Mental status return to baseline
- Source control
- Central venous oxygen saturation ($ScvO_2$) $\geq$ 70% or SvO_2 $\geq$ 65% (if CVP or PA line is available)
- CVP (if available), 8–12 mmHg

Differentiation of Infection, Sepsis, and Septic Shock Answers

Match the condition in the left-hand column with the clinical signs of patients in the right-hand column, each of which has a documented infection.

A. Infection
B. Sepsis
C. Septic shock

1. __B__ B/P 78/36 before fluids, 102/58 after a 500 mL fluid bolus, BE –5, pH 7.30, lactate 3 mmol/L, acute abdomen

2. __A__ B/P 110/80, BE –1, pH 7.34, lactate 1.5 mmol/L, temperature 39°C, WBC 15,000, acute abdomen

3. __C__ B/P 78/40 before fluids, 88/49 after a 500 mL fluid bolus × 4, BE –5, pH 7.31, lactate 6 mmol/L, acute abdomen

ANAPHYLACTIC SHOCK

- Anaphylaxis is an allergic reaction that is rapid in onset and may cause death.
- Usually occurs after previous exposure to the substance
- Hives, angioedema in ~ 88% of cases
- Respiratory tract involvement in ~ 50% of cases
- Shock occurs in ~ 30% of anaphylaxis cases.

Etiology

- **IgE-mediated** immediate hypersensitivity reaction to **protein** substances
  - Penicillin, contrast media, bee sting, foods, latex

An anaphylactoid response looks the same clinically but is NOT IgE-mediated. Previous exposure is not necessary (Figure 6-5).

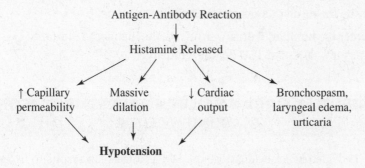

Antigen-Antibody Reaction

Histamine Released

↑ Capillary permeability   Massive dilation   ↓ Cardiac output   Bronchospasm, laryngeal edema, urticaria

Hypotension

Figure 6-5. Pathophysiology of anaphylactic shock

Treatment

- Removal of offensive agent, if able
- O_2
- 0.3–0.5 mg of 1:1,000 epinephrine **IM** (more rapid absorption than subcutaneous) to decrease dilation, bronchospasm
- Aggressive fluid resuscitation (1–4 L) to treat the relative hypovolemia
- Antihistamine: diphenhydramine (Benadryl) 25–50 mg IV to decrease allergic response
- Inhaled beta-adrenergic agents to decrease bronchospasm
- Steroids IV (high-dose): peaks in 4–6 hours, give ASAP to get "on board" to decrease inflammatory response

MULTIPLE ORGAN DYSFUNCTION SYNDROME (MODS)

- Multiple organ dysfunction syndrome (MODS), which is sometimes referred to as multi-organ dysfunction syndrome, is the progressive insufficiency of 2 or more organs in an acutely ill patient, such that homeostasis cannot be maintained without intervention (Table 6-6).

Table 6-6. Markers of Multiple Organ Dysfunction Syndrome (MODS)

Cardiovascular	Pulmonary	Renal
Hypotension	Tachypnea	Elevated creatinine
Tachycardia	Dyspnea	Decreased GFR
Dysrhythmias	Hypoxemia	Oliguria
Need for vasopressor support		Life-threatening electrolyte imbalances
Decreased systemic vascular resistance	**Neurological**	**Endocrine**
Abnormal CVP (low or high)	Confusion	Hyperglycemia or hypoglycemia
Positive troponin	Delirium	Adrenal insufficiency
	Disorientation	
	Lethargy, coma	
	Seizure	
Hepatic	**Hematologic**	**Metabolic**
Elevated liver enzymes	Thrombocytopenia	Metabolic acidosis
Hypoglycemia	Coagulopathy	Elevated lactate
Decreased albumin	Increased D-dimer levels	
Jaundice	Decreased protein C levels	

- MODS may be the result of any type of shock.
  - The greater the number of organs involved, the higher the mortality
  - Accounts for $\sim$ 80% of all ICU deaths annually

SEQUENTIAL ORGAN FAILURE ASSESSMENT (SOFA) SCORING SYSTEM

- Unlike the bedside qSOFA evaluation, the SOFA utilizes lab results to assess the extent of a patient's organ dysfunction. Six organ systems are evaluated, and each is assigned a score from 0 to 4 based on results to obtain the total score:
  1. Hypotension (cardiovascular)
  2. Glasgow Coma Scale score (neurological)
  3. PaO_2/FiO_2 (pulmonary)
  4. Serum creatinine or urine output (renal)
  5. Bilirubin level (hepatic)
  6. Platelet count (hematologic)

- The total score may be useful for predicting the clinical outcome of critically ill patients. Studies have shown that mortality rates are associated with the SOFA score: the mortality rate is 50% if the score increases in the first 96 hours after admission; the mortality rate is 25% if the score remains the same in the first 96 hours after admission; and the mortality rate is less than 27% if the score decreases in the first 96 hours after admission.

TRAUMA

- Trauma is included in the Adult CCRN test blueprint. However, questions related to trauma are generally very straightforward.
- Make sure you know the trauma first-line assessment and second-line assessment.

Trauma First-Line Assessment (A, B, C, D, E)

- **A**irway: ensure a patent airway—consider intubation (stabilize the cervical spine if a spinal cord injury is suspected).
- **B**reathing: provide 100% oxygen and ventilation.
- **C**irculation: two large bore IVs with warm isotonic lactated Ringer's
- **D**isability: perform a quick neurological exam—LOC, motor, pupils.
  - Glasgow Coma Scale score is part of the neurological exam, not ALL of it.
- **E**xpose/**E**nvironmental: remove the patient's clothes, provide warmth/cooling as needed.

Trauma Second-Line Assessment (F, G, H, I)

- **F**ull set of vital signs
  - Focused adjuncts: ECG monitor, pulse oximeter, CO_2 detector, urinary catheter, gastric tube, radiography, FAST, CT, DPL, labs
  - Family presence
- **G**ive comfort measures (pain management)
- **H**istory
- **I**nspect posterior: turn the patient over!

PROVIDING SEDATION TO THE CRITICALLY ILL

The Adult CCRN test blueprint has included treatment of pain and the use of sedation agents in the multisystem section; management of agitated behavior is also included in the behavioral/psychosocial section of the blueprint.

Overview of Sedation

- A patient who is agitated (even a patient with a medical, rather than a surgical, diagnosis) should first receive an analgesic (**analgesia-first sedation**) before receiving anxiolytics. (Analgesic agents will be covered in the next section of this chapter after the following discussion of anxiolytics.)

- The degree of sedation (the sedation goal) should be based on the needs of the patient and should be agreed upon by and communicated to all members of the health care team. This sedation goal applies to the sedation provided during a procedure and to the sedation provided as part of the therapeutic plan of care.

- Maintaining **light levels** of sedation in adult ICU patients is associated with improved clinical outcomes (i.e., a shorter duration of mechanical ventilation and a shorter ICU length of stay).

- When sedation is provided on an as-needed, PRN basis, there is less of a possibility of oversedation than there is when sedation is provided with a continuous infusion.

- Daily interruptions of continuous infusions of sedation agents allows for an assessment of further need for the sedation agent and a neurological assessment of the patient.

- Nonpharmacological treatment (massage, music, cold therapy, and relaxation techniques) should be considered before using an anxiolytic agent, especially for mild anxiety and agitation.

- The levels of sedation are:

  - **Minimal (Light) Sedation:** The patient responds normally to verbal commands.
  - **Moderate Sedation:** The patient responds purposefully to verbal commands, either alone or accompanied by light tactile stimulation. The patient is able to maintain a patent airway.
  - **Deep Sedation:** The patient cannot be easily aroused but responds purposefully to repeated or painful stimulation. The patient may require assistance in maintaining a patent airway. Deep sedation is generally only used during a procedure by providers with specialized privileging.
  - **General Anesthesia:** This is a loss of consciousness during which patients are not arousable, even by painful stimulation.

- The level of sedation may exceed the level intended; therefore, the RN needs to be able to identify when this occurs and act accordingly.

Assessment of Agitation and Sedation

■ Rule out hypoxemia, hemodynamic instability, and pain as causes of agitation. If any of these is present, treat accordingly.

■ Assess for additional etiologies (Table 6-7).

Table 6-7. Causes of Agitation in Critically Ill Patients

Physiological	Pharmacological	Emotional	Environmental
Hypoxemia	Anesthetics	Preexisting anxiety disorders	Noise, alarms
Hemodynamic instability (shock)	Sedatives	Preexisting psychoses	Lights
Pain	Analgesics	Dementia	Too cold or warm
DELIRIUM (hyperactive)	Steroids	Fear	Restraints
Withdrawal from ETOH, drugs	Bronchodilators	Anger	Tubes, lines
Dyspnea			Odors
Immobility			Isolation
Sleep deprivation			Sensory deprivation
			Sensory overload

■ Use a valid and reliable sedation assessment tool for measuring the quality and depth of sedation before and after treatment.

○ The Richmond Agitation-Sedation Scale (RASS) and the Sedation-Agitation Scale (SAS) are valid and reliable sedation assessment tools that are used for adult critical care patients.

Treatment with Select Sedation Agents

■ See Table 6-8 for select sedation agents that are commonly used for an acute/critically ill patient. **The dose that is given may vary depending upon unit protocols.**

Table 6-8. Dosing and Nursing Implications for Select Sedation Agents

Agent	Start Dose	Titration Time/Dose	Usual Dose Range	Nursing Implications
Dexmedetomidine (Precedex)	**Continuous Infusion:** Begin at 0.2–0.4 mcg/kg/hr, titrate to goal RASS score	If goal RASS score is not achieved, titrate by 0.1 mcg/kg/hr q 15 min	0.2–1.7 mcg/kg/hr	• Loading dose not recommended due to risk of hypotension and bradycardia • Do NOT paralyze patients while they're on dexmedetomidine • The patient may not need to be mechanically ventilated while on this medication • Sedation vacation may not be indicated
Ketamine (Ketalar)	**IV Bolus:** 1–2 mg/kg IV over 1 min followed by 0.25–0.5 mg/kg IV q 5–10 min if needed **Continuous Infusion:** 0.5–1 mg/kg/hr	**Continuous Infusion:** Titrate by 0.25 mg/kg/hr q 30 min; max infusion dose 3 mg/kg/hr for sedation	**Sedation:** 0.5–2 mg/kg/hr **Refractory Status Epilepticus:** 0.5–5 mg/kg/hr	• Give slow IV push over at least 1 min; faster rates of administration may cause respiratory depression • May cause increase in B/P and/or HR or hypersalivation • May produce psychosis, including auditory and visual hallucinations; pretreatment with a benzodiazepine reduces incidences of psychosis
Lorazepam (Ativan)	**Loading Dose:** 1–4 mg IVP q 30 min until goal RASS score or CIWA score **Continuous Infusion:** 1–2 mg/hr	**Intermittent Bolus:** Titrate by 1–2 mg/hr q 1 hr until sedation goal is achieved; if RASS score or CIWA score is not achieved, re-bolus with MIDAZOLAM 2 mg IV q 10 min to a max infusion rate of 10 mg/hr	1–20 mg/hr	• Contact the physician if a rate > 10 mg/hr is needed • Turn off daily and assess unless a contraindication exists for sedation vacation; attempt to manage sedation with PRN dosing with midazolam; if you need to resume the infusion, resume at half the previous dose • Use a 0.22-micron filter for continuous infusions • Consider checking the serum osmolarity if > 10 mg/hr is needed • Doses > 20 mg/hr have been associated with metabolic acidosis and renal insufficiency due to solvent, propylene glycol

(continued)

Table 6-8. Dosing and Nursing Implications for Select Sedation Agents (*Continued*)

Agent	Start Dose	Titration Time/Dose	Usual Dose Range	Nursing Implications
Midazolam (Versed)	**Loading Dose:** 1–4 mg IV q 5–15 min until goal level of sedation is achieved **Continuous Infusion:** 1–2 mg/hr	**Intermittent Bolus:** Titrate by 1–2 mg/hr every hour until goal sedation score is achieved; if RASS score or CIWA score is not achieved, re-bolus 2 mg IV q 10 min to a max infusion rate of 10 mg/hr	1–20 mg/hr	• Contact the physician if a rate > 10 mg/hr is needed • Turn off daily and assess unless a contraindication exists for sedation vacation • Attempt to manage sedation with PRN dosing with midazolam; if you need to resume the infusion, resume at half the previous dose
Propofol (Diprivan)	**Continuous Infusion:** 10 mcg/kg/min **Loading Dose:** Not recommended due to risk of hypotension	Titrate by 5 mcg/kg/ min q 10 min until goal sedation score is achieved	5–80 mcg/kg/min **Status Epilepticus:** Rates up to 150 mcg/kg/ min may be appropriate	• Turn off daily and assess unless a contraindication exists for sedation vacation; attempt to manage sedation with PRN dosing with midazolam; if you need to resume the infusion, resume at half the previous dose • Only use for ventilated patients • Do not paralyze • No analgesic properties • Propofol infusion syndrome may occur with prolonged use or in higher doses • Monitor triglycerides at baseline and q 48 hours during the infusion • Change the tubing every time a bottle is changed OR a minimum of q 12 hours • Count as a source of calories (lipids)

*Note that memorization of exact dosing is not generally needed for this exam. You need to understand how to care for a patient who requires procedural and continuous sedation and how to deal with adverse effects.

Benzodiazepine Reversal with Flumazenil (Romazicon)

- Reverse the effects of benzodiazepines with flumazenil (Romazicon) 0.2 mg IV over 15 seconds for moderate sedation/over 30 seconds for overdosage.

- Repeat doses, 0.2 mg at 1-minute intervals, maximum of 4 doses, until patient awakens.

- For resedation, give repeat doses at 20-minute intervals as needed, 0.2 mg per minute to a maximum of 1 mg total, and 3 mg total in 1 hour.

- Onset of action of flumazenil is 1–2 minutes, 30% response within 3 minutes, peak effect in 6–10 minutes.

- Resedation occurs after approximately 1 hour; the duration of flumazenil is related to the dose given and the benzodiazepine plasma concentrations.

☆ Note that the reversal effects of flumazenil may wear off before the effects of the benzodiazepine. Therefore, monitor for a return of sedation and respiratory depression for at least 2 hours and until the patient is stable and resedation is unlikely.

- Use with caution for those with a history of prolonged use. A seizure may occur with reversal.

Daily Sedation Withdrawal (Spontaneous Awakening Trial)

An evidence-based strategy for preventing oversedation and its complications is to withhold the sedation for patients who are receiving a **continuous drip** in order to perform a neurological assessment and determine whether the continuous sedation drip is still clinically beneficial. The daily spontaneous awakening trial (SAT), or sedation vacation, is best done in conjunction with the daily spontaneous breathing trial (SBT). Suggested guidelines for performing the daily SAT are as follows:

1. Screen the patient prior to the spontaneous awakening trial.

   - No myocardial ischemia
   - No active seizures
   - No alcohol withdrawal
   - No paralytic drip
   - Stable intracranial pressure
   - No recent increase in the sedation drip dose to maintain the goal RASS score

2. Turn off the sedation drip.

   - If the sedation agent is propofol, consider weaning down every 5 minutes to prevent sudden agitation.

3. Monitor the patient for awakening and tolerance to drug withdrawal.
   - Assess the patient's neurological status, discomfort, and pain.
   - Assess the level of sedation/agitation with a sedation tool.
   - Signs of SAT failure include:
     - Dangerous agitation
     - Sustained tachypnea, increased work of breathing
     - Sustained drop in SpO_2 to < 90%
     - Acute arrhythmia
     - Hypotension

4. Determine whether the sedation drip should be discontinued and replaced with PRN dosing, restarted at half the dose, or returned to the pre-SAT dose.

Overview of Pain

- Pain has adverse physiological and psychological effects, including activation of the physiological stress response, depression, and delirium.
- Etiologies of pain in the acutely and critically ill include the obvious sources and the not-so-obvious sources (Table 6-9).

Table 6-9. Causes of Pain/Discomfort in an Acutely or Critically Ill Patient

Obvious Causes of Pain	Less Obvious Causes of Pain
Incisions	Monitoring and therapeutic devices (catheters, drains,
Invasive procedures	endotracheal tubes, noninvasive ventilating devices)
Trauma, fractures	Routine nursing care (airway suctioning, dressing
Prolonged immobility	changes, physical therapy)

Pain Assessment

- It is recommended that pain be routinely assessed in all adult ICU patients.
- Attempt to obtain the patient's self-report of pain using the Numerical Rating Scale (NRS), pointing, and head nodding.
- The Behavioral Pain Scale (BPS) is recommended for a patient who is receiving mechanical ventilation and is unable to self-report pain. The Critical-Care Pain Observation Tool (CPOT) is recommended for assessing the pain of a patient who is unable to self-report pain, with or without mechanical ventilation.
- Vital signs alone should not be used for pain assessment in critically ill adults, but they can be used as a cue to assess pain further.
- Consider asking a family member or friend who knows the patient well (a proxy reporter) whether the patient's behavior may indicate the presence of pain.

Pain Management

- Intravenous (IV) opioids are the first-line choice to treat non-neuropathic pain in critically ill patients. All available IV opioids, when titrated to similar pain intensity endpoints, are equally effective (Table 6-10). **The dose that is given may vary depending upon unit protocols.**
- **Prevent** pain as you are able to by using:
  - Preemptive analgesia prior to procedures that are likely to cause pain
  - Nonpharmacological interventions (distraction, relaxation therapy)
- If the patient is agitated, treat pain first and then sedate.

Opioid Reversal with Naloxone

- Give 0.4 to 2 mg IV every 2 minutes until effect to a maximum of 10 mg.
- Duration of naloxone action is 1 to 2 hours; repeated doses may be needed for a long-acting opioid.

Table 6-10. Pharmacology of Select Opioid Analgesics

Agent	Start Dose	Titration Time/Dose	Usual Dose Range	Nursing Implications
Fentanyl (Sublimaze)	**Loading Dose:** 25–100 mcg slow IV push over 1–2 min q 10–15 min until pain is controlled (using NRS or BPS) **Continuous Infusion:** 25–50 mcg/hr	If the goal pain score is not achieved, give 25–50 mcg IV push and then increase the rate of infusion by 25 mcg/hr; contact the physician if the rate exceeds 200 mcg/hr or if higher doses are needed	25–200 mcg/hr	• If a patient is receiving this agent regularly for > 1 week, do not suddenly stop; taper gradually by ~ 10–25% daily in order to prevent withdrawal • Weaning is not needed if fentanyl is replaced with an equianalgesic dose by an alternate route • If the patient is not mechanically ventilated, decrease dosing requirements for those with sleep apnea, those with significant cardiovascular/pulmonary disease, those who are elderly, and those who are obese (correlates with sleep apnea) • Consider a sedation vacation, if appropriate
Hydromorphone (Dilaudid)	**Loading Dose:** 0.2–0.5 mg q 5–15 min until pain is controlled (using NRS or BPS) **Continuous Infusion:** 0.2–0.5 mg/hr; Caution: 1 mg of hydromorphone is equivalent to 7–10 mg of morphine	If the goal pain score is not achieved, give 0.2–0.5 mg IV push and then increase the infusion by 0.2–0.3 mg/hr q 30 min; contact the physician if the rate exceeds 3 mg/hr or if higher doses are needed	0.2–3.0 mg/hr	• If a patient is receiving this agent regularly for > 1 week, do not suddenly stop; taper gradually by ~ 10–25% daily in order to prevent withdrawal • Weaning is not needed if hydromorphone is replaced with an equianalgesic dose by an alternate route • If the patient is not mechanically ventilated, decrease dosing requirements for those with sleep apnea, those with significant cardiovascular/pulmonary disease, those who are elderly, and those who are obese (correlates with sleep apnea) • Consider a sedation vacation, if appropriate

(continued)

Table 6-10. Pharmacology of Select Opioid Analgesics (Continued)

Agent	Start Dose	Titration Time/Dose	Usual Dose Range	Nursing Implications
Morphine	**Loading Dose:** 2–4 mg IV push q 5–15 min until pain is controlled (using NRS or BPS) **Continuous Infusion:** 1–2 mg/hr	If the goal pain score is not achieved, give 2–4 mg IV push and then increase the rate by 1–2 mg/hr q 30 min; contact the physician if the rate exceeds 10 mg/hr or if higher doses are needed	1–10 mg/hr	• If a patient is receiving this agent regularly for > 1 week, do not suddenly stop; taper gradually by ~ 10–25% daily in order to prevent withdrawal • Weaning is not needed if morphine is replaced with an equianalgesic dose by an alternate route • If the patient is not mechanically ventilated, decrease dosing requirements for those with sleep apnea, those with significant cardiovascular/pulmonary disease, those who are elderly, and those who are obese (correlates with sleep apnea) • Consider a sedation vacation, if appropriate • If the patient is elderly, active metabolite may accumulate, resulting in renal insufficiency and increased sedation • Monitor the duration of therapy; possibly consider an alternate opioid

TARGETED TEMPERATURE MANAGEMENT (TTM)

Overview

- Targeted Temperature Management (TTM) is a treatment that lowers the patient's core body temperature in order to prevent the neurological effects of an ischemic injury in the brain of survivors of sudden cardiac death.
- Assess patients after cardiac arrest for inclusion criteria and exclusion criteria (Table 6-11).

Table 6-11. Inclusion Criteria and Exclusion Criteria for the Use of Targeted Temperature Management

Inclusion Criteria	Exclusion Criteria
Cardiac arrest with a return of spontaneous circulation	Pregnancy
Unresponsive or not following commands after cardiac arrest	Core temperature of less than 35°C
Witnessed arrest with downtime of less than 60 minutes	Age < 18 or > 85
	Existing DNR status or terminal disease
	Chronic renal failure
	Sustained refractory ventricular arrhythmias
	Active bleeding
	Shock
	Hemodynamic instability
	Drug intoxication

This therapy involves 3 phases:

1. Induction phase: lower the patient's temperature to 32–36°C (as ordered by the provider); start this cooling ASAP.

   ○ The RN should initiate this cooling within 90 minutes of the patient going into arrest; the cooling may last for as long as 6 hours after the arrest.

2. Maintenance phase: keep the patient at the target temperature (32–36°C) for 24 hours.

3. Rewarming phase: slowly increase the patient's temperature to 36.5–37°C (as ordered by the provider).

Induction Phase

- Set the goal time to the target temperature.
- Monitor the core temperature (bladder, rectal).
- Apply the device (external pads or internal central venous catheter).
- The goal systolic B/P is generally > 90 mmHg, and the goal MAP is generally > 70 mmHg.
- Obtain baseline labs and generally complete a metabolic panel, a complete blood count, a coagulation panel, a check of the patient's serum magnesium and phosphorus levels, and an arterial blood gas.
- Get a baseline bedside blood glucose measurement.
- Obtain a 12-lead ECG.
- Initiate deep sedation.
- Manage shivering by covering the head, hands, and feet or by using meperidine (Demerol); use a neuromuscular agent if shivering is not controlled with meperidine (Demerol).
- Monitor/manage the systemic effects of hypothermia.

SYSTEMIC EFFECTS OF HYPOTHERMIA

- Insulin resistance → hyperglycemia
- Electrolyte and fluid shifts
- Shivering
- Skin breakdown
- Pupil and corneal reflexes may be absent due to hypothermia
- Decreased cardiac output
  - Up to 25%
- Alteration in coagulation
  - Platelet dysfunction
- Increased risk for infection
  - Neutrophil and macrophage functions decrease at temperatures less than 35°C.

Maintenance Phase (Duration 24 Hours)

- Continuously monitor the core temperature (bladder, rectal); the core temperature should not be lower than the specified goal (32–36°C).
- Monitor vital signs (at least hourly).
- Obtain routine bedside blood glucose measurements and initiate an insulin drip as needed.
- Monitor train-of-four (TOF) every hour if a paralytic is used and ensure a goal of 1–2 twitches to prevent prolonged paralysis.
- Repeat labs (same as baseline labs) every 8 hours until the patient is rewarmed.

Rewarming Phase

- Perform passive rewarming to 36.5–37°C.
- Program the cooling unit to increase the target temperature by 1 degree per hour.
- Stop all potassium administration 8 hours prior to rewarming.
  - Rewarming causes rebound hyperkalemia.
- Discontinue paralytics (if they were being used) after the patient is warmed to 36.5°C.
- Repeat labs (same as baseline) when the patient is rewarmed.
- Perform a close neurological assessment; pupil and corneal reflexes may continue to be absent for a time.

TOXIN/DRUG EXPOSURE

The Adult CCRN exam may include 1 question related to toxin/drug exposure.

General Points

- Toxin/drug exposure may be accidental or intentional.
  - ☆ Initial management—always assess ABCs (airway, breathing, circulation).
- If the patient is comatose, be prepared to give 50% dextrose 50 mL, thiamine 50–100 mg, naloxone 2 mg IV.

- To prevent absorption of the toxin/drug, give activated charcoal 1 gm/kg via gastric lavage.
  - Contraindicated with hydrocarbon or corrosive ingestions
  - Not necessary for the ingestion of iron, lithium, or alcohols
- Facilitate the removal of the drug—urine alkalization, hemodialysis.
- Administer an antidote, if indicated (e.g., naloxone).
- Monitor for arrhythmias.
- Monitor the urine output.
- If there is a **chemical exposure**, give an antidote (if possible), remove the chemical (if it is a powder, brush it away; if it is a liquid, flush it with saline or water), do not rub the affected area, and cover the affected area with a sterile damp dressing.

Management of Toxin/Drug Exposure

- See Table 6-12 for the management of specific toxin/drug exposure.

Table 6-12. Signs, Symptoms, and Treatment of Specific Toxic Agents

Drug	Signs/Symptoms	Treatment
Acetaminophen (Tylenol)	Nausea, vomiting, perhaps none early on	N-acetylcysteine dosing is effective for 8 hours after ingestion • 140 mg/kg loading dose, then • 70 mg/kg every 4 hrs for 17 doses • Give ALL drug doses, regardless of drug level
	Later RUQ pain, abnormal liver function test results, mental status changes	GI lavage with activated charcoal within 4 hours after ingestion
Benzodiazepines	Drowsiness, confusion, slurred speech, respiratory depression, hypotension, aspiration	Support the airway
		Flumazenil (Romazicon) 0.2 mg slow IV push; then 0.3 mg IV; then 0.5 mg IV at 1-minute intervals, total 3 mg
		Short half-life; watch for reoccurrence of symptoms
		Gastric lavage with activated charcoal
		Fluid resuscitation
Beta blockers	Bradycardia	Glucagon, epinephrine, insulin plus dextrose, sodium bicarbonate
	Hypotension	
	CV collapse	
Calcium channel blockers	Bradycardia	Calcium gluconate, epinephrine, insulin plus dextrose, sodium bicarbonate
	Hypotension	
	CV collapse	

(continued)

Table 6-12. Signs, Symptoms, and Treatment of Specific Toxic Agents (*Continued*)

Drug	Signs/Symptoms	Treatment
Cocaine	Seizure activity, agitation, hyperthermia, rhabdomyolysis	Activated charcoal
		Fluids, glucose, thiamine IV
		Benzodiazepines for sedation, seizures
		Vasopressin is preferred over epinephrine in full arrest
		Vasodilators for hypertension
		Nitrates, calcium channel blockers for ischemia; NO beta blockers
		Cooling for hyperthermia
Ethylene glycol	Intoxication behavior	Gastric lavage
	Vomiting	Sodium bicarbonate
	Metabolic acidosis, anion gap	Antidotes: ethanol or fomepizole
	Renal failure	Dialysis
ETOH	Stupor, respiratory depression, aspiration risk	Support, protect the airway
		Fluid resuscitation
		Multivitamin and thiamine 100 mg IV
		Electrolyte replacement PRN (Mg^{++}, Ph^{++}, K^+)
	Intermittent agitation	Prevention of delirium tremens: benzodiazepines, CIWA protocol
Methamphetamine	Fever, tachycardia, hypertension, seizure, agitation, renal failure	Fluids, cooling
		Benzodiazepines, haloperidol
		Physical restraints: protect self and others
Opioids	Drowsiness, hypoventilation, hypotension, hypothermia, deep sedation, pinpoint pupils	Support the airway
		Naloxone (Narcan) 0.4–2 mg IV every 2 minutes until effect to a maximum of 10 mg
		Gastric lavage with activated charcoal
Phencyclidine (PCP)	Blank stare, rapid involuntary eye movement, hallucinations, severe mood disorder, flushing, sweating, hypertension, tachycardia, seizure, coma	Support the airway
		Provide a calm environment; do not leave the patient alone due to a high possibility of harm to self and others
		Benzodiazepines for agitation
		Fluids, cooling, monitor renal function
Salicylates	Vomiting, tinnitus, confusion, hyperthermia, respiratory alkalosis, metabolic acidosis, multiple organ failure	Activated charcoal
		Urine alkalization
		Dialysis, regardless of admission renal function, to PREVENT acute kidney injury
Tricyclic antidepressants	CV signs: arrhythmias, shock	Sodium bicarbonate, activated charcoal, fluids, cardiac monitoring
	Neurological signs: drowsiness, delirium, seizures, coma	
	Anticholinergic signs: blurred vision, fever, twitching	

Healthcare-associated infections (HAIs), also known as healthcare-associated conditions, were recently added to the Adult CCRN test blueprint. Be prepared to understand the role of the nurse in the prevention of these infections, which are considered indicators of the quality of care that is provided to patients. In general, an infection that develops more than 48 hours after admission to the hospital is considered healthcare-associated; if the infection is identified within 48 hours after admission to the hospital, it is considered community-acquired. Hospitals are now required to report cases of HAIs to government agencies, and some cases are publicly reported.

Guidelines for the prevention of ventilator-associated pneumonia (VAP), central line-associated bloodstream infections (CLABSIs), and catheter-associated urinary tract infections (CAUTIs) have been provided by several national organizations, including the Centers for Disease Control and Prevention (CDC), the Society for Healthcare Epidemiology of America (SHEA), the Infectious Diseases Society of America (IDSA), and the Association for Professionals in Infection Control and Epidemiology (APIC). "Care bundles" are sets of evidence-based practices that lead to improved outcomes **if** all elements are completed.

Ventilator-Associated Event (VAE)

- VAE is a term that was created by the CDC to better describe an occurrence of ventilator-associated pneumonia (VAP). VAP is a type of VAE. For the Adult CCRN exam, you will be expected to understand VAP and strategies to prevent VAP; you will not be expected to understand the complex VAE algorithm.
- Refer to page 90 of the Respiratory Concepts chapter of this book for a review of the ways to prevent VAP.

Central Line-Associated Bloodstream Infection (CLABSI)

A central line-associated bloodstream infection (CLABSI) is a laboratory-confirmed bloodstream infection that develops within 48 hours of a central line placement and is not related to an infection at any other sites. A CLABSI results in longer hospital stays, increased costs, and an increased risk of death. CLABSI mortality rates of 12% to 25% have been reported.

The guidelines for the prevention of CLABSIs are as follows:

- Develop standardized, evidence-based policies/procedures with indications for central line use, insertion, and maintenance.
- Insertion
  - Ensure that processes are in place for insertion according to the guidelines (e.g., central line cart, checklists).
  - Optimize site selection (subclavian vein) as able; avoid femoral or internal jugular site if at all possible.
  - Ensure that the team utilizes aseptic technique during insertion.
  - Utilize maximal barrier precautions and personal protective equipment during insertion.
  - Prepare the skin using chlorhexidine skin antisepsis.
  - Use chlorhexidine patch/gel dressing over the insertion site (unless there is an allergy).

- Maintenance
  - Practice hand hygiene prior to line manipulation/care.
  - Provide a head-to-toe chlorhexidine bath daily for ICU patients.
  - Disinfect catheter hubs, needleless connectors, and injection ports with mechanical friction for no less than 5 seconds with an antiseptic before accessing the catheter.
  - Ensure the patency of the dressing, and change the dressing and tubing according to hospital policy.
  - Do not routinely replace central lines (e.g., every 72 hours) unless it is known that the insertion was performed emergently without antisepsis.
  - Discontinue a central line if there are signs of an infection.
  - Perform a daily review of line necessity.
  - Use aseptic technique for dressing changes, ensuring dressing patency at all times.
  - Ensure that there is an appropriate nurse-to-patient ratio and limit the use of float nurses in ICUs.
- Monitoring
  - Perform root cause analyses on line infections and develop action plans for improvement accordingly.
  - Develop processes for measuring compliance with policies/procedures.
  - Share quality monitoring and infection results with the staff.
  - Assess competency of the staff who insert/care for lines.
- Require that all health care personnel, who are involved in the insertion, care, and maintenance of central venous catheters (CVCs), be educated about CLABSI prevention.

Catheter-Associated Urinary Tract Infection (CAUTI)

The Centers for Disease Control and Prevention (CDC) defines a catheter-associated urinary tract infection (CAUTI) as an infection of the urinary tract, where an indwelling urinary catheter was in place for more than 2 consecutive days in an inpatient location on the date of event, with day of device placement being Day 1 AND an indwelling urinary catheter in place on the date of event or the day before.

The guidelines for the prevention of CAUTIs are as follows:

- Develop standardized, evidence-based policies/procedures with criteria for catheter use.
- Utilization practices
  - Avoid inserting an indwelling urinary catheter, if at all possible.
  - Develop standardized, evidence-based reasons for insertion such as select operative procedures, acute urinary retention or bladder outlet obstruction, gross hematuria, a need for an accurate measurement of urine output, to assist in the healing of open sacral or perineal wounds in incontinent patients, or for patients who require prolonged immobilization (e.g., potentially unstable thoracic or lumbar spine, multiple traumatic injuries such as pelvic fractures).
  - Perform a daily review of catheter need based on agreed upon hospital standardized criteria.
  - Remove catheters as soon as they are no longer necessary; as per the CDC, when a catheter is placed during surgery and remains in place post-op, remove the catheter as soon as possible, preferably within 24 hours, unless there are appropriate indications for continued use.

- Implement a nurse-driven protocol to empower nurses to evaluate and discontinue unnecessary urinary catheters.
- Utilize alternative strategies (external catheters, intermittent straight catheterization as able).

■ Insertion and maintenance practices

- Use aseptic technique during insertion
- Make insertion a 2-person activity to reduce breaks in aseptic technique during insertion.
- Practice hand hygiene prior to/following catheter manipulation/care.
- Utilize standard precautions, including the use of gloves and gowns, as appropriate.
- Employ routine catheter care, cleansing the meatal area (antiseptic solution is not needed); replace basin bathing with plain wipes.
- Maintain an unobstructed urine flow (e.g., ensure proper securement of the catheter, maintain tubing free of kinks or dependent loops, maintain the collection bag below the level of the bladder).
- Do not disconnect/reconnect system components.
- Collect urine samples from the sampling port using aseptic technique.

■ Process measures

- Assess the competency of the clinicians who insert catheters; provide periodic training and competency assessments.
- Identify unit "CAUTI champions," whose role is to monitor patients with indwelling urinary catheters and ensure that standards for infection prevention are utilized by caregivers.
- Develop quality measures and share outcomes with the staff.
- Perform a root cause analysis for each infection and implement action plans based on those analyses.

Multi-Drug Resistant Organisms (MDROs)

■ Patients who are vulnerable to colonization and an infection with MDROs include the critically ill, especially those with compromised host defenses from underlying medical conditions, recent surgery, or the presence of indwelling medical devices (e.g., urinary catheters, central lines).

■ The following are the most common organisms that are found in hospitals, long-term care facilities, and at times, in the community:

- Methicillin-resistant *Staphylococcus aureus* (MRSA)
- Vancomycin-resistant enterococci (VRE)
- *Clostridium difficile* (*C. diff*)
- Carbapenem-resistant enterobacteriaceae (CRE)

■ The following strategies are used to prevent infections caused by multi-drug resistant organisms (MDROs):

- Establish a culture where hand hygiene is expected of all caregivers.
- Develop an antibiotic stewardship and an antibiotic de-escalation program.
- Provide universal decolonization of ICU patients through chlorhexidine bathing and nasal decolonization.

- Focus on the rapid identification of MDROs and the development of a strong containment program.
- Utilize team rounding/huddles to ensure that VAP/CLABSI/CAUTI evidence-based interventions (bundles) are followed and that antibiotic stewardship is practiced.
- Conduct a root cause analysis of infections that occur.
- Develop a process to assess that clinicians utilize contact precautions according to hospital policy.
- Develop processes for reliable cleaning of equipment and surfaces.
- Provide education regarding hand hygiene and when **soap and water** (rather than hand gel) is required: following contact with patients with *C. difficile*: when the clinician's hands are visibly soiled, after the clinician has used the restroom, and before the clinician eats.

PALLIATIVE CARE, HOSPICE CARE, AND END-OF-LIFE CARE

Palliative Care

- Palliative care is the prevention and treatment of the symptoms and side effects of a serious illness. Physiological, emotional, social, and spiritual problems are considered.
  - Palliative care can be initiated anytime during a disease or life-threatening illness.
  - This type of care has been found to be most beneficial when it is initiated early.
  - Symptom management may include the management of pain, anxiety, dyspnea, urticaria, nausea/vomiting, constipation, and diarrhea, among other symptoms.
- Aggressive treatment may be continued.
- All critically ill patients deserve palliative care.
- Palliative care has been shown to improve survival, decrease resource utilization, and decrease hospital readmissions and the cost of care.

Hospice Care

- Hospice care is the provision of symptom management for those with a **terminal** illness. It includes palliative care, but disease-modifying treatments are discontinued unless they may provide symptom management.
- Grief and bereavement services are included.

End-of-Life Care

- End-of-Life (EOL) care supports the needs of patients and their families at the time of imminent death. It is always a part of hospice care, and it may or may not be a part of palliative care. It is provided to all patients who are at the end of their lives, regardless of whether or not palliative care or hospice care were initiated.
  - EOL care avoids prolongation of the dying process.
  - EOL care provides support to the patient's family.

Similarities Between Palliative Care, Hospice Care, and End-of-Life Care

All three of these types of care involve:

- Advance care planning
- Focusing on patient/family wishes
- Optimizing quality of life

> Now that you have reviewed the key multisystem concepts, go to the Multisystem Practice Questions. Answer the questions, and then check your answers. Continue to review the information until you answer 80% of the practice questions correctly.

MULTISYSTEM PRACTICE QUESTIONS

1. Which medications are most often prescribed for anaphylaxis after initial therapy with IM epinephrine?

   (A) antihistamines and corticosteroids
   (B) vasopressors and inotropes
   (C) antihistamines and antibiotics
   (D) corticosteroids and vasopressors

2. Which of the following would most likely result in an SvO_2 of 82%?

   (A) hypovolemic shock
   (B) anaphylactic shock
   (C) septic shock
   (D) cardiogenic shock

3. The initial management of any drug intoxication is to:

   (A) prevent further absorption of the drug.
   (B) increase excretion of the drug.
   (C) administer an antidote when appropriate.
   (D) ensure a patent airway and adequate breathing.

4. A patient is being treated for sepsis with fluid resuscitation, but the MAP is 55 mmHg and norepinephrine is ordered. What primary beneficial effect will norepinephrine provide for this patient?

   (A) It will maintain renal blood flow.
   (B) It will increase coronary artery blood flow.
   (C) It will increase venous return and preload.
   (D) It will restore vascular tone and afterload.

5. Which of the following would be an indicator that fluid resuscitation is adequate?

   (A) The CVP is 2 mmHg.
   (B) The heart rate is decreasing.
   (C) The pulse pressure is narrowing.
   (D) The serum lactate is 4.1 mmol/L.

6. Which of the following is TRUE in regard to shock?

   (A) The MAP is adequate in the compensatory phase of shock.
   (B) The blood pressure is maintained in Class III hemorrhagic shock.
   (C) An elevated lactate level occurs late in septic shock.
   (D) Serum bicarbonate is elevated in shock.

7. A patient with upper GI bleeding received procedural sedation with midazolam during his endoscopy procedure. He required higher doses to maintain sedation and screened positive for obstructive sleep apnea (OSA). Which of the following is TRUE regarding this patient's plan of care?

   (A) Respiratory depression will generally precede sedation.
   (B) Pulse oximetry will detect early hypoventilation.
   (C) Waveform capnography monitoring is indicated for this patient post-procedure.
   (D) The maximum dose of flumazenil (Romazicon) for midazolam reversal is 0.2 mg IV.

8. A patient is receiving a continuous sedation infusion of propofol (Diprivan) at 30 mcg/kg/min. Which of the following is an appropriate intervention for this patient?

   (A) Reverse the side effects with flumazenil (Romazicon).
   (B) Provide a daily spontaneous awakening trial.
   (C) Avoid administering analgesia.
   (D) Monitor the patient closely for hypertension.

9. Which of the following statements is TRUE in relation to the treatment of sepsis?

   (A) Special protocols, "bundles" of interventions, are indicated for the presence of an infection with evidence of organ dysfunction.
   (B) Administering pressors is required for treating sepsis.
   (C) By definition, a patient with systemic inflammatory response syndrome (SIRS) has an infection.
   (D) Positive cultures are required in order to make the diagnosis of septic shock.

10. Which of the following statements regarding targeted temperature management (TTM) is CORRECT?

   (A) TTM should be provided for all patients status post ventricular fibrillation.
   (B) Potassium infusions will most likely be required during rewarming.
   (C) Shivering is expected and is generally self-limiting.
   (D) Insulin infusions are often required during the maintenance phase.

11. A patient who has sustained traumatic injuries, including a pelvic fracture and soft tissue injuries, has required a transfusion of 7 units of packed red blood cells (PRBCs). Which of the following is TRUE related to the care of this patient?

(A) Pressors will most likely be required.
(B) The patient will need to be monitored for hypercalcemia.
(C) Blood products and crystalloids should be warmed.
(D) Platelets will need to be given if the platelet count drops.

12. A patient is receiving mechanical ventilation and is able to write notes to communicate. Which of the following is the most appropriate intervention related to the management of pain for this patient?

(A) Coach the patient in the use of self-reporting with the numerical rating scale (NRS).
(B) Initiate pain medication during procedures when the patient first demonstrates pain behaviors.
(C) Disregard the use of nonpharmacological interventions for pain since the patient is receiving mechanical ventilation.
(D) Ensure that the mean arterial pressure (MAP) is greater than 60 mmHg before providing intravenous opiates.

13. A 38-year-old female patient was admitted with multiple traumatic injuries, including flail chest, a ruptured spleen, and a crush injury to her left leg. She is receiving mechanical ventilation. The nurse considers requesting a palliative care consult, knowing that the benefits of palliative care include all of the following EXCEPT:

(A) improved survival.
(B) symptom management.
(C) improved quality of care.
(D) increased cost of care.

14. It is usually important to decrease the number of days that a patient has an indwelling urinary catheter in place. Which of the following statements presents a valid reason for maintaining this type of catheter?

(A) The patient is receiving mechanical ventilation.
(B) The catheter was inserted yesterday during renal surgery.
(C) It is painful for the patient to use the bedpan.
(D) The patient is receiving medications that may cause urine retention.

15. A patient requires the insertion of a chest tube, and the physician plans for moderate sedation with fentanyl. During the procedure, the RN notices that the patient only responds to repeated vigorous shaking. Which of the following choices provides an accurate assessment of this situation and describes the proper intervention that is indicated?

(A) A patient assessment reveals a level of general anesthesia; the proper intervention is to call the anesthesiologist for intubation.

(B) A patient assessment reveals a level of moderate sedation; the proper intervention is to ask for a flumazenil (Romazicon) order.

(C) A patient assessment reveals a level of deep sedation; the proper intervention is to assess the patient's oxygenation/ventilation.

(D) The proper interventions are to alert the physician to the level of sedation and to begin assisting the patient's ventilation with a bag/mask.

16. Which of the following is true for a patient who has SIRS (meaning that the patient has 2 or more of the 4 criteria) or has a positive qSOFA score (meaning that the patient has 2 or 3 of the criteria)?

(A) An assessment of the qSOFA score requires laboratory testing.

(B) Both SIRS and the qSOFA score are markers of an infection.

(C) SIRS is a component of the Sepsis-3 definitions, and the qSOFA score is a component of the Sepsis-2 definitions.

(D) SIRS is a marker of inflammation, and the qSOFA score is a marker of organ dysfunction.

17. Within the past 2 weeks, 3 patients developed VRE in 1 critical care unit. Which of the following strategies has been demonstrated to be effective in the prevention of additional cases of VRE?

(A) Perform a root cause analysis of the 3 known cases of VRE.

(B) Screen all newly admitted patients for VRE.

(C) Administer vancomycin prophylactically to all patients within the unit.

(D) Tape posters about hand washing on the doors of all patient rooms.

18. A patient is being treated for a confirmed salicylate overdose. Which of the following interventions should the nurse anticipate?

(A) Closely monitor for respiratory depression.

(B) Prepare for hemodialysis.

(C) Administer thiamine 100 mg IV.

(D) Administer all doses of N-acetylcysteine, regardless of subsequent salicylate levels.

19. If a patient's death appears imminent, which of the following should be the focus of care for the health care team?

(A) a palliative care consult

(B) hospice placement

(C) completion of an advance directive

(D) supporting the patient/the patient's family

20. A patient is being treated for septic shock. Four hours after the identification of sepsis, the serum lactate is 5.2 mmol/L. Based on this information, which of the following steps is indicated?

(A) Perform a passive leg raise.
(B) Initiate vasopressin.
(C) Reevaluate the choice of antibiotic.
(D) Increase FiO_2.

21. Which of the following strategies is used to reduce central line-associated bloodstream infections (CLABSIs)?

(A) Avoid the subclavian insertion site.
(B) Ensure that the patient's chest is covered with sterile towels during insertion of the central line.
(C) If possible, avoid frequent blood draws from the central line.
(D) Always wash your hands with soap and water before entering the room.

ANSWER KEY

1.	**A**	5.	**B**	9.	**A**	13.	**D**	17.	**A**
2.	**C**	6.	**A**	10.	**D**	14.	**B**	18.	**B**
3.	**D**	7.	**C**	11.	**C**	15.	**C**	19.	**D**
4.	**D**	8.	**B**	12.	**A**	16.	**D**		

20. **A**
21. **C**

ANSWERS AND EXPLANATIONS

1. **(A)** An antihistamine will help halt the allergic response, and a corticosteroid will help halt the inflammatory response. Vasopressors, inotropes, and antibiotics are not helpful for anaphylactic shock.

2. **(C)** The normal SvO_2 is 60% to 75%. In septic shock, oxygen delivery (DO_2) is adequate, but oxygen utilization (VO_2) at the cellular level is low. A sign of poor oxygen utilization when oxygen delivery is adequate is an elevated SvO_2. Oxygen is not being used, despite its availability, and blood is returning to the pulmonary artery with more oxygen than expected. The other 3 types of shock result in poor oxygen delivery, which causes low oxygen utilization with a low SvO_2. In summary, poor oxygen utilization may result in a low SvO_2 when delivery of oxygen is low and an elevated SvO_2 when the oxygen delivery is adequate or high.

3. **(D)** If the intoxication affects the patient's airway and breathing, the other 3 interventions listed will be of no use since the patient will not survive.

4. **(D)** The problem in sepsis/septic shock is massive dilation (low SVR) and capillary leak (resulting in relative hypovolemia). If needed, pressors (such as norepinephrine) cause vasoconstriction and increase SVR (afterload). Although pressors may also increase preload and renal blood flow, these are secondary effects. The primary effect of pressors is the restoration of afterload. Although septic shock may result in ventricu-

lar damage with resultant elevated troponin, myocardial damage is not due to a drop in coronary artery blood flow; rather, the damage is due to the effects that endotoxins have on cardiac muscles.

5. **(B)** As vascular volume is restored and preload is increased, there is less need for compensatory mechanisms (an increase in heart rate). A CVP of 2 mmHg, narrowing of the pulse pressure, and an elevated lactate (anaerobic metabolism) are all signs that filling pressures have not been optimized.

6. **(A)** Since compensatory mechanisms are working, the MAP is maintained in the compensatory phase. If these mechanisms fail, the MAP drops and hypotension results (progressive phase). In Class III hemorrhagic shock, the blood pressure decreases and is no longer maintained. In septic shock, lactate rises early on during sepsis, not later on. Serum bicarbonate is decreased (not elevated) in shock due to lactic acidosis.

7. **(C)** Waveform capnography is indicated during and after procedural sedation in order to identify EARLY hypoventilation. Longer monitoring may be required for a patient with a history of obstructive sleep apnea (OSA). Sedation usually precedes respiratory depression. SpO_2 will not decrease until the $PaCO_2$ is very high. Flumazenil reverses benzodiazepines. However, resedation may occur, and subsequent doses of flumazenil may be necessary.

8. **(B)** Studies have shown improved patient outcomes, shorter ventilator times, and less risk of oversedation when "awakening trials" are done for a patient who is on a continuous sedation infusion. Propofol is not reversed with flumazenil. Analgesia should be used for agitation, not avoided. Propofol is more likely to cause hypotension, not hypertension.

9. **(A)** "Sepsis bundles" are indicated for the presence of an infection with signs of organ dysfunction, since these cases result in increased mortality. Sepsis, by definition, does not require pressor administration. SIRS may be present without an infection (e.g., trauma, pancreatitis). In addition, only 30–50% of patients with sepsis/septic shock present with positive cultures.

10. **(D)** Targeted temperature management (TTM) may result in hyperglycemia, which will necessitate insulin infusions to maintain normoglycemia during the maintenance phase of TTM. Targeted temperature management is only indicated for an unresponsive patient s/p cardiac arrest, not for ALL patients. Potassium is required during the maintenance phase of TTM to correct hypokalemia. However, during rewarming, potassium replacement needs to be stopped. Shivering will prevent temperature reduction, is not self-limiting, and will need to be treated with either meperidine or neuromuscular blocking agents.

11. **(C)** It is important to prevent hypothermia and its resultant adverse consequences during fluid/transfusion resuscitation. Therefore, fluids and blood products need to be warmed. Pressors are not indicated in hypovolemic shock since the afterload in hypovolemic shock is already abnormally high due to compensation for volume loss. The problem needs to be addressed by "filling up the tank" to restore circulation volume. HYPOCALCEMIA (not hypercalcemia) secondary to calcium binding to citrate in stored blood is a potential problem related to the transfusion of PRBCs. Platelets are

not in PRBCs and should be replaced regardless of platelet count when a large volume of PRBCs is administered. Replacing platelets will prevent thrombocytopenia and coagulation problems.

12. **(A)** Self-reporting pain is always preferred. In the scenario described, the patient is capable of providing a pain intensity number. Preemptive analgesia is preferred for procedures that are likely to be painful rather than waiting until pain is experienced. Nonpharmacological interventions are always appropriate. Hypotensive patients still require pain management. Pain should not be used to "keep up the B/P." An opiate (such as fentanyl) may be used because it is less likely to cause a further drop in blood pressure, and the hypotension can be treated as needed.

13. **(D)** Palliative care consults have been shown to decrease, not increase, the cost of care, especially when they occur early during a hospital stay. Choices (A), (B), and (C) ARE benefits of palliative care consults.

14. **(B)** A patient who is only 1 day post-op renal surgery needs an indwelling catheter until the surgeon has determined that the patient's condition would not be adversely impacted by removing the catheter. Mechanical ventilation (choice (A)) itself is not a criterion for an indwelling urinary catheter; the need for an indwelling urinary catheter should be based on further assessments for one of the CDC criteria for catheter use. Pain with mobility (as described in choice (C)) could be controlled, and the risks associated with a Foley catheter outweigh patient discomfort, which can be managed. If the patient is receiving medications that may lead to acute urine retention (choice (D)), the patient should be monitored for urine retention. Even if that does occur, the patient may be a candidate for intermittent straight catheterization, or the medications may be able to be changed to alternative agents.

15. **(C)** The need for vigorous shaking in order to elicit a response is evidence of deep sedation, and the first priority is for the nurse to ensure that the patient has adequate ventilation and oxygenation. This patient is not evidencing general anesthesia (choice (A)), and intubation is most likely not going to be needed since a reversal agent could be given and the patient's ventilation could be temporarily assisted. The patient assessment would not reveal moderate sedation (choice (B)), and flumazenil is not the reversal agent for fentanyl. Naloxone (Narcan) is the reversal agent for the opioid fentanyl. This scenario does not describe the signs of inadequate ventilation that require immediate assistance (choice (D)), although the physician does need to be alerted to the level of sedation.

16. **(D)** SIRS is a marker of inflammation and is not necessarily associated with organ dysfunction or an infection. The qSOFA score is a marker of organ dysfunction. The remaining choices are not true.

17. **(A)** It is important to understand the reason for MDRO infections in order to look for patterns and to correct gaps in infection control so as to prevent future infections. A root cause analysis, led by quality improvement staff, often provides the answers in terms of the cause of these infections. The remaining 3 strategies have not been demonstrated to prevent the development of MDROs. Screening for VRE (choice (B)) has not been demonstrated to be successful, nor is it cost-effective. Providing vancomycin

(choice (C)) is not good antibiotic stewardship. Displaying posters has not been shown to be an enduring strategy; there may be an initial impact, but over time, the posters are not often noticed by clinicians.

18. **(B)** Salicylate toxicity will require dialysis in order to prevent acute renal failure, even if the renal lab values are normal upon admission. The remaining 3 choices are not anticipated interventions for a salicylate overdose.

19. **(D)** When the health care team expects that a patient's death is imminent, the focus of care shifts to end-of-life care. Family support, avoiding the prolongation of death, and bereavement services become the focus. A palliative care consult (choice (A)) is done as early as possible in the event of an acute, severe illness. Hospice placement (choice (B)) is indicated as soon as the disease is determined to be terminal, not when death is imminent. Completing an advance directive (choice (C)) should ideally be done by all patients (with their primary care provider) prior to developing an acute illness.

20. **(A)** A component of the 3-hour bundle for sepsis is to remeasure the lactate 2–4 hours after the initial lactate if the initial lactate is > 2 mmol/L. If the second lactate is ≥ 4 mmol/L (or if the MAP remains ≤ 65 mmHg), the patient's fluid status should be reassessed. A passive leg raise is a strategy that is used to evaluate whether or not the patient will respond to additional fluids. Vasopressin administration (choice (B)) is indicated when the MAP is not responsive, despite the infusion of higher doses of a vasopressor. Reevaluating the choice of antibiotic (choice (C)) is not generally indicated until cultures are available or until further testing indicates an infectious source that is different than what was initially suspected. An increase in FiO_2 (choice (D)) is indicated as soon as hypoxemia is identified, but it is not determined by serum lactate.

21. **(C)** Manipulating the central line may increase the risk of contamination. Even if the central line is completely flushed, blood draws may result in increased colonization. The subclavian insertion site (choice (A)) is the preferred location for the insertion of a central line, whereas the femoral site is the least preferred site of insertion. During the insertion of a central line, full body draping with sterile towels, not just covering the patient's chest with sterile towels (choice (B)), is preferred. Hand hygiene should be practiced with either gel **or** soap and water. The use of soap and water is required after working with a patient with *C. difficile* or a known infectious diarrhea (norovirus), after using the restroom, when hands are visibly dirty, and before eating. Other than these instances, gel may be used for hand hygiene, and soap and water do not need to be used.

Hemodynamics Concepts

7

One of the most important keys to Success is having the discipline to do what you know you should do, even when you don't feel like doing it.

—Unknown

Hemodynamics is included in the Cardiovascular section of the Adult CCRN test blueprint. However, this topic has been placed after the Cardiovascular Concepts, Respiratory Concepts, and Multisystem Concepts chapters in this book because each of these content areas includes hemodynamic concepts.

Although most critically ill patients do not receive invasive hemodynamic monitoring, ALL patients have hemodynamics that reflect their specific problems. These, to a degree, determine the plan of care. Hemodynamics and invasive hemodynamic monitoring are included in numerous Adult CCRN exam questions.

☆ The equation in Figure 7-1 is the foundation of hemodynamics. The cardiac output (CO) is equal to the heart rate (HR) times the stroke volume (SV). The SV is dependent upon the preload, afterload, and contractility of the ventricles of the heart.

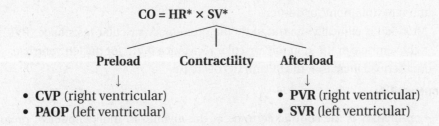

$$CO = HR^* \times SV^*$$

Preload	Contractility	Afterload
↓		↓

- **CVP** (right ventricular)
- **PAOP** (left ventricular)

- **PVR** (right ventricular)
- **SVR** (left ventricular)

*Heart rate (HR); stroke volume (SV); central venous pressure (CVP); pulmonary artery occlusive pressure (PAOP); pulmonary vascular resistance (PVR); systemic vascular resistance (SVR)

Figure 7-1. Regulation of hemodynamics

CRITICAL POINTS

- The normal cardiac output (CO) is 4 L to 8 L per minute. If it becomes critically low, the blood pressure will decrease.

  ○ Cardiac index (CI) takes into account the body surface area (BSA) and is **a more meaningful value than CO**.

  ○ The normal CI is 2.5 to 4.0 L/min/m^2.

- As **heart rate** (HR) increases, CO increases up to a point. The point is determined by the patient's age or the condition of his or her ventricles. Generally, 130–170 beats per minute is the maximal heart rate originating from the sinoatrial (SA) node that is attainable for most people.
  - Extreme bradycardia results in low CO and hypotension.
  - An increase in HR is the first sign of compensation for a low CO. This will occur before the B/P drops. Patients on beta blocker drugs, or any drug that decreases heart rate, may not be able to compensate as well for a problem that is decreasing cardiac output.
  - Conversely, extreme tachycardia will also decrease the CO no matter the patient's age or the condition of his or her ventricles. Why? A loss of diastolic filling time occurs. If diastolic filling time is decreased, the ventricles do not have time to fill, ventricular preload drops, and ultimately the ventricle cannot put out what is not delivered.
- As **stroke volume** increases, CO increases. The stroke volume (SV) is how many mL per beat the left ventricle ejects. It is determined by the preload, afterload, and contractility. The normal SV is 50–100 mL per beat.
- **Preload**
  - Preload is the volume/pressure in the ventricle at the end of diastole after the AV valves close, just prior to ejection. The right atrial (RA) pressure or central venous pressure (CVP) reflects the right ventricular preload. The PAOP reflects the left ventricular preload.
  - As preload increases, the SV and CO increase up to a point.
  - Too high of a preload may lead to heart failure.
  - In general, preload will seldom be elevated if the heart is disease-free and if there are no metabolic abnormalities.

- **Afterload**
  - Afterload is the pressure (resistance) against which the ventricle must pump to open the valve (pulmonic or aortic).
  - Afterload is clinically measured by the pulmonary vascular resistance (PVR) for the right ventricle or the systemic vascular resistance (SVR) for the left ventricle.
  - As afterload increases, the SV and CO decrease.

- **Contractility**
  - Contractility is the contractile force of the myofibrils, independent of preload and afterload.
  - As contractility increases, the SV and CO increase.

☆ For the Adult CCRN exam, you need to know normal hemodynamic values and how various drugs and therapies affect preload, afterload, and contractility. Therefore, you need to know how these drugs and therapies affect stroke volume and, ultimately, cardiac output.

Table 7-1 summarizes normal hemodynamics, and Table 7-2 outlines how various clinical problems affect hemodynamics. Table 7-3 lists the hemodynamic effects of various cardiovascular agents. You **must** have an understanding of this information, as it is the foundation for patient management.

☆ **Table 7-1. Normal Hemodynamic and Oxygenation Parameters**

Parameter	Normal	Formula
Heart rate (HR)	60–100 beats/minute	Direct measurement
Blood pressure (B/P)	90/60–140/90 mmHg	Direct measurement
Mean arterial pressure (MAP)	70–110 mmHg	SBP + 2(DBP) ÷ 3
Cardiac output (CO)	4–8 L/min	Direct measurement
Cardiac index (CI)	2.5–4.0 L/min/m^2	CO ÷ BSA
Stroke volume (SV)	50–100 mL/beat	Direct measurement
Stroke index (SI)	25–45 mL/beat/m^2	SV + BSA
Right atrial pressure (RAP) [also known as central venous pressure (CVP)]	2–6 mmHg 3–8 cm H_2O	Direct measurement
Pulmonary artery pressure (PAP)	20/8–30/15 mmHg Mean: < 20 mmHg	Direct measurement
Pulmonary artery occlusion (wedge) pressure (PAOP)	8–12 mmHg (although it varies depending upon the LV function)	Direct measurement
Systemic vascular resistance (SVR)	800–1200 dynes/s/cm^{-5}	(MAP − CVP) ÷ CO × 80
Pulmonary vascular resistance (PVR)	50–250 dynes/s/cm^{-5}	(MPAP − PAOP) ÷ CO × 80
Coronary artery perfusion pressure (CAPP)	60–80 mmHg	DBP - PAOP
Mixed venous oxygen saturation (SvO$_2$)	60–75%	Direct measurement (pulmonary artery)
Central venous oxygen saturation (ScvO$_2$)	> 70%	Direct measurement (superior vena cava)
Arterial oxygen saturation (SaO$_2$)	95–99% on room air	Direct measurement
Arterial oxygen content (CaO$_2$)	12–16 mL/dL	(Hgb × 1.39 × SaO$_2$) + (PaO$_2$ × 0.003)
Oxygen delivery (DO$_2$)	900–1,100 mL/min	CaO$_2$ × CO × 10
Oxygen consumption (VO$_2$)	250–350 mL/min	(SaO$_2$ − SvO$_2$) × Hgb × 13.9 × CO

- "Normal" differs somewhat from resource to resource. Those values listed in Table 7-1 are generally accepted.
- You do not need to memorize formulas for the Adult CCRN exam.

☆ Table 7-2. Hemodynamic Profiles for Select Abnormal Conditions

Condition	B/P	RAP (CVP)	PAP	PAOP	CO/CI	SV/SI*	SVR	PVR	SvO₂**	Comments
Shock States										
Cardiogenic	↓	↑	↑	↑	↓	↓	↑	~ or ↑	↓	
Hypovolemic	↓	↓	↓	↓	↓	↓	↑	~	↓	
Septic, early	↓	↓	↓	↓	↑	↑	↓	~	↑	Lactate may ↑ before B/P ↓
Septic, late	↓	↓	↓	~ or ↑	↓	↓	↑	~	↓	
Cardiogenic pulmonary edema (left ventricular failure)	~ or ↑	↑	↑	↑	↓	↓	~	~ or ↑	↓	
Noncardiogenic pulmonary edema (ARDS)	~ or ↓	~ or ↑ or ↓	↑	~ or ↓	~	~	~	↑	~ or ↓	PAP↑ due to hypoxemia
Pulmonary hypertension (PE, COPD, hypoxemia)	~	↑	↑	~	~	~	~	↑	↑	B/P, CO may ↓ if PE
Cardiac tamponade	↓	↑	↑	↑	↓	↓	↑	~ or ↑	↓	Pressures equalize

Key: ↓ = decrease; ↑ = increase; ~ = no change

Table 7-3. Hemodynamic Effects of Various Cardiovascular Agents

Drug	B/P	RAP (CVP)	PAP	PAOP	CO/CI	SV/SI	SVR	PVR	Heart Rate
Dopamine									
• Low dose (1-3 mcg/kg/m)	~	~	~	~	~	~	~	~	~
• Medium dose (4-10 mcg/kg/m)	~ or ↑	~	~ or ↑	~ or ↑	↑↑	↑	~	~	↑
• High dose (11-20 mcg/kg/m)	↑	~ or ↑	↑	↑	↑	↑	↑	↑	↑↑
Norepinephrine (Levophed)	↑	↑ or ~	↑	↑	↑	↑	↑↑	~ or ↑	↓
Phenylephrine (Neo-Synephrine)	↑	~	~	~ or ↑	~	↑	↑	~	↓
Epinephrine drip	↑	↑ or ~	↑	↑	↑	↑	↑↑	~ or ↑	↑
Nitroglycerin									
• Doses up to 1 mcg/kg	~ or ↓	↓	↓	↓↓	~	~	~	~ or ↓	↑ or ~
• Doses > 1 mcg/kg*	↓	↓	↓	↓	~ or ↑	~ or ↑	↓	↓	↑ or ~
Nesiritide (Natrecor)*	~ or ↓	↓	↓	↓	~ or ↑	~ or ↑	↓	↓	~
Nitroprusside (Nipride)*	↓↓	~	↓	↓↓	~ or ↑	~ or ↑	↓↓	↓	~ or ↑
ACE inhibitors	~ or ↓	~	↓	~ or ↓	↑	↓ or ↑	↓	↓	~
Dobutamine (Dobutrex)	~ or ↓ or ↑	↓	~	↓	↑	↑	~ or ↓	~	↑
Milrinone (Primacor)	~ or ↓	~ or ↓	↓ or ~	↓	↑	↑	↓ or ~	~	↓
Labetalol (Normadyne)	↓	~	~	~	↓	↓	↓ or ~	~	↓
Morphine	↓	↓	↓	↓	~	~	~	↓	~

Key: ↓ = decrease; ↑ = increase; ~ = no change

*High-dose NTG, nesiritide, and nitroprusside are afterload reducers, not positive inotropes, but they may increase CO indirectly by decreasing afterload.

There will be questions that test your knowledge on appropriate interventions for various abnormal hemodynamics and the significance of various oxygenation parameters. Table 7-4 summarizes therapies for alterations in hemodynamics, and Table 7-5 outlines oxygenation parameters.

⭐ **Table 7-4. Therapies for Alterations in Hemodynamics***

PRELOAD Therapies	
Increases	**Decreases**

Volume expanders
• Crystalloids
• Colloids
Pressors
	Diuretics
	Dilators
	   • Nitrates
	   • Nitroprusside
	   • Nesiritide
	Morphine

AFTERLOAD Therapies	
Increases	**Decreases**
Norepinephrine Phenylephrine High-dose dopamine (11–20 mcg/kg/min) Epinephrine drip	Nitroprusside ACE inhibitors Hydralazine Calcium channel blockers IABP Nitroglycerin (high doses)
CONTRACTILITY Therapies	
Increases	**Decreases**
Positive inotropes • Dobutamine • Dopamine 5–10 mcg/kg/min • Primacor • Epinephrine drip	Negative inotropes • Beta blockers • Calcium-channel blockers Metabolic problems (i.e., metabolic acidosis, endotoxins of sepsis)

*For all abnormalities, attempt to identify the underlying cause(s) and, if able, correct them.

Table 7-5. Hemodynamic Oxygenation Parameters

Parameter	Normal	How it's Calculated/ Measured	Clinical Relevance
Mixed venous oxygen saturation (SvO_2)	60–75%	Direct measurement, intermittent or continuous (pulmonary artery)	Most sensitive indicator of cellular oxygenation
Central venous oxygen saturation ($ScvO_2$)	> 70%	Direct measurement, intermittent or continuous (superior vena cava)	Used to monitor therapy for septic shock
Oxygen delivery (DO_2)	900–1,100 mL/min	$CaO_2 \times CO \times 10$	Pump problems (heart) will decrease DO_2
Oxygen consumption (VO_2)	250–350 mL/min	$(SaO_2 - SvO_2) \times Hgb \times 13.9 \times CO$	Low with septic shock
Oxygen extraction	$\sim$ 50% of O_2 delivery	$(CaO_2 - CvO_2)$	Myocardial oxygen extraction is > than that of any other muscle; increases with a drop in CO

- You do not need to memorize formulas for the Adult CCRN exam, but you should know the normal values and their clinical relevance.
- SvO_2: normal is 60% to 75% (too low or too high is **BAD**)
- Sustained changes, not brief changes (e.g., during position change), are significant (Table 7-6).

Table 7-6. SvO_2 Changes

Increased	Decreased
Septic shock Hypothermia Paralysis	Low cardiac output Decreased PaO_2 Increased O_2 demand (fever, shivering, seizures, increased WOB)
If SvO_2 is increased: • Assess for sepsis, septic shock • Assess for hypothermia	If SvO_2 is decreased: • Assess for hypoxemia, increased WOB • Assess for hypotension • Assess for hypovolemia • Assess hemoglobin (drop) • Assess temperature (fever) • Assess for arrhythmias

☆ For the Adult CCRN exam, concentrate on studying the normal and abnormal hemodynamic ranges. Also, study the therapies that affect hemodynamics. Note that printed waveform strips, such as the one in Figure 7-2, are seldom included on this exam.

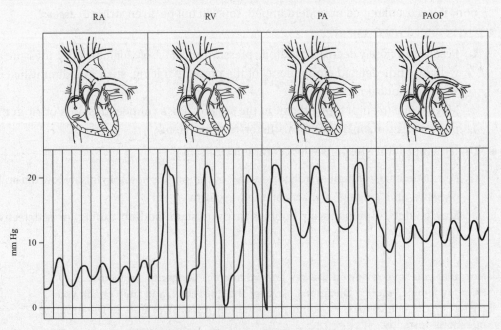

Figure 7-2. Normal pulmonary artery waves

Acute mitral valve insufficiency: In the presence of mitral valve insufficiency, the PAOP waveform changes appearance. When the PA catheter balloon is inflated, **giant V-waves** appear on the PAOP tracing (see Figure 7-3).

- The PAOP is read at the A-wave, not at the V-wave.

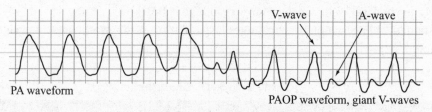

Figure 7-3. Giant V-waves on the PAOP waveform

If you see the term "giant V-waves" on the exam, the problem is mitral valve insufficiency (regurgitation). As you should recall from the Cardiovascular Concepts chapter, this is often associated with acute inferior wall myocardial infarction/papillary muscle dysfunction/ rupture.

Square Wave Test (Dynamic Response Test)

- The **dynamic response test**, also called the "square wave test," is performed to assess the accuracy of the hemodynamic monitoring system. This is done immediately after catheter insertion, at the beginning of each shift after zeroing the system and whenever values are questionable. The strip recorder is started. Then, the flush device is squeezed and immediately released. The dynamic response that is documented on the strip is then examined.
- For the exam, you will only need to know what the square wave test is and the implications if it is overdamped or underdamped. You will not be given strips to assess.
- Overdamped wave response:
  - Results in a falsely decreased systolic pressure and a falsely high diastolic pressure as well as poorly defined components of the pressure tracing, such as a diminished or absent dicrotic notch
  - May be due to air or a blood clot in the system, loose connections, loss of air in the pressure bag, or kinking of the catheter/tubing system
- Underdamped wave response (less common clinically):
  - Results in a falsely high systolic pressure (overshoot), a possibly falsely low diastolic pressure, and "ringing" artifacts on the waveform
  - May be due to pinpoint air bubbles in the system, add-on tubing, or a defective transducer

> Now that you have reviewed the key hemodynamics concepts, go to the Hemodynamics Practice Questions. Answer the questions, and then check your answers. Continue to review the information until you answer 80% of the practice questions correctly.

HEMODYNAMICS PRACTICE QUESTIONS

<u>For questions 1–3</u>

The following hemodynamic profile has been obtained for a patient:

B/P	112/60 mmHg	RA	3 mmHg
PA	44/24 mmHg	PAOP	22 mmHg
SVR	1,600 dynes/s/cm^{-5}	CI	1.9 L/min/m^2
SVI	23 mL/m^2	SvO$_2$	0.58

1. Based on this hemodynamic profile, which of the following conclusions is correct?

   (A) The patient is hypovolemic.
   (B) The patient has evidence of left ventricular failure.
   (C) The patient seems to have sepsis.
   (D) The patient has developed ARDS.

2. Shortly after obtaining the values above, the nurse inflated (wedged) the catheter balloon and observed giant V-waves on the PAOP tracing. What is the most likely problem?

   (A) The patient has evidence of mitral valve regurgitation.
   (B) The PA catheter has fallen back into the RV.
   (C) The PA catheter needs to be advanced.
   (D) The PAOP seems to be 40 mmHg.

3. What would be the most appropriate intervention for this patient?

   (A) Call the physician for possible catheter repositioning.
   (B) Document the strip, administer the PRN order for furosemide (Lasix) for a PAOP > 16 mmHg, and reassess in 1 hour.
   (C) Label the balloon "do not wedge."
   (D) Document the strip, interpret the pressure, and notify the physician.

   ---

4. A patient with continuous SvO$_2$ monitoring has a sustained a decrease in SvO$_2$ to 0.50. Priority interventions would include each of the following EXCEPT:

   (A) checking the urine output.
   (B) checking the B/P and the CO/CI.
   (C) checking O$_2$ sat with a pulse oximeter (SpO$_2$).
   (D) checking the temperature.

For questions 5–8

It is important to integrate hemodynamic parameters with each other and not evaluate parameters individually in isolation. Assess the following hemodynamic profiles. Match each profile with the clinical problem listed below that is most likely associated with it.

(B/P = blood pressure; HR = heart rate; CVP = central venous pressure; PAOP = pulmonary artery occlusion pressure; SVR = systemic vascular resistance; CI = cardiac index; SV = stroke volume)

	Profile 5	**Profile 6**	**Profile 7**	**Profile 8**
B/P	78/40	78/40	78/40	78/40
HR	120	120	120	120
CVP	5	2	15	1
PAOP	19	4	5	4
SVR	1,697	453	1,300	1,387
CI	2.0	5.5	2.5	3.0
SV	29	75	27	25
	5._____	6._____	7._____	8._____

5. (A) hypovolemic shock.
   (B) cardiogenic shock
   (C) acute right ventricular failure
   (D) septic shock

6. (A) hypovolemic shock
   (B) cardiogenic shock
   (C) acute right ventricular failure
   (D) septic shock

7. (A) hypovolemic shock
   (B) cardiogenic shock
   (C) acute right ventricular failure
   (D) septic shock

8. (A) hypovolemic shock
   (B) cardiogenic shock
   (C) acute right ventricular failure
   (D) septic shock

Match the drug with its **primary** hemodynamic effect. Consult Table 7-3.

9. ____ Dopamine 5–10 mcg/kg/min

10. ____ Dopamine > 10 mcg/kg/min

11. ____ Dobutamine

12. ____ Nitroglycerin 20 mcg/min

13. ____ Norepinephrine

14. ____ Beta blockers

15. ____ Nitroprusside (choose 2)

16. ____ ACE inhibitors

17. ____ Furosemide

18. ____ Fluid bolus

19. ____ Milrinone

20. ____ Morphine

(A) increase preload
(B) decrease preload
(C) increase afterload
(D) decrease afterload
(E) increase contractility
(F) decrease contractility

For questions 21 and 22

Mr. A, a 66-year-old male, presents S/P colectomy for colon cancer. He has the following results upon examination:

MAP of 58 mmHg (↓ from 70) after 2 L of 0.9 normal saline; heart rate of 112 beats/minute; respiratory rate of 34 breaths/minute; temperature of 38.9°C; urine output < 0.5 mL/kg for the past 2 hours; lungs are clear; skin is warm and dry; WBC is 20,000; 66% segs; 24% bands; 7% lymphs; blood cultures are positive for gram-negative organisms

21. This patient does not have a pulmonary artery catheter. If he did, and his systemic vascular resistance was measured, what SVR should the nurse anticipate this patient would have?

(A) 2,550 dynes/s/cm^{-5}
(B) 1,550 dynes/s/cm^{-5}
(C) 550 dynes/s/cm^{-5}
(D) 900 dynes/s/cm^{-5}

22. What hemodynamic changes are consistent with this patient's clinical status?

(A) increase in preload and decrease in afterload
(B) decrease in preload and increase in afterload
(C) decrease in preload and decrease in afterload
(D) decrease in CO due to impaired contractility

---

23. Ms. B, a 78-year-old female, is admitted with the following clinical findings:

- Chief complaint of SOB and fatigue
- Bibasilar crackles noted with S3 gallop
- Chest radiograph shows venous congestion and cardiomegaly
- Weight increase of 20 pounds over the last 2 weeks

Which of the following hemodynamic alterations is found with her presenting problems, and what treatment and rationale for that treatment are indicated?

(A) increased afterload, decreased contractility, and decreased preload; nesiritide to increase contractility
(B) decreased afterload, decreased contractility, and increased preload; furosemide (Lasix) to increase afterload
(C) decreased afterload, increased contractility, and increased preload; amiodarone to decrease preload
(D) increased afterload, decreased contractility, and increased preload; dobutamine to increase contractility

For questions 24 and 25

Mr. C, a 54-year-old male, presents with near-syncope. He has no significant past medical history. He sought medical help today after almost fainting in the shower. Clinical findings include:

- Blood pressure of 98/58 mmHg; heart rate of 108 beats/minute with S1 and S2 heart sounds; respiratory rate of 18 breaths/minute; temperature of 37.1°C
- Alert and orientated × 3; lungs are clear; skin is cool and dry; neck veins are flat
- Thirsty with dry oral mucous membranes; abdomen is soft/non-tender with hyperactive bowel sounds

24. The next vital sign assessment reveals a blood pressure of 88/60 mmHg. Which of the following does Mr. C seem to need?

(A) Volume expansion is needed to increase preload and increase myocardial stretch.
(B) Pressors are needed to increase afterload and increase myocardial stretch.
(C) Volume expansion is needed to decrease afterload and increase myocardial stretch.
(D) Pressors are needed to decrease preload and decrease myocardial stretch.

25. The nurse suspects that the arterial line waveform appearance has changed. The recommended method for assessing the adequacy of the catheter/tubing system is to:

(A) perform a square wave test.
(B) zero balance.
(C) check a cuff pressure.
(D) calibrate the monitor.

ANSWER KEY

1. **B**	6. **D**	11. **E**	16. **D**	21. **C**
2. **A**	7. **C**	12. **B**	17. **B**	22. **C**
3. **D**	8. **A**	13. **C**	18. **A**	23. **D**
4. **A**	9. **E**	14. **F**	19. **E**	24. **A**
5. **B**	10. **C**	15. **B, D**	20. **B**	25. **A**

ANSWERS AND EXPLANATIONS

1. **(B)** Although there are several hemodynamic abnormalities, the key here is the PAOP of 22 mmHg. Left heart failure is the only problem of those listed that would result in an elevated PAOP. Since the LV is in failure and is not emptying normally, there is a backup of volume, reflected as a higher pressure on the left side of the heart. This, in turn, causes the pulmonary capillary pressures to exceed 18 mmHg and cause pulmonary edema. The low CI causes the elevated PAOP. However, other problems, such as hypovolemia, may also result in a low CI. The SVR is high due to compensatory vasoconstriction, which in this case seems to be maintaining the blood pressure.

2. **(A)** The giant V-waves are due to mitral valve insufficiency or regurgitation, which may be acute or chronic. The PAOP is measured, however, at the A-wave.

3. **(D)** If the patient develops acute mitral valve insufficiency, the physician needs to be notified. There is no problem with the PA catheter. The patient does not automatically require a diuretic (but he might). The balloon is OK, so it doesn't need to be labeled.

4. **(A)** The SvO_2 is low; therefore, the reason for that needs to be determined. A drop in blood pressure or cardiac output, a decrease in the arterial oxygen saturation, or a fever are possible causes. Urine output is not directly associated with a decrease in the SvO_2.

5. **(B)** The key indicator is the elevated PAOP with the low CI. The SVR is elevated as a compensatory response.

6. **(D)** The key indicator is the low SVR (massive dilation) with the higher-than-normal CI.

7. **(C)** The key indicator is the high CVP with a low PAOP due to poor RV output. Since volume is not getting to the left heart, the left heart pressure (PAOP) is low and the CI is low.

8. **(A)** The key indicator is the low CVP and PAOP with the elevated SVR as a compensatory response to the hypovolemia.

9. **(E)** "Midrange" dopamine stimulates the beta-1 receptors in the heart to increase contractility.

10. **(C)** High-dose dopamine stimulates the alpha receptors in the arteries to cause vasoconstriction and to increase afterload.

11. **(E)** Dobutamine stimulates the beta-1 receptors in the heart and increases contractility.

12. **(B)** Nitroglycerin at lower doses causes venodilatation and results in a decrease in preload. Only at higher doses does it dilate the arterial vessels.

13. **(C)** Norepinephrine is a potent vasoconstrictor as it stimulates the alpha receptors of the arteries and increases afterload.

14. **(F)** Beta blockers block the beta-1 receptors of the heart, blocking the adrenergic effects of the autonomic nervous system from affecting the heart. This results in decreased contractility as well as a decrease in heart rate.

15. **(B, D)** Nitroprusside dilates both the venous and arterial sides of the vascular system, resulting in a decrease in both preload and afterload.

16. **(D)** ACE inhibitors (or angiotensin-converting enzyme inhibitors) block the conversion of angiotensin I to angiotensin II. Angiotensin II is a potent constrictor. By blocking its formation, the arterial vessels dilate more, resulting in a decrease in afterload.

17. **(B)** Furosemide is a potent loop diuretic and venodilator. The resulting diuresis and venodilation cause a reduction in preload.

18. **(A)** A fluid bolus increases volume in the vasculature, thereby increasing the preload.

19. **(E)** Milrinone, in the class of phosphodiesterase inhibitors, stimulates cardiac muscle contraction and increases contractility.

20. **(B)** Morphine mildly dilates the venous bed, thereby reducing preload. It may be used in low doses to treat heart failure.

21. **(C)** The scenario describes a patient with septic shock as evidenced by an infection and hypotension, despite 2 L of fluid. The endotoxins cause massive vasodilation, which results in a loss of vascular tone, which leads to a low SVR.

22. **(C)** Septic shock causes massive vasodilation, which decreases afterload. It also causes capillary leakage with a loss of volume in the vasculature, resulting in a decrease in preload.

23. **(D)** The patient scenario reflects heart failure. To compensate for the reduced cardiac output, a patient with heart failure vasoconstricts. Therefore, afterload is high. The heart muscle loses contractility, so contractility is decreased. Due to a low ejection fraction, the left heart pressure increases, resulting in lung crackles, S3 heart sound, and increased preload. A positive inotropic drug, such as dobutamine (as well as other drugs), may be indicated.

24. **(A)** The patient scenario is one of hypovolemia. Fluid administration will increase preload (fill up the tank), which will in turn improve myocardial stretch. This increase in stretch to increase output is the Frank-Starling law of the heart. Since the patient is volume depleted, the systemic vascular resistance (SVR) is most likely high because vasoconstriction occurs as a compensatory response to maintain the arterial blood pressure. Pressors should not be used in the presence of hypovolemia.

25. **(A)** The square wave (or dynamic response) test provides information as to whether the catheter/tubing system is optimally damped, overdamped, or underdamped. Then, troubleshooting needs to be done accordingly. Cuff pressures should not be used to verify the accuracy of intra-arterial pressures.

Neurological Concepts

8

You have brains in your head. You have feet in your shoes. You can steer yourself any direction you choose.

—Dr. Seuss

NEUROLOGICAL TEST BLUEPRINT

Neurological 10% of total test   **15 questions***

→ Acute spinal cord injury
→ Brain death
→ Delirium (e.g., hyperactive, hypoactive, mixed)**
→ Dementia**
→ Encephalopathy
→ Hemorrhage
   ○ Intracranial (ICH)
   ○ Intraventricular (IVH)
   ○ Subarachnoid (traumatic or aneurysmal)
→ Increased intracranial pressure (e.g., hydrocephalus)
→ Neurologic infectious disease (e.g., viral, bacterial, fungal)
→ Neuromuscular disorders (e.g., muscular dystrophy, CP, Guillain-Barré, myasthenia)
→ Neurosurgery (e.g., craniotomy, Burr holes)
→ Seizure disorders
→ Space-occupying lesions (e.g., brain tumors)
→ Stroke
   ○ Hemorrhagic
   ○ Ischemic (embolic)
   ○ TIA
→ Traumatic brain injury (TBI): epidural, subdural, concussion

*The number of questions and percentages in this category may vary slightly from test to test.

**This topic is covered in the Behavioral/Psychosocial Concepts chapter of this book.

NEUROLOGICAL TESTABLE NURSING ACTIONS

☐ Recognize indications for and manage patients requiring neurologic monitoring devices and drains (e.g., ICP, ventricular or lumbar drain)

☐ Use a swallow evaluation tool to assess dysphagia

☐ Manage patients requiring:

○ Neuroendovascular interventions (e.g., coiling, thrombectomy)

○ Neurosurgical procedures (e.g., pre-, intra-, post-procedure)

○ Spinal immobilization

Neurological concepts comprise approximately 10% of the Adult CCRN test blueprint with approximately 15 questions. Therefore, you will need to study for approximately 15 hours.

NEUROLOGICAL ANATOMY

The brain is enclosed within the skull, with the "higher" centers above the transtentorial shelf and the brain stem below the transtentorial shelf (Figure 8-1). Although the skull protects the brain, the inner surface and shelf have jagged edges that can tear brain tissue in the event that a traumatic injury causes movement of the brain within the skull. If brain swelling occurs, the brain has nowhere to expand except down toward the foramen magnum.

■ There are 2 "holes" in the skull, the transtentorial notch (small) and the foramen magnum (large), through which the brain stem is attached to the spinal cord.

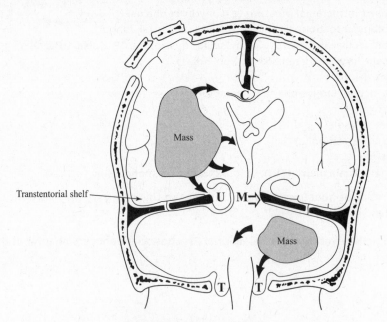

Figure 8-1. Brain anatomy

Cranial Nerves

- You do not need to memorize all of the cranial nerves for the Adult CCRN exam. However, several cranial nerves may be incorporated into the questions. Review Figure 8-2 to study the 12 cranial nerves.

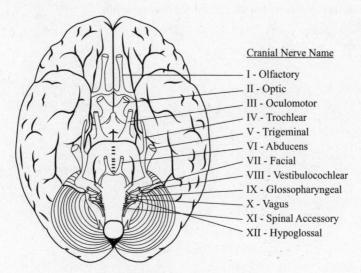

Cranial Nerve Name

I - Olfactory
II - Optic
III - Oculomotor
IV - Trochlear
V - Trigeminal
VI - Abducens
VII - Facial
VIII - Vestibulocochlear
IX - Glossopharyngeal
X - Vagus
XI - Spinal Accessory
XII - Hypoglossal

Figure 8-2. Cranial nerves

- I (olfactory): smell, often affected with a basilar skull fracture
- II (optic): sight, NOT pupil reaction
- III (oculomotor): pupillary function, flows out of midbrain (in brain stem) and traverses the transtentorial notch; therefore, with an increase in intracranial pressure, parasympathetic stimulation is blocked, sympathetic stimulation predominates = dilated pupil on the side of the injury
- V (trigeminal): corneal reflex, chewing
- VIII (vestibulocochlear): intactness of this cranial nerve is tested by doll's eyes and cold caloric exams
- IX (glossopharyngeal): swallow, gag
- X (vagus): pharyngeal/laryngeal movement

- All cranial nerves arise from the brain stem except cranial nerves I and II, which arise from the cerebrum above the brain stem.

Blood Supply to the Brain

- The 2 vertebral arteries come together and form the basilar artery, which supplies the lower areas of the brain and the brain stem (refer to Figure 8-3).
- The carotids supply the upper areas of the brain.
  - The left internal carotid is dominant for most people.

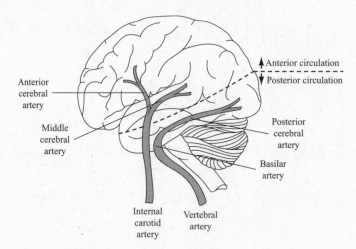

Figure 8-3. Blood supply to the brain

Brain Function Based on Anatomic Location

- Frontal lobe: Personality, abstract thought, long-term memory
- Temporal lobe: Hearing, sense of taste and smell, interpretations
- Occipital lobe: Vision, visual recognition, reading comprehension
- Parietal lobe: Object recognition by size, weight, shape; body part awareness
- Cerebellum: Coordination, balance, gait
- The Circle of Willis is a circulatory anastomosis comprised of various arteries that supply blood to the brain. A well-developed Circle of Willis allows collateral blood flow to one area from another area in the event of an occlusion (Figure 8-4).

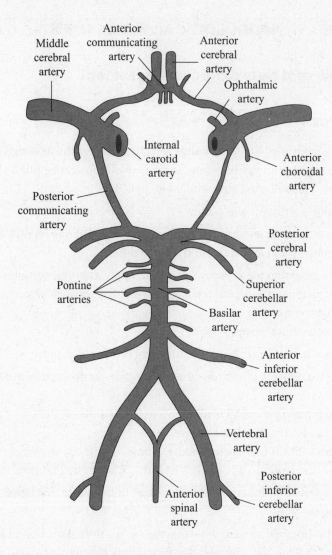

Figure 8-4. Circle of Willis

- Less than 50% of the population has a well-developed, intact Circle of Willis, which accounts for the varied clinical symptoms that may occur for 2 individuals who have a stroke in the same area of the Circle of Willis.
- The following arteries compose the Circle:
  - Anterior cerebral artery (left and right)
  - Anterior communicating artery
  - Internal carotid artery (left and right)
  - Posterior cerebral artery (left and right)
  - Posterior communicating artery (left and right)
- The basilar artery and middle cerebral arteries (MCA) are **not** part of the Circle of Willis.

Components of a Neurological Assessment

MENTAL STATUS

- Level of consciousness (LOC): **a change in LOC is always the first sign of a neurological problem** (except for an epidural hematoma, which may cause pupil changes before an LOC change). The following are included in an LOC assessment:
  - Arousability—voice, shake, pain
    - Each of these should be applied one at a time in order to identify any subtle change (i.e., don't shout and shake at the same time).
    - When assessing for a response to pain, apply a central stimulus (e.g., sternal rub, trapezius squeeze, orbital pressure) for a full 30 seconds before you state that there is no response.
  - Orientation—time, place, person
    - Generally, the first to become abnormal is time, then place, and lastly person.
  - The RAS is a network of neurons that connect the brain stem (lower RAS) to the cortex (upper RAS).
  - The upper part of the RAS is responsible for awareness; the lower part of the RAS is responsible for the sleep-wake cycle.
  - If the lower RAS is damaged, a coma occurs; if only the upper portion of the RAS is damaged, the patient loses awareness but still wakes up and goes to sleep.
- Speech/language: dysfunction in the dominant hemisphere (left hemisphere for most of the population)
  - Expressive (Broca's) aphasia—dysfunction in the dominant frontal lobe
  - Receptive (Wernicke's) aphasia—dysfunction in the dominant temporal lobe
- Memory: short-term usually becomes abnormal before long-term.
- Attention span/thought content/judgment
- Personality: occasionally the first sign of a problem; before the LOC changes, the patient's personality may change (e.g., in brain tumors).

MOTOR FUNCTION

- **Decussation** (crossing) of motor fibers occurs in the medulla; motor problems are contralateral to the brain problem (e.g., stroke, tumor).
- Strength and movement are indicators of motor function.
- Pronator drift may be evident before strength changes are detected.
  - Ask the patient to close his or her eyes, hold out both arms with palms up, and hold for 15 seconds.
  - If one arm drifts down, that arm has weakness.
- Abnormal flexion or distention (Figure 8-5)

TIP

☆ **Consciousness depends upon an intact cerebral cortex and reticular activating system (RAS).**

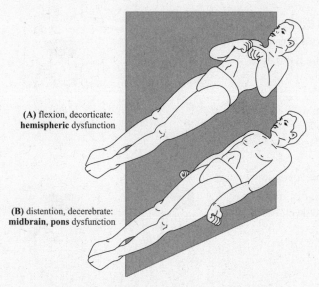

(A) flexion, decorticate: **hemispheric** dysfunction

(B) distention, decerebrate: **midbrain, pons** dysfunction

Figure 8-5. Abnormal flexion or distention

- Flaccid: **medulla** dysfunction

SENSORY FUNCTION

- Sensory deficits are generally on the same side as motor deficits and, like motor deficits, are contralateral to the side of the brain injury.

PUPILLARY ASSESSMENT

- Pupillary response assesses **cranial nerve III** (oculomotor) function and pupil constriction and accommodation.
- Sympathetic effect on pupils: dilate
- Parasympathetic effect on pupils: constrict
- 17% of the population have unequal pupils.
- Changes occur on the side of the injury (ipsilateral).

REFLEXES

- Babinski: positive is abnormal in adults (toes flare up toward the head when the bottom of the foot is stroked); this reflex is due to pressure on the pyramidal/motor tracts in the cerebrum; a Babinski reflex is found on the opposite side of the brain injury.
- Brain stem reflexes are assessed if all other reflexes are absent and brain death is suspected.

  - Cough, gag, corneal
  - Oculocephalic reflex assessment: "doll's eyes"

    - Doll's eyes assesses cranial nerves III, VI, and VIII.
    - The C-spine is cleared first; the patient's eyes are held open and eye movement is watched as the head is rapidly turned from side to side.
    - Positive: eyes move in the opposite direction of the head turn.
    - Positive reflex is good: "it's good to be a doll" (Figure 8-6).

A is normal: eyes reflexively turn opposite of the side the head is turned

B is abnormal: eyes stay midpoint, do not move to either side when head is turned

C is abnormal: eyes turn to the same side the head is turned

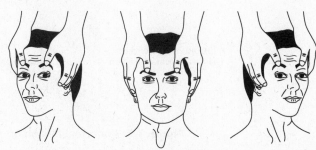

Figure 8-6. Assessment of oculocephalic reflex (doll's eyes)

○ Oculovestibular reflex assessment (Figure 8-7)

  – The patient's eyes are held open while ice water is injected slowly into the ear canal and the eye response is observed (cold calorics).

  – Positive: eyes move toward the side of the ice water injection.

  – Positive reflex is good.

A is normal

B is abnormal

C is abnormal, absent response

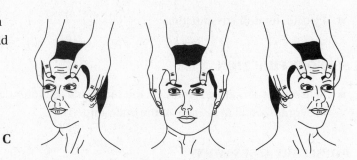

Figure 8-7. Assessment of oculovestibular reflex (cold calorics)

VITAL SIGN CHANGES ARE A LATE SIGN OF NEUROLOGICAL INJURY, BRAIN STEM INVOLVEMENT

- **Cushing's triad** is a sign of herniation of the brain:

  1. ↑ Systolic pressure, **widening** pulse pressure
  2. ↓ Heart rate
  3. ↓ Respiratory rate

- Respiratory patterns associated with brain stem abnormalities (Figure 8-8):

  ○ Midbrain problem—hyperventilation
  ○ Pontine problem—apneustic breathing
  ○ Medulla problem—ataxic breathing, leads to respiratory ARREST!

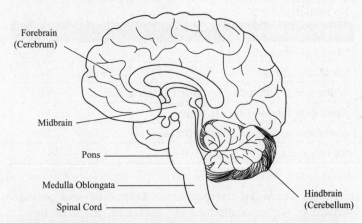

Figure 8-8. Brain stem (midbrain, pons, medulla oblongata)

MISCELLANEOUS ASSESSMENTS

- Trauma, drainage
- Meningeal irritation
- Abnormal ICP waveforms
- Radiology studies
- Chemistries, ABGs, urine osmolality
- Cerebrospinal fluid (CSF) assessment

There **may be a test question** related to the assessment of the Glasgow Coma Scale (GCS), as shown in Table 8-1. The patient is scored for the BEST response. The score may vary from 15 (best) to 3 (worst). If the score is 8 or less, the outcome is poor.

Table 8-1. Glasgow Coma Scale

Best Eye Opening	Score
Spontaneously	4
To speech	3
To pain	2
No response	1
Best Verbal Response	**Score**
Oriented	5
Confused conversation	4
Inappropriate words	3
Garbled sounds	2
No response	1
Best Motor Response	**Score**
Obeys commands	6
Localizes stimuli	5
Withdrawal from stimulus (normal flexion)	4
Abnormal flexion (decorticate)	3
Abnormal extension (decerebrate)	2
No response	1

Which is worse: obtunded or stuporous? Stuporous—the patient cannot speak. Remember: "O" comes before "S"; therefore, "O" is better!

➤ Obtunded = the patient can speak, mumbles words

➤ Stuporous = the patient cannot speak, but he or she may moan or grimace

Homonymous Hemianopsia

■ Homonymous hemianopsia is a loss of vision in half the field of each eye (*hemi* = half, *anopia* = of each field); see Figure 8-9.

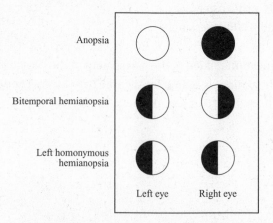

Figure 8-9. Examples of visual field defects

■ Indicates damage to the **optic nerve** (cranial nerve II)

■ Occurs opposite the side (contralateral) of the problem (e.g., stroke, tumor)

- Results in neglect of the affected side
- Initially, approach the patient from the unaffected side to increase environmental awareness and to prevent confusion; as the patient's condition improves, approach the patient from the affected side to expand awareness of the neglected visual field.

Summary of Neurological Assessment

- Whether the pathology is a tumor, a hematoma, an infarct, or swelling, several general assessment principles apply:
  - Eyes deviate toward the pathology.
  - Pupil changes are ipsilateral (same side as the pathology).
  - Visual changes (homonymous hemianopsia) are contralateral (opposite side of the pathology).
  - Motor changes are contralateral (opposite the side of the pathology).
  - Babinski is contralateral (opposite side of the pathology).
  - If the pathology is on both sides, the patient has a bilateral Babinski reflex.

BRAIN HERNIATION

- Brain herniation occurs when swelling within the brain becomes so severe that structures of the brain are squeezed to the point where blood cannot get up into the brain; death may occur.
- Although there are several types of brain herniation, the Adult CCRN exam generally focuses on either **uncal or transtentorial (central) herniation** (Figure 8-10).

1. **Uncal***
2. **Central***
3. Cingulate
4. Transcalvarial
5. Upward
6. Tonsillar

*Most likely to be covered on the CCRN Exam

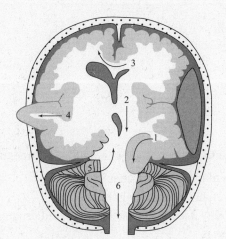

Figure 8-10. Types of brain herniation

Uncal Herniation

- Displacement of the temporal lobe (uncus) against the brain stem and the third cranial nerve (oculomotor)
- Lateral shift, **no** initial change in LOC
- Compresses (knocks off) parasympathetic innervation to the affected side, blown (dilated) pupil on the same side (ipsilateral) seen **before** change in LOC

- Babinski: on opposite side (contralateral)
- Slight weakness and pronator drift on opposite side
- Could progress to a stupor, a coma, abnormal posturing, bilateral fixed and dilated pupils, or even death
- Most often caused by **epidural hematoma** (which occurs in the temporal area) and some strokes

Central Herniation

- Swelling on both sides, downward displacement of hemispheres
- Usually due to diffuse edema, slower development
- Slight change in LOC and then could lead to a coma
- First, both pupils are small (1–3 mm), and then parasympathetic innervation on both sides is suppressed and both pupils dilate.
- Babinski: bilaterally
- Could lead to death
- May be caused by cerebral edema secondary to encephalopathy or a stroke

ENCEPHALOPATHY

- Encephalopathy is a nonspecific term for any diffuse disease of the brain that alters brain function or structure.

Etiology

- Hypoxic
- Metabolic
- Hepatic
- Drugs
- Infection

Signs

- Minor to major, can result in swelling, ↑ intracranial pressure (ICP)
  - Loss of memory and cognitive ability
  - Personality changes, agitation
  - Inability to concentrate, lethargy, and progressive loss of consciousness
  - Seizures
  - Coma
  - Brain death

Treatment

- Identify the etiology and treat it.
- Keep the patient safe.
- Avoid conditions that may increase the ICP (which are described later in the Increased Intracranial Pressure (ICP) section of this chapter).

STROKE

Questions on the Adult CCRN exam that are related to a stroke generally focus on the clinical presentation that is typical of a right-sided or left-sided stroke (Table 8-2) and key nursing interventions.

Table 8-2. Types of Stroke

Embolic, Ischemic	Hemorrhagic
TIA (transient ischemic attack) within 24 hours Cerebral infarct	Intracerebral Subarachnoid AV malformation

Stroke Assessment

RIGHT BRAIN BLEED, INFARCT

- Eyes deviate toward the pathology—RIGHT
- LEFT-sided muscle weakness, paralysis
- LEFT homonymous hemianopsia
- LEFT Babinski
- Emotional lability

LEFT BRAIN BLEED, INFARCT

- Eyes deviate to the LEFT
- RIGHT-sided muscle weakness, paralysis
- RIGHT homonymous hemianopsia
- RIGHT Babinski
- Aphasia (expressive, receptive, or global) if the left hemisphere is dominant
- In most people, the dominant internal carotid artery is on the left.

Treatment of an Acute Ischemic Stroke

NEUROLOGICAL EMERGENCY! "TIME IS BRAIN"

- Rule out hypoglycemia (which may mimic stroke symptoms).
- Assess the ABCs.
- Assess the B/P: do not treat acutely unless the systolic B/P is > 220 mmHg or the diastolic B/P is > 120 mmHg.
  - A sudden decrease in blood pressure will decrease perfusion to an area of the brain that has already lost perfusion; this may increase the size of the ischemic area.
- IV, O_2, cardiac monitoring
- Baseline labs
- CT scan within 25 minutes of arrival (or symptom onset)

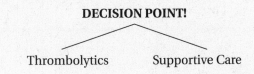

DECISION POINT!

Thrombolytics   Supportive Care

Eligibility Criteria for the Use of Recombinant Tissue Plasminogen Activator (rtPA) for an Acute Ischemic Stroke

INCLUSION CRITERIA FOR THE USE OF rtPA

- Onset of signs/symptoms was less than 4.5 hours ago.
- CT scan is negative.
- No contraindications

EXCLUSION CRITERIA FOR THE USE OF rtPA

- Evidence of a hemorrhage
- Stroke or head trauma in the past 3 months
- Any history of an intracranial hemorrhage
- Major surgery in the past 14 days
- Active bleeding in the past 21 days
- MI in the past 3 months
- Seizure at the onset of stroke (history of a seizure disorder is OK)
- Platelets $< 100,000/mm^3$
- Serum glucose < 50 mg/dL
- INR > 1.7 if the patient is taking warfarin or if the patient has a noncompressible arterial puncture
- Spontaneous clearing of symptoms or only minor (NIH Stroke Score 1) symptoms
- Persistent blood pressure elevation (systolic is ≥ 185 mmHg; diastolic is ≥ 110 mmHg)

rtPA (Alteplase) Administration

NOTE

Dosing is not usually included on the exam.

- Administer rtPA 0.9 mg/kg total (maximum 90 mg), with 10% of total dose as a bolus.
  - 75 kg: 0.9 mg $\times 75 = 67.5$ total (or 68)
  - Bolus = 10% of 68 = 6.8 mg
  - Infuse the remainder (61.2 mg) over 60 min.
- Goal B/P for first 24 hours after rtPA: systolic < 180 mmHg and diastolic < 105 mmHg (IV labetalol is usually the drug of choice for B/P control for this patient population)

Post-rtPA Infusion Care

- Complete a close neurological assessment: what is the worst complication?
  - Intracerebral hemorrhage: watch for a change in the level of consciousness (LOC).
- Complete a close B/P assessment: goal is systolic < 180 mmHg and diastolic < 105 mmHg.
- Initiate bleeding precautions, and do NOT administer antiplatelets (such as ASA) or anti-coagulants (such as heparin) for 24 hours.
- Provide supportive care (the patient will probably be left with some neurological deficits, although those deficits will not be as severe as they would have been if rtPA had not been used).

Treatment Post-Ischemic Stroke

The following interventions apply to all patients who have had an ischemic stroke (including those who received rtPA and those who did not receive rtPA).

- Maintain adequate oxygenation.
- Treat hypotension.
- Address any fevers (temperatures > 37.5°C).
- Maintain the serum glucose level at 80–150 mg/dL.
- Elevate the head of the bed to 45° or more.
- Use a Dysphagia Screening Tool to assess for signs of dysphagia which include: decreased LOC; facial, tongue, and/or palatal asymmetry/weakness; throat clearing, coughing, and/or vocal changes following water consumption.

  - Keep the patient NPO until a swallow screening is completed and if the screen is positive.
  - Refer the patient to a speech pathologist if there is a positive screen.
  - Utilize dysphagia precautions as advised by the speech pathologist (e.g., assist the patient with meals and use thickened liquids when oral intake can be resumed).

Pontine Infarct Stroke Characteristics . . . Think "P"!

- **Ap**neustic breathing pattern
- **P**inpoint **p**upils
- **P**arasympathetic innervation (if the patient has a pontine stroke, he or she loses sympathetic nervous system innervation)

SUBARACHNOID HEMORRHAGE (SAH)

- An SAH may be caused by trauma, a rupture of an aneurysm, or a tumor—SAH is the cause of 5% of all strokes.
  - An aneurysm, often of the middle cerebral artery, is the most common cause (Figure 8-11).

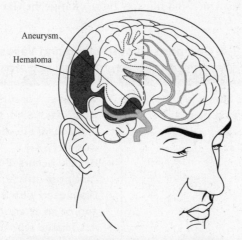

Aneurysm

Hematoma

Figure 8-11. Subarachnoid hemorrhage

- When caused by an aneurysm, SAHs are usually seen in those who are 50 to 70 years of age, and incidences increase with age.
- The patient's Hunt and Hess scale score, which provides a grade/score based on the patient's neurological status at the time of presentation of the SAH, helps predict the outcome and the immediate treatment; refer to Table 8-3.

Table 8-3. Hunt and Hess Scale

Grade/Score	Neurological Status
I	Asymptomatic or mild headache, slight nuchal rigidity
II	Awake, alert, severe headache, stiff neck, cranial nerve palsy*
III	Drowsy or confused, stiff neck, mild focal neurological deficit
IV	Stuporous, moderate or severe hemiparesis, perhaps mild posturing
V	Coma, posturing

*Diplopia, ptosis, dilation

- Note that LOC does not change until the score is III or greater.

Classic Triad of Symptoms for a Ruptured Aneurysm

1. Sudden explosive headache
2. Decreased LOC
3. Nuchal rigidity, positive Kernig's sign (explained in the Meningitis section of this chapter)

- The patient may have prominent U-waves on the ECG.
- Surgery?

    o Within 48 hours if the patient exhibits a Grade I, II, or III on the Hunt and Hess scale
    o Perhaps delayed if the patient exhibits a Grade IV or V on the Hunt and Hess scale

Complications of Subarachnoid Hemorrhage (SAH)

- **Hydrocephalus** may develop since the chorionic villi in the subarachnoid space reabsorb CSF. If the chorionic villi are blocked, CSF may not be able to be reabsorbed.
- Rebleed and vasospasm are manifested by a **change in the level of consciousness** (Table 8-4).

Table 8-4. Comparison of Rebleed and Vasospasm

Rebleed	Vasospasm
• Possible 7 to 10 days after the initial bleed, peak incidence on days 4–8 • Greatest cause of death • Confirmed with a CT scan	• Vasospasm occurs in 40–60% of all cases of SAH; the symptoms of vasospasm are seen in 20–30% of all cases of SAH • Usually occurs 5–7 days **post-bleed** (not post-op) • Diagnosed with a Transcranial Doppler and/or an arteriogram • Associated with hyponatremia

- Vasospasm results in brain ischemia, which can be a devastating complication.
- Figure 8-12 depicts blood flow via a normal cerebral artery and via a vasospastic artery.

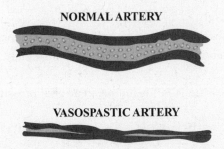

NORMAL ARTERY

VASOSPASTIC ARTERY

Figure 8-12. Comparison of a normal artery and a vasospastic artery

TREATMENT OF VASOSPASM

- Transluminal balloon angioplasty for select cases of vasospasm
- Prevent vasospasm by:

  ○ Providing the calcium channel blocker nimodipine (Nimotop), 60 mg every 4 hours for an aneurysmal SAH
  ○ Maintaining the cerebral perfusion pressure (CPP) at 60–70 mmHg with fluids, pressors, and inotropes; **AVOID** hypotension
  ○ Monitoring for and treating hyponatremia (which may precede vasospasm)

BRAIN TUMORS

- The principles of pathology (right hemisphere, left hemisphere) that were already discussed earlier in this chapter (in the section on strokes) also apply to brain tumors.
- Seizures are an early manifestation.
- Mortality remains high.
- Benign tumors may cause death.
- A brain tumor is the one neurological problem that includes **steroid therapy**, such as dexamethasone (Decadron), in the treatment plan. Steroids can prevent elevated ICP for a patient with a brain tumor.

INCREASED INTRACRANIAL PRESSURE (ICP)

The concept of increased ICP is very likely to be included on the exam. It is important to remember that there are many causes of increased ICP: medical, surgical, and trauma. Therefore, any patient with a neurological problem may develop signs of increased ICP.

- The first sign of an increase in ICP is a **change in the level of consciousness (LOC)** since the "higher" centers of the brain show symptoms first and then symptoms progress down toward the brain stem.

Intracranial Pressure Overview

- Normal is ∼ 0–10 mmHg.
- 11–20 mmHg is moderately high.

- Increased is > 20 mmHg.
- Cerebral perfusion pressure (CPP), especially in the presence of elevated ICP, is more important than ICP alone and demonstrates the important relationship between the MAP and the ICP.
- Cerebral perfusion pressure (CPP) is the mean arterial pressure (MAP) minus the intra-cranial pressure (ICP):

$$CPP = MAP - ICP$$

- ○ Average CPP is 80–100 mmHg.
- ○ Minimum for perfusion is 50 mmHg.
- ○ Brain death is < 30 mmHg.
- ○ With elevated ICP, maintain CPP ~ 70 mmHg.
- ○ Hypotension in the presence of elevated ICP can be devastating.

> **Examples:** Note that with the same ICP, a patient with hypotension (Patient B) has poor brain perfusion, whereas a patient with a higher MAP (Patient A), even with an ICP of 30 mmHg, has better cerebral perfusion.
>
> | A | B |
> |---|---|
> | MAP = 110 | MAP = 55 |
> | ICP = 30 | ICP = 30 |
> | CPP = 80 | CPP = 25 |

Signs and Symptoms of Increased ICP

- Altered LOC
- Restlessness/agitation
- Headache
- Nausea and vomiting
- Seizures
- Cranial nerve palsies (most commonly III, VI–X)
- Visual dysfunction
- Papilledema
- Pupillary changes
- Motor dysfunction (weakness, flexor and/or extensor posturing, flaccidity)
- Cushing's triad

ICP MONITORING

- ICP monitoring may be done with a fiber-optic catheter or a fluid-filled system.
- Indications include head trauma (with a GCS of 8 or less upon presentation) and post-op neurosurgery.
- When using the fluid-filled system, the level of the transducer should be at the external auditory meatus, which is at the level of the foramen of Monro.

- In addition to the pressure value, there are 3 types of ICP waves (Figure 8-13):

   1. C waves
   2. B waves
   3. A waves

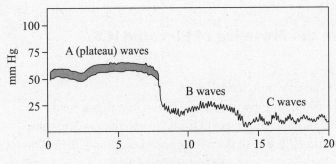

Figure 8-13. ICP waves

Wave Interpretation

- A waves are "awful."
- B waves are "bad."
- C waves are "common."
- In order to be significant, pressure and wave changes need to be sustained over several minutes.
- Cerebral vasospasm results in A waves and high ICP.

Strategies to Lower ICP

- Decrease volume: mannitol/furosemide/3% saline, patient position (upright to facilitate venous drainage from the brain).
- Prevent dilation of cerebral vessels: prevent acidosis (a low pH causes dilation of the arteries).
- Reduce cerebrospinal fluid (CSF): ventriculostomy.
- Prevent secondary brain injury.

   ○ Airway: control the pH
   ○ Breathing: prevent hypoxemia
   ○ Circulation: prevent hypotension

- Prevent agitation, pain.

   ○ Propofol has been demonstrated to reduce ICP by as much as 15 mmHg.

- Why would 0.45 NS or D5W be contraindicated for a patient with ↑ ICP?

   ○ These are hypotonic fluids. Therefore, they would rapidly leave the vascular compartment and go intracellular. In the brain, which already has an increase in ICP, cell "swelling" would exacerbate the problem.
   ○ Use isotonic fluids.

- Should hyperventilation be used to decrease the ICP?

  - No! Hyperventilation will cause an alkalosis (pH will rise). This will result in cerebral vasoconstriction, which WILL lower the ICP. The bad news, however, is that the vasoconstriction also reduces cerebral blood flow.
  - Keep the pH low normal, $\sim$ 7.35.

Summary—In the Presence of Elevated ICP

- Avoid:

  - Acidosis—causes vasodilation, $\uparrow$ ICP
  - Alkalosis—causes vasoconstriction, $\downarrow$ blood flow to the head
  - Hypotonic solution—fluid moves from the vasculature into cells
  - Hyperextension, flexion of the neck—prevents optimal jugular venous outflow
  - PEEP—$\uparrow$ thoracic pressure, prevents optimal jugular venous outflow
  - Low protein—$\downarrow$ serum oncotic pressure, fluid displaced from vasculature into the intracellular space; feed!
  - Restraints—$\uparrow$ agitation
  - Agitation, noxious stimuli—$\uparrow$ ICP
  - Fever—could lead to cerebral hypermetabolism, $\uparrow$ ICP

  These may all contribute to elevated ICP.

TRAUMATIC BRAIN INJURY (TBI)

Overview

- A **traumatic brain injury (TBI)** is a blunt (closed) or penetrating insult to the brain from an external mechanical force.

  - Causes primary brain injury and potential secondary brain injury
  - Results in temporary or permanent impairments of cognitive, physical, and psychosocial function

- Etiologies of TBI: **falls** (40%); **blunt trauma** (16%); **motor vehicle accidents** (14%); **assaults** (11%); **unknown/other** (19%)
- Severity according to GCS score within first 48 hours:

  - Severe TBI   3–8
  - Moderate TBI   9–12
  - Mild TBI   13–15

- Types of TBI

  - Diffuse: concussion, diffuse axonal injury (DAI)
  - Focal: contusions, intracranial hematomas, skull fractures, open head injuries

- CT scan of the head is the diagnostic test of choice.

Intracranial Hematomas, Hemorrhage

Hematomas may develop above the dura (epidural, Figure 8-14), below the dura (subdural, Figure 8-15), and within the brain tissue itself (intracerebral). Usually at least 1 question on the Adult CCRN exam involves intracranial hematomas.

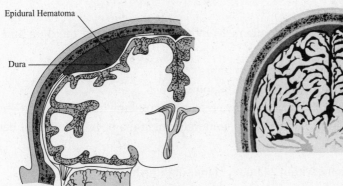

Figure 8-14. Epidural hematoma

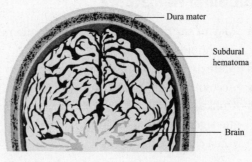

Figure 8-15. Subdural hematoma

☆ Epidural Hematoma

- Usually due to middle meningeal artery bleed secondary to temporal bone trauma with bleeding between the skull and the dura (Figure 8-16)

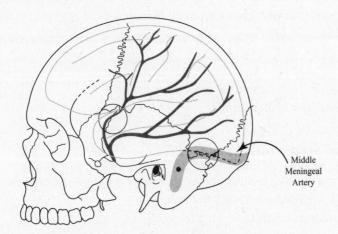

Figure 8-16. Middle meningeal artery

- **Rapidly** developing symptoms
- More common in younger population, not common in the elderly population
- Accounts for 20–30% of all intracerebral hematomas

CLINICAL PRESENTATION

- Headache
- Irritability—confusion
- Vomiting
- Ipsilateral pupil dilation, often BEFORE decreased LOC
- Contralateral hemiparesis/hemiplegia
- Decreasing LOC

NOTE

What type of herniation results from an epidural hematoma? Uncal!

TREATMENT

- Emergent surgery to evacuate the hematoma (burr hole)
- Monitor and treat increasing ICP.

Subdural Hematoma

- May occur due to trauma or spontaneously with bleeding between the dura and the arachnoid membrane
- More prevalent in the elderly or alcoholics (falls)
- Accounts for 50–70% of all intracerebral hematomas
- Unlike an epidural hematoma, which is always acute, a subdural hematoma may generate signs/symptoms more slowly than an epidural hematoma does. A subdural hematoma can be classified as:

  - Acute (signs/symptoms within 24 hours of the subdural hematoma)
  - Subacute (signs/symptoms within 2 weeks of the subdural hematoma)
  - Chronic (signs/symptoms more than 2 weeks after the subdural hematoma)

CLINICAL PRESENTATION

- Similar to epidural hematoma, although less vomiting and pupil change does not usually precede change in the LOC
- May develop more slowly than an epidural hematoma

TREATMENT

- Close neurological assessment for signs of increased ICP
- Surgery to evacuate the hematoma

Intracerebral Hematoma

- May be due to a gunshot wound, a severe acceleration-deceleration injury, or a laceration of the brain from a depressed skull fracture
- May be nontraumatic (stroke)
- 2–20% of all hematomas

CLINICAL PRESENTATION

- Varies greatly due to the area of the brain that is involved
- May or may not have increased ICP

TREATMENT

- Surgery if the hematoma is large and if the patient's neurological status is deteriorating

Types of Skull Fractures

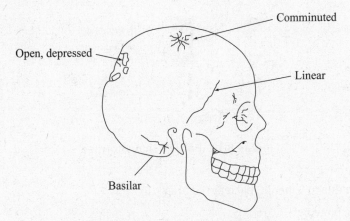

Figure 8-17. Types of skull fractures

- A linear skull fracture does not require surgery.
- Open, depressed:

    ○ Most surgeons prefer to elevate depressed skull fractures if the depressed segment is **greater than 5 mm** below the inner table of the adjacent bone.

    ○ Indications for immediate elevation are gross contamination, a dural tear with pneumocephalus, and an underlying hematoma.

    ○ A comminuted skull fracture is a fracture with bone fragmentation, usually depressed.

- ☆ A basilar skull fracture is a linear fracture that occurs in the floor of the cranial vault (skull base), resulting in a **meningeal tear**.

    ○ Most likely to be covered on the Adult CCRN exam

    ○ Requires more force to cause than for other areas of the neurocranium

    ○ Rare—occurs in approximately 4% of patients with severe head injuries

Signs/Symptoms of a Basilar Skull Fracture

- Raccoon eyes (Figure 8-18)—manifested as periorbital edema and ecchymosis

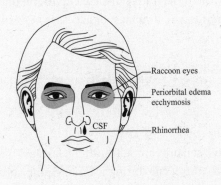

Figure 8-18. Raccoon eyes, rhinorrhea

- Battle's sign (Figure 8-19)—manifested as a discoloration at the back of the ear

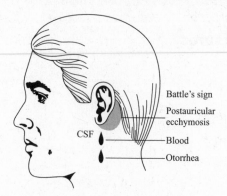

Figure 8-19. Battle's sign, otorrhea

- Rhinorrhea due to a meningeal tear (Figure 8-18)
  - No nose blowing!
- Otorrhea, fluid from the ear, due to a meningeal tear (Figure 8-19)
- Damage to cranial nerve I often occurs, resulting in a loss of the sense of smell (which may be temporary or permanent).

Nursing Implications

- Determine whether ear or nose drainage is cerebrospinal fluid:
  - Check for sugar; if positive, it is cerebrospinal fluid.
  - Put the drainage on a 4 × 4.
    - If the drainage is cerebrospinal fluid, you will see a clot surrounded by a **yellow halo** (**"halo sign"**).
- Cover the ear or nose with dry, sterile gauze: do not pack in.

Treatment

- Don't block CSF drainage.
- Surgical repair ONLY if CSF leakage is persistent
- Risk of meningitis—monitor for infection; antibiotics ONLY if there is a sign of infection.
- Do not insert a nasogastric tube. It may displace up to the brain. Use an orogastric tube instead if gastric decompression, drainage, or access is needed.

SEIZURES

Overview

- Most general tonic-clonic seizures are self-limiting, last less than 3 minutes.
- Normal ventilation does not occur during a tonic-clonic seizure; therefore, the $PaCO_2$ may be elevated immediately post-seizure.

- Protect the patient's airway, turn the patient to his or her side.
- Maintain patient safety.
- STOP the seizure.
  - Lorazepam (Ativan): 0.05–0.15 mg/kg at 1 mg/min, max ~ 8 mg OR
  - Diazepam (Valium): 0.25 mg/kg at 2–5 mg/min, max ~ 30 mg
  - Lorazepam, which is longer-acting, is preferred.
- PREVENT seizures.
  - Phenytoin (Dilantin): 15–20 mg/kg at 50 mg/min, max 1 gram
  - Fosphenytoin sodium (Cerebyx)
  - Carbamazepine (Tegretol)
  - Phenobarbital
- A seizure may be followed by a postictal period with transient signs of decreased LOC.
- What if the phenytoin (Dilantin) level is therapeutic and the patient seizes?
  - Give lorazepam (Ativan)!
- How are benzodiazepines reversed?
  - Flumazenil (Romazicon)! Romazicon has a shorter half-life than some benzodiazepines; therefore, sedation effects may recur and flumazenil (Romazicon) may need to be repeated.
- After a generalized tonic-clonic seizure, the patient may experience a postictal state of decreased level of consciousness.

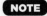

NOTE

Dosages are not usually covered on this exam.

Status Epilepticus

- Seizure activity of **5 minutes** (time revised from 30 minutes) or more caused by a single seizure or a series of seizures with no return of consciousness between seizures

☆ **Table 8-5. Pathophysiology of Status Epilepticus**

Early	Late (30 minutes)
↑ Cerebral blood flow Tachycardia, hypertension $PaCO_2$ ↑, PaO_2 ↓ ↑ Glucose (stress response) ↑ K^+ (destruction of skeletal muscle cells)	Cerebral blood flow is unable to meet demands Arrhythmias (hyperkalemia) Hypoglycemia ↑ ↑ K^+ and CKs Rhabdomyolysis (extremely high CKs) Ventricular fibrillation
☆ Death is due to **cerebral hypermetabolism**.	

- The patient is not responsive to usual therapy and may require barbiturates, intubation/ventilation, or a short-acting anesthetic.
- Causes
  - Withdrawal from anticonvulsant medications
  - Acute alcohol withdrawal
  - Toxic levels of drugs
  - CNS infections
  - Brain tumors/CNS trauma

- ○ Metabolic disorders—hypoglycemia, hepatic failure, hyponatremia, hypocalcemia, hypomagnesemia, hypoxic encephalopathy
- ○ Stroke

- **Note:** An EEG may be needed to identify nonconvulsive status epilepticus or status epilepticus in a patient who requires therapeutic neuromuscular blockade.

MENINGITIS

Cerebrospinal Fluid (CSF) Overview

- CSF is produced in the choroid plexus (4th ventricle) and is absorbed by arachnoid villi.
- Normal CSF glucose is 60% of serum glucose.
- Normal CSF protein is 20–45 mg/dL protein.
- Normal LP pressure is 80–180 cm H_2O.

For this exam, you will need to know the signs of meningeal irritation and the differences between bacterial and viral meningitis (Table 8-6).

Table 8-6. Differences Between Bacterial Meningitis and Viral Meningitis

Bacterial Meningitis	Viral Meningitis
↑↑ Protein	↑ Protein
↓ Glucose	Normal glucose (60% of serum glucose)
↑↑ WBCs	↑ WBCs
Purulent CSF	Clear CSF
Opening lumbar puncture pressure > 180 cm H_2O	Opening lumbar puncture pressure is often normal

Signs of Meningeal Irritation

Both bacterial meningitis and viral meningitis have 1 or more signs of meningeal irritation:

Headache + nuchal rigidity + Brudzinski's sign + Kernig's sign

Nuchal rigidity

- Flex the patient's head to his or her chest; if pain and stiffness occur, the patient is positive for nuchal rigidity.

Brudzinski's sign (Figure 8-20 (A))

- Move the patient's chin to his or her chest; if the patient's legs come up, the patient has a positive Brudzinski's sign.

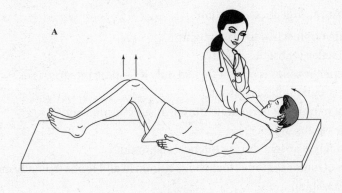

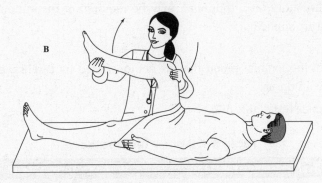

Figure 8-20. Brudzinski's sign (A) and Kernig's sign (B)

Kernig's sign (Figure 8-20 (B))

■ Move the patient's legs up and out; if doing so leads to pain in the neck and leg, the patient has a positive Kernig's sign.

Treatment: Administer antibiotics for bacterial meningitis.

BRAIN DEATH

Brain death is the complete, irreversible cessation of function of the cerebrum, cerebellum, and brain stem.

Determination of Brain Death

■ First, confirm the following:

○ Coma is irreversible and the cause is known.

○ Neuroimaging explains the coma.

○ The effects of any CNS depressant drugs are absent (as indicated by the toxicology screen).

○ No evidence of residual paralytics (verify that a twitch response is not present with peripheral nerve stimulation if paralytics were used)

○ Absence of severe acid-base, electrolyte, or endocrine abnormality

○ Normothermia or mild hypothermia (core temperature is ~ 36°C)

○ Systolic blood pressure is 100 mmHg or greater.

○ No spontaneous respirations

- Then, perform a clinical examination:
  - Pupils are nonreactive to bright light.
  - Corneal reflex is absent.
  - Oculocephalic reflex is absent (tested only if C-spine integrity is ensured).
  - Oculovestibular reflex is absent.
  - No facial movement to noxious stimuli at supraorbital nerve
  - Gag reflex is absent.
  - Cough reflex is absent during tracheal suctioning.
  - Absence of motor response to noxious stimuli in all 4 limbs (spinally mediated reflexes are permissible)
- Perform confirmatory tests (optional, may be required at institutions where "whole-brain" criteria are applied).
  - EEG
  - Absence of intracranial blood flow as demonstrated by cerebral angiography or a Transcranial Doppler
- Perform an apnea test (Table 8-7).

Table 8-7. Apnea Test Protocol

Apnea Test Prerequisites	When to Terminate the Test Early
Core temperature > 36.5°C SBP > 90 mmHg $PaCO_2$ > 35 mmHg Absence of drugs that could cause respiratory depression Preoxygenation prior to use of a ventilator; disconnection for 20 minutes at 100% PaO_2 may be normal or supranormal after the preoxygenation period	Spontaneous respiratory movements are noted SBP < 90 mmHg SpO_2 falls below 85% Unstable cardiac arrhythmias occur

☆ After 8–12 minutes, get an ABG, reconnect the ventilator, and interpret the test results.

Interpretation of Apnea Test Results

Apnea test is **positive**—supports brain death.

- Absent respiratory movements
- $PaCO_2 \geq 60$ mmHg or $PaCO_2 \geq 20$ mmHg over baseline

Apnea test is **negative**—does not support brain death.

- Respiratory movements are observed.

Apnea test is **indeterminate**.

- The test was terminated prior to achieving a $PaCO_2 \geq 60$ mmHg or a $PaCO_2 \geq 20$ mmHg over the baseline.
- $PaCO_2$ is < 60 mmHg or < 20 mmHg over baseline.

Management of Brain Death

- Provide support to the patient's family.
- Consider organ donation.
- If the patient's family consents to organ donation, and the patient meets donation criteria, assist the organ transplant team in maintaining hemodynamic support until the donation is complete.

GUILLAIN-BARRÉ SYNDROME (GBS)

Etiology

- An autoimmune response to a viral infection (parainfluenza type 2, measles, mumps, herpes zoster) is the cause of ~ 50% of GBS cases.
- A recent vaccination (flu shot) is the cause of ~ 15% of GBS cases.
- A recent surgical procedure is the cause of ~ 5% of GBS cases.

Clinical Features

- Demyelination of the lower motor neurons affects the spinal nerves and the cranial nerves.
- GBS results in **ascending** paralysis (of the feet, legs, diaphragm, or arms), which is usually symmetrical.
- A return of motor movement (of the feet, legs, diaphragm, or arms) occurs proximally.
- Diaphragmatic involvement may result in ventilatory failure.
- A lumbar puncture may demonstrate protein in the patient's CSF.
- No alteration in consciousness

Treatment

- Monitor:
  - Vital capacity for impending respiratory failure
  - Urine OP for urinary retention
- Intubation, mechanical ventilation for respiratory failure
- Corticosteroids
- IV immunoglobulin (IVIG) over 2 to 5 days
- Plasma exchange or plasmapheresis (if IVIG is not used) for 5 treatments—this is the complete exchange of plasma with the removal of abnormal circulating antibodies that affect the myelin sheaths; the removal of these antibodies will lessen the severity and duration of GBS.
- Monitor for dysphagia.

- Myasthenia gravis (MG) is an autoimmune attack of the neuromuscular junction, resulting in "grave muscular weakness."
- Clinical presentation:
  - Progressive skeletal muscle weakness
  - Early: easily fatigued
  - Later: paralysis
  - 70% of patients with MG have ocular dysfunction.
    - Ptosis, diplopia, difficulty keeping an eye closed
  - Dysarthria, dysphagia
- Myasthenia gravis crisis
  - Treatment of myasthenia gravis crisis depends upon which of the 2 types of crises the patient is experiencing (Table 8-8).

Table 8-8. Myasthenic Crisis vs. Cholinergic Crisis in Myasthenia Gravis

Myasthenic Crisis	Cholinergic Crisis
• Due to being undiagnosed/undertreated or due to an acute exacerbation • Deficiency of acetylcholine (an excitatory neurotransmitter)	• Due to being overtreated • Excess of acetylcholine

How are the 2 types of crises differentiated? The patient is given the Tensilon test (Table 8-9).

Table 8-9. Tensilon Test

Myasthenic Crisis	Cholinergic Crisis
Tensilon 2 mg IV ↓ Clinical improvement	Tensilon 2 mg IV ↓ Increased muscle weakness ↓ SLUDGE • Salivation • Lacrimation • Urination • Defecation • Gastrointestinal distress • Emesis

During the administration of the tensilon, the patient is asked to hold his or her arms out in order to detect weakness (Figure 8-21).

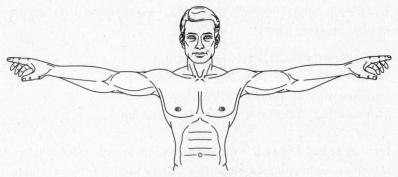

Arms raised to fatigue the muscles

Figure 8-21. Tensilon administration

Treatment

- Pyridostigmine (Mestinon)—an acetylcholinesterase inhibitor; it prevents cholinesterase from breaking down acetylcholine
- Corticosteroids, immunosuppressants
- Removal of the thymus gland
- Plasmapheresis
- IV immune globulin

Now that you have reviewed the key neurological concepts, go to the Neurological Practice Questions. Answer the questions, and then check your answers. Continue to review the information until you answer 80% of the practice questions correctly.

NEUROLOGICAL PRACTICE QUESTIONS

1. Which of the following statements about pupillary response is TRUE?

   (A) Pupil change is the first sign of an increase in intracranial pressure.
   (B) Sympathetic stimulation produces dilation of the pupil.
   (C) The optic nerve is responsible for pupil size.
   (D) Bilateral dilation of the pupil is an early sign of increased intracranial pressure.

2. Consciousness is dependent upon an intact:

   (A) reticular activating system (RAS) and cerebral cortex.
   (B) occipital lobe and midbrain.
   (C) medulla and meningeal artery.
   (D) cerebellum and pons.

3. A patient presented with a **left** cerebral hemispheric ischemic stroke. This patient would most likely have which of the following?

   (A) left Babinski reflex
   (B) eye deviation to the right
   (C) left homonymous hemianopsia
   (D) right pronator drift

4. Which of the following interventions would a nurse consider to be inappropriate for a patient with increased ICP?

   (A) maintaining the PaCO$_2$ level at ~ 35 mmHg
   (B) feeding the patient via a feeding tube
   (C) logrolling when turning the patient
   (D) administering 5% dextrose/water at 83 mL an hour

5. A patient has a history of a fall while skiing, hitting the right side of his head. He presented with a nose fracture, developed a sudden episode of emesis, and had a dilated right pupil followed by a decrease in his level of consciousness. Which of the following should the nurse anticipate?

   (A) emergent lumbar puncture to assess his pressure
   (B) emergent surgery for septal deviation
   (C) emergent treatment for uncal herniation
   (D) emergent treatment for a subdural hematoma

6. An examination of the CSF in bacterial meningitis will reveal all of the following EXCEPT:

   (A) cloudiness.
   (B) decreased glucose.
   (C) decreased protein.
   (D) increased pressure.

7. Five days after a subarachnoid hemorrhage, the patient experienced a decrease in her level of consciousness. The CT scan is negative for rebleed. This patient will most likely benefit from:

   (A) a trip to the operating room.
   (B) aggressive fluid administration.
   (C) a diltiazem (Cardizem) infusion.
   (D) an osmotic diuretic (e.g., mannitol).

8. A 71-year-old female presented with a possible stroke. She was responsive to verbal stimuli, her blood pressure was 180/110, and her pupils were equal and reactive. Her level of consciousness suddenly decreases. Upon examination of her eyes, the nurse notices that the left pupil is large and nonreactive to light. Her blood pressure is now 192/114, and her blood glucose level is 90 mg/dL. Based on this information, what has likely occurred?

   (A) Second (optic) cranial nerve compression has occurred.
   (B) The patient is having a hypoglycemic reaction.
   (C) Increased MAP (mean arterial pressure) has decreased the cerebral perfusion pressure.
   (D) Increased ICP has compressed the third (oculomotor) cranial nerve.

9. A 32-year-old is admitted with raccoon eyes. The nurse notices clear fluid draining from his nose. The most appropriate intervention would be to:

(A) tape rolled sterile gauze under his nose.
(B) insert a nasogastric tube to prevent vomiting.
(C) suction the nasopharynx as needed.
(D) insert nasal packing until the physician arrives.

10. A patient presented with a scalp laceration, a 6 mm depressed skull fracture, and no neurological changes. Which of the following is true regarding the care of this patient?

(A) The patient should be held for observation for 24 hours before being discharged.
(B) The patient may be discharged with instructions to return in 48 hours.
(C) The patient needs a prescription for antibiotic therapy.
(D) The patient needs immediate surgery.

11. A 53-year-old woman presents with complaints of "the worst headache I have ever had." The physician determines that she has had a Grade I aneurysm. Which of the following describes a Grade I aneurysm?

(A) minimal headache, no neurological deficits
(B) mild to severe headache, minimal neurological deficits
(C) stuporous, moderate to severe hemiparesis
(D) coma, decerebrate posturing

12. Which of the following is TRUE of brain tumors?

(A) Benign tumors cannot cause death.
(B) Steroids are contraindicated.
(C) Seizures are often an early symptom.
(D) Mortality has been dramatically reduced.

13. A nurse suspects brain death for a patient 3 days after he was admitted with hepatic encephalopathy. Which of the following is most definitive of brain death?

(A) coma
(B) absent corneal, cough, or gag reflexes
(C) positive Babinski
(D) posturing

14. Increased intracranial pressure may be caused by many disorders—ischemic or hemorrhagic stroke, traumatic brain injury, hypoxic encephalopathy, intracranial hematoma, tumor, and infection, among others. Which of the following would most likely prevent a further increase in intracranial pressure or a decrease in the cerebral perfusion pressure?

(A) maintaining the $PaCO_2$ between 25 mmHg and 35 mmHg
(B) maintaining neck flexion
(C) preventing/treating agitation/pain
(D) keeping the head of the bed flat

15. Priority interventions for a patient with a generalized tonic-clonic seizure with a normal serum phenytoin level include:

(A) turning the patient to the side and administering phenytoin (Dilantin).
(B) monitoring the seizure duration and assessing the level of consciousness.
(C) monitoring the seizure duration and inserting a bite block.
(D) turning the patient to the side and administering lorazepam (Ativan).

16. A patient has had a right hemispheric stroke. Which of the following clinical presentations is most typical for this patient?

(A) eyes deviate right, left homonymous hemianopsia, left-sided weakness, right pupil dilation
(B) eyes deviate right, right homonymous hemianopsia, left-sided weakness, right pupil dilation
(C) eyes deviate left, left homonymous hemianopsia, right-sided weakness, left pupil dilation
(D) eyes deviate left, right homonymous hemianopsia, right-sided weakness, left pupil dilation

17. Which of the following patients would most likely require neurosurgery?

(A) a patient with metabolic encephalopathy
(B) a patient with a subdural hematoma
(C) a patient with meningitis
(D) a patient with a basilar skull fracture

18. A patient has been diagnosed with Guillain-Barré syndrome and is anxiously asking numerous questions. Which of the following would be CORRECT regarding this diagnosis?

(A) A coma will be prevented with plasmapheresis.
(B) Weakness will occur on one side of the body.
(C) Guillain-Barré syndrome was most likely caused by a recent bacterial infection.
(D) The patient's lung vital capacity will be closely monitored.

ANSWER KEY

1. **B**	4. **D**	7. **B**	10. **D**	13. **B**	16. **A**
2. **A**	5. **C**	8. **D**	11. **A**	14. **C**	17. **B**
3. **D**	6. **C**	9. **A**	12. **C**	15. **D**	18. **D**

ANSWERS AND EXPLANATIONS

1. **(B)** The reason why an increase in ICP will eventually cause pupil dilation is that compression of the oculomotor nerve (on the side of the injury or pathology) decreases parasympathetic stimulation, which allows sympathetic stimulation to predominate, resulting in pupil dilation. Pupil changes occur AFTER a change in the level of consciousness (except for uncal herniation). The optic nerve is responsible for vision. Bilateral pupil dilation is a late (not early) sign of an increase in ICP.

2. **(A)** The lower end of the reticular activating system is in the brain stem and is responsible for the sleep-wake cycle. If the RAS is damaged, a coma will occur. The cerebral cortex is also responsible for consciousness. Choices (B), (C), and (D) are responsible for functions other than consciousness.

3. **(D)** Reflex, motor, and vision changes are contralateral to the injury or pathology. Eyes deviate toward the side of an injury. A pronator drift is a subtle, early sign of motor weakness.

4. **(D)** 5% dextrose/water is a hypotonic solution that will easily leave the vascular space. By osmosis, the solution will displace to the intracellular space, resulting in cell swelling (including brain cell swelling) and an increase in ICP. The other choices are all appropriate for a patient with increased ICP and will not make the ICP worse.

5. **(C)** This patient has signs of an epidural hematoma, most likely to the right temporal area, and possible uncal herniation. This is one neurological problem that causes pupil dilation BEFORE a sustained change in the level of consciousness.

6. **(C)** Protein is increased, not decreased, in bacterial meningitis. Cloudiness, decreased glucose, and increased pressure—choices (A), (B), and (D), respectively—are all typical of bacterial meningitis.

7. **(B)** The 2 major complications of a subarachnoid hemorrhage are rebleed and vasospasm. In this case, rebleed was ruled out. This patient most likely has vasospasm, and aggressive fluid administration is indicated. Choice (A) does not help vasospasm. Choice (C) may cause hypotension and is not indicated for cerebral vasospasm. A diuretic—choice (D)—will decrease vascular volume and may worsen vasospasm.

8. **(D)** Left pupil dilation is a sign of cranial nerve III (oculomotor) compression on the side of the pathology due to an increase in ICP. Choice (A), optic nerve compression, affects vision. Choice (B), a hypoglycemic reaction, would not result in pupil dilation. Choice (C), an increase in MAP, would increase, not decrease, the cerebral perfusion pressure (CPP).

9. **(A)** This patient most likely has a basilar skull fracture, which causes a meningeal tear with potential for CSF drainage from the nose (or ear). The CSF should be allowed to drain. Choices (B), (C), and (D) may be harmful.

10. **(D)** With a skull depression of 6 mm, the patient will require surgery to elevate the skull from brain tissue. The other three choices will not prevent the potential complications that might occur.

11. **(A)** This patient has signs of a subarachnoid hemorrhage secondary to an aneurysm. The Hunt and Hess scale score for a Grade I aneurysm is choice (A). Choice (B) is a Grade II. Choice (C) is a Grade IV. Choice (D) is a Grade V. This patient's prognosis, according to the Hunt and Hess scale score, is good.

12. **(C)** Seizures are often an early symptom of brain tumors. The other three choices are NOT truly related to brain tumors.

13. **(B)** A cough reflex, gag reflex (cranial nerve IX), and corneal reflex (cranial nerve V) are brain stem reflexes, and an absence of them reflects a loss of brain stem activity, all of which are present in brain death. While a coma is present in brain death, it represents a loss of function of the reticular activating system, which is higher than the brain stem. Babinski reflex and posturing are not present in brain death.

14. **(C)** When an increase in ICP is suspected, it is important to prevent anything that may worsen the ICP. Agitation and/or pain will further increase the ICP. The other 3 choices are not indicated when an increase in ICP is suspected or known. Choice (A), hyperventilation, may decrease the ICP by causing alkalosis and cerebral vasoconstriction. However, it will decrease the cerebral perfusion pressure. Choice (B) will prevent venous drainage from the head. Choice (D) will not optimize venous drainage from the head.

15. **(D)** Turning the patient helps to protect the airway and to prevent pulmonary aspiration. Lorazepam will help stop the current seizure. Choice (A), which includes the administration of phenytoin, is not an immediate priority. However, it will be given to prevent future seizure activity after the current seizure is controlled. Monitoring the seizure duration, as stated in choice (B), is correct. However, an assessment of the level of consciousness is not possible during a generalized tonic-clonic seizure. Choice (C) is not correct because an attempt to insert a bite block may cause more problems by displacing the tongue back and occluding the airway.

16. **(A)** Eyes deviate to the side of the pathology. Visual and motor problems occur opposite the side of the pathology. Pupil change occurs on the side of the pathology. The other 3 choices are not completely accurate.

17. **(B)** A subdural hematoma requires evacuation unless it is very small without clinical signs. Metabolic encephalopathy, meningitis, and a basilar skull fracture are all managed medically, not surgically.

18. **(D)** A patient with Guillain-Barré syndrome develops ascending, bilateral weakness/paralysis, which may affect the main muscle of ventilation: the diaphragm. Therefore, the patient's lung vital capacity is monitored regularly in order to identify impending respiratory failure. Choice (A) is not correct since a coma is not typical of Guillain-Barré syndrome. Choice (B) is not correct because weakness is bilateral, not unilateral. Choice (C) is not correct because a bacterial infection does not usually lead to Guillain-Barré syndrome. Viral infections have been associated with this problem.

Gastrointestinal Concepts

9

Luck is what happens when preparation meets opportunity.

—Darrell Royal

GASTROINTESTINAL TEST BLUEPRINT

Gastrointestinal 6% of total test　　　　　　　　　　　**9 questions***

→ Abdominal compartment syndrome
→ Acute abdominal trauma
→ Acute GI hemorrhage
→ Bowel infarction, obstruction, perforation (e.g., mesenteric ischemia, adhesions)
→ GI surgeries (e.g., Whipple, esophagectomy, resections)
→ Hepatic failure/coma (e.g., portal hypertension, cirrhosis, esophageal varices, fulminant hepatitis, biliary atresia, drug-induced)
→ Malnutrition and malabsorption
→ Pancreatitis

*The number of questions and percentages in this category may vary slightly from test to test.

GASTROINTESTINAL TESTABLE NURSING ACTIONS

☐ Monitor patients and follow protocols for procedures pre-, intra-, post-procedure (e.g., EGD, PEG placement)
☐ Intervene to address barriers to nutritional/fluid adequacy (e.g., chewing/swallowing difficulties, alterations in hunger and thirst, inability to self-feed)
☐ Recognize indications for, and manage, patients requiring:

   ○ Abdominal pressure monitoring
   ○ GI drains
   ○ Enteral and parenteral nutrition

Gastrointestinal concepts comprise approximately 6% of the Adult CCRN test blueprint with approximately 9 questions. Therefore, you will need to study these concepts for approximately 9 hours.

Although there will not be questions on abdominal anatomy, the Adult CCRN exam may have questions on physical assessment findings. The GI concepts are easier to follow if you have a good understanding of abdominal structures (Figure 9-1).

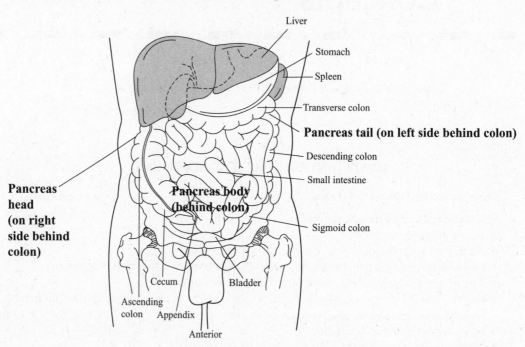

Figure 9-1. Anatomy of the abdomen

Midline Urinary bladder Urethra (female)	
Right Upper Quadrant Pylorus Duodenum Liver Right kidney and adrenal gland Hepatic flexure of the colon Head of the pancreas	**Left Upper Quadrant** Stomach Spleen Left kidney and adrenal gland Splenic flexure of the colon Body of the pancreas
Right Lower Quadrant Cecum Appendix Right ovary and fallopian tube (female) Right ureter and lower kidney pole Right spermatic cord (male)	**Left Lower Quadrant** Sigmoid colon Left ovary and fallopian tube (female) Left ureter and lower kidney pole Left spermatic cord (male)

- Acute GI hemorrhage may be divided into 2 broad categories: upper and lower.
  - ○ Upper GI bleeding accounts for approximately 80% of acute GI bleeding.
    - – Peptic ulcer disease (gastric, duodenal) ~ 50%
    - – Esophageal ~ 10–20%
    - – Stress ulcers
    - – Mallory-Weiss tear
    - – Cancer
  - ○ Lower GI bleeding accounts for approximately 20% of acute GI bleeding.
    - – Diverticulosis
    - – Angiodysplasia (AVMs)
    - – Tumor
    - – Radiation
    - – Colitis
    - – Inflammatory
      - • Crohn's disease
    - – Infectious
      - • *Clostridium difficile*
      - • *E. coli*
- Which has higher mortality? **UPPER**
  - ○ Seldom do patients with lower GI bleeding require admission to the ICU.

General Management of Upper GI Bleeding

- Address the CAUSE.
- Isotonic fluid resuscitation as for hypovolemic shock
- PRBCs
- Replace clotting factors (fresh frozen plasma, platelets).
- Medications
  - ○ Vasopressin constricts the splanchnic arteriolar bed, decreases portal venous pressure; watch for chest pain, ST elevation.
  - ○ Octreotide (Sandostatin) reduces splanchnic blood flow, gastric acid secretion, and GI motility.
  - ○ Osmotic laxatives (lactulose) remove nitrogenous materials (blood) out of the gut to prevent ammonia conversion; these are important to administer in the presence of liver disease.
  - ○ Beta blockers constrict mesenteric arterioles, reducing portal venous flow.

Esophageal Varices

- Common cause is portal hypertension secondary to liver disease.
- Venous drainage of the GI tract (Figure 9-2)

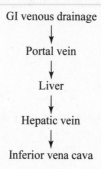

GI venous drainage

↓

Portal vein

↓

Liver

↓

Hepatic vein

↓

Inferior vena cava

Figure 9-2. Venous drainage of the GI tract

Liver cirrhosis prevents normal drainage through the liver. Pressure backs up into the esophageal vein, like "hemorrhoids of the esophagus."

TREATMENT OF ESOPHAGEAL VARICES

- General management as described previously
- Endoscopy procedure with banding or sclerosing of varices
- Esophageal balloon tamponade (Sengstaken-Blakemore tube)

  ○ A gastric balloon (200–500 mL) is attached to suction and empties the stomach.
  ○ An esophageal balloon (20–40 mmHg) is prescribed by the physician to control bleeding.
  ○ If the esophageal balloon is displaced up, the inflated balloon may occlude the airway.

  ☆ Cut the esophageal balloon if there is respiratory distress.

ACUTE PANCREATITIS

- The pancreas has both exocrine functions and endocrine functions.

Table 9-1. Exocrine Functions and Endocrine Functions of the Pancreas

Exocrine Functions	Endocrine Functions
Secretion of:	Alpha cells → secrete **glucagon**
Bicarbonate to neutralize stomach acid	Beta cells → secrete **insulin**
• H_2O	Delta cells → **inhibit** the secretion of glucagon and insulin
• Na⁺, K⁺	
• Digestive enzymes → trypsin, amylase, lipase	
Secretion ↑ by:	
• Parasympathetic stimulation	
• Ingestion of food (secretin and choleycystokinin)	

Acute pancreatitis is the diffuse inflammation, destruction, and auto-digestion of the pancreas from premature activation of exocrine enzymes. It is NOT usually caused by an infection!

- Up to 6 L of fluid may be secreted into the interstitial space.
- Activation of inflammatory mediators (cytokines, kinins, histamine, clotting factors)
- Results in systemic inflammatory response syndrome (SIRS)

  - ↑ Vascular permeability
  - Vasodilatation
  - Vascular stasis
  - Microthrombosis

Etiology of Acute Pancreatitis

- Alcoholism
- Obstruction (gallstones)
- Abdominal surgery
- Drugs
- Hyperlipidemia
- Trauma
- Infection (although it is seldom an infection)

☆ Pulmonary Complications of Acute Pancreatitis

- Atelectasis, left lower lobe
- Left-sided pleural effusion
- Bilateral crackles
- ARDS

Signs and Symptoms of Acute Pancreatitis

- Abdominal pain—boring
- Pain radiates to all quadrants and the lumbar area.
- Nausea/vomiting, rigid abdomen, no rebound tenderness
- ↓ or absent bowel sounds
- Low-grade fever
- ↑ WBC
- ↑ Amylase—peaks in 4–24 hours, returns to normal in 4 days.
- ↑ Lipase—stays elevated longer than amylase.
- ↓ Calcium
- ↑ Blood sugar

RATIONALE FOR THE SIGNS AND SYMPTOMS OF ACUTE PANCREATITIS

- Calcium is used up for auto-digestion, which precipitates hypocalcemia → Trousseau's sign, prolonged QT, seizures.
  - Trousseau's sign: during inflation of the blood pressure cuff, the brachial artery is occluded. The absence of blood flow, the patient's hypocalcemia, and subsequent neuromuscular irritability will induce **spasms of the muscles of the hand and forearm**.

- Beta cell injury → hyperglycemia, hyperosmolar hyperglycemic state (HHS)
- Phospholipase A is released → "kills" type II alveolar cells → ↓ surfactant → ARDS
- Pancreatic inflammation and capillary leak may block the pancreatic duct and cause left diaphragmatic lifting, left atelectasis, and/or left pleural effusion.

☆ Signs of Hemorrhagic Pancreatitis

- Cullen's sign—bluish discoloration and ecchymosis of the periumbilical area (Cullen's . . . umbilicus)
  - In acute pancreatitis, **methemalbumin** forms from digested blood and tracks around the abdomen from the inflamed pancreas; this is a sign of intra-abdominal bleeding.
- Grey Turner's sign—bluish discoloration of the flanks (**Turn**er's . . . turn the patient to see the flank)
  - Sign of retroperitoneal bleeding

Ranson's Criteria for the Severity of Acute Pancreatitis

- The more criteria present, the more severe the acute pancreatitis and increased morbidity (Table 9-2).

Table 9-2. Ranson's Criteria for the Severity of Acute Pancreatitis

At Admission	During the Next 48 Hours
Age > 55 years old WBC > 16,000/mm³ Glucose > 200 mg/dL LDH > 350 IU/L AST > 250 U/L	Hct decrease of > 10% BUN increase of > 5 mg/dL Fluid sequestration > 6 L Ca⁺⁺ < 8 mg/dL PaO₂ < 60 mmHg Base deficit > 4 mEq/L

☆ Treatment for Acute Pancreatitis

- Fluid replacement
- Calcium, K+, and Mg⁺⁺ replacement
- H2 blockers or proton-pump inhibitors (PPIs) to decrease the gastric pH
- NG suction to decrease gastric secretion
- Pain management, morphine
- Glucose control
- Enteral feeding below the duodenum
- ☆ Monitor for pulmonary complications:
  - ARDS
  - Elevation of the diaphragm and bilateral basilar crackles
  - Atelectasis (especially left base)
  - Left-sided pleural effusion

HEPATIC FAILURE

- Most common cause of **acute** hepatic failure → acetaminophen (Tylenol) OD, which may lead to fulminant hepatitis
- Most common cause of **chronic** hepatic failure → alcohol abuse

Hepatic Failure Lab Abnormalities

- ↓ Serum protein
- ↓ Serum albumin and ascites
- ↑ NH_3
- Pancytopenia (↓ WBC, RBC, platelets)
- Coagulopathies (↑ PT, PTT)
- ↑ AST, ALT, alkaline phosphatase, GGT
- ↑ Serum bilirubin
- ↓ Blood sugar
- Hyperventilation, respiratory alkalosis → ↑ lactate—metabolic acidosis
- ↑ Serum creatinine, BUN—late

Clinical Findings for Hepatic Failure

- Mental status change due to hepatic encephalopathy secondary to elevated NH_3
- **Asterixis** (a flapping hand tremor seen in hepatic failure) due to elevated NH_3
- Ascites due to low albumin and protein, risk of spontaneous bacterial peritonitis
- Jaundice due to elevated bilirubin
- Renal failure (hepatorenal syndrome)—not fully understood, but high mortality (~ 80%), usually due to bleeding or infection
- Sepsis (bacterial or fungal) due to decreased immune function
- The liver becomes enlarged/tender during the **acute inflammatory** state.
- The liver becomes non-palpable as hepatocellular necrosis progresses.

Stages of Hepatic Encephalopathy

- Stage I: Mild confusion, forgetfulness, irritability, change in sleep patterns, EEG is normal
- Stage II: Lethargy, confusion, apathy, aberrant behavior, asterixis, EEG is normal
- Stage III: Severe confusion, semi-stupor to stupor, hyperactive deep tendon reflexes, hyperventilation, EEG is abnormal
- Stage IV: No response to stimuli, posturing, positive Babinski, areflexia except for pathologic reflexes, EEG is abnormal

NOTE

Anything that increases the ammonia level causes hepatic encephalopathy and may ↑ ICP.

☆ Factors That Increase Serum NH₃ (Which Worsens Hepatic Encephalopathy)

- Hypokalemia: triggers ammoniagenesis in the kidneys (the mechanism is entirely unclear)
- ↑ BUN: breakdown of nitrogen
- ↑ Protein: breakdown of nitrogen
- ↑ Lactic acidosis: may be precipitated by the administration of Ringer's lactate—normally, it is converted into bicarbonate by a healthy liver (that is not the case in hepatic failure)

Management of Hepatic Failure

- Prevent anything that will increase the serum NH₃; attempt to decrease serum NH₃.

  ○ Prevent low K⁺ level, which worsens NH₃; use Aldactone (a potassium-sparing diuretic) to treat ascites.
  ○ Prevent ↑ BUN, which increases NH₃.
  ○ Prevent GI bleeding because a breakdown of protein in the gut increases NH₃.
  ○ Prevent acid buildup (lactic acidosis due to a low B/P and no administration of Ringer's lactate), which increases NH₃.

- Restrict protein **only** if hepatic encephalopathy is present.
- Administer clotting factors.
- Lactulose—for increased serum ammonia
- Neomycin—kills bacteria in the gut that produce NH₃

  ○ Complication of neomycin therapy—vitamin K deficiency
  ○ Bacteria (*E. coli*) in the gut help produce folic acid, riboflavin, and vitamin K.

- Adjust doses of medication that are metabolized by the liver.
- Monitor glucose.
- Administer acetylcysteine (Mucomyst) or Acetadote for **all** suspected acetaminophen ODs.

  ○ Give all doses if confirmed, not related to acetaminophen levels.

- Perform a close neurological assessment.
- Transjugular intrahepatic portosystemic shunt (TIPS procedure)

  ○ Procedure for select patients with cirrhosis to relieve esophageal varices or ascites
  ○ A complication of this procedure is hepatic encephalopathy—why?

    – The stent inserted during the procedure allows shunting of blood directly from the hepatic veins into the portal vein, **bypassing the liver** (which decreases portal hypertension but decreases detoxification of the blood).

- It might be necessary to decrease the diameter of the stent.

SPLEEN

Remember 2 concepts related to the spleen:

1. A patient with a history of a splenectomy has reduced immune function since the spleen is thought to "filter" the blood.
2. Signs of splenic rupture

   ○ Sharp left shoulder pain—**Kehr's sign** (diaphragmatic irritation causes referred pain)
   ○ Abdominal distension with absent bowel sounds

ABDOMINAL TRAUMA

Clinical Signs

- Ecchymosis over the left upper quadrant → soft tissue trauma or splenic injury
- Ecchymosis around the umbilicus (**Cullen's sign**) → intraperitoneal bleeding
- Ecchymosis of the flank (**Grey Turner's sign**) → retroperitoneal bleeding
- Left shoulder pain (**Kehr's sign**) → ruptured spleen (referred pain due to diaphragmatic irritation)
- Absence of bowel sounds with abdominal distension and guarding → visceral injury
- Bowel sounds in the chest → diaphragmatic rupture
- Free air in the abdomen as confirmed by an X-ray → disruption of the GI tract
- Diagnostic peritoneal lavage positive for blood → intra-abdominal bleeding

Intra-abdominal Hypertension and Abdominal Compartment Syndrome

ETIOLOGY

- Massive fluid resuscitation
- Trauma
- Emergent abdominal surgery

PATHOPHYSIOLOGY

- If pressure in the abdominal cavity becomes greater than the pressure in the capillaries that perfuse the abdominal organs, ischemia and infarction may result.
- Increased intra-abdominal pressure may result in reduced cardiac output, increased systemic vascular resistance, reduced venous return, and decreased renal perfusion.
- Affects multiple organ systems: cardiovascular, pulmonary, renal, liver, GI
- May occur without obvious clinical abdominal distension

DEFINITIONS

- Intra-abdominal hypertension (**IAH**) = intra-abdominal pressure (IAP) > 12–15 mmHg
- Abdominal perfusion pressure (**APP**) = the difference between MAP and IAP

    - APP 60 mmHg or > is associated with improved survival.
    - APP 50 mmHg or < is associated with increased mortality.

- Abdominal compartment syndrome (**ACS**) is a sustained IAP of > 20 mmHg, with or without an APP of 60 mmHg, and is associated with new organ dysfunction or failure.

ASSESSMENT

- Measure the bladder pressure; it most closely approximates the intraperitoneal pressure.
- Place the transducer at the level of the symphysis pubis to get an accurate pressure.

    - Physiologic compromise begins at a pressure of 12–15 mmHg.
    - A decompressive laparotomy should be considered if the pressure exceeds 20 mmHg.

TREATMENT

- For an IAP of 12 mmHg or greater:
  - Optimize the patient position by placing the patient in reverse Trendelenburg and maintaining head of bed elevation at 20 degrees or less.
  - Loosen constrictive clothing, dressings, and/or binders.
  - Manage pain and agitation.
  - Prevent overhydration.
  - Place a nasogastric tube to low intermittent suction to decompress the abdomen.
  - Optimize stool management, assess for impaction and treat, and consider a rectal tube or an enema.
  - Discuss with the physician whether gastro/colon prokinetic agents are appropriate for the patient.
- For an IAP ≥ 20 mmHg:
  - This is considered abdominal compartment syndrome.
  - Decompression surgery may be indicated.

BARIATRIC COMPLICATIONS

Complications of Bariatric Surgery

- Malabsorption—vitamin supplements are needed.
  - Vitamin deficiencies: protein, calcium, iron, B12, folate
  - Symptoms include vomiting, headache, diplopia, and memory loss.
- Wound-related
- Enteric leakage from anastomosis
- Gallstones—52% of patients who have had bariatric surgery have gallstones within 1 year.
- Bowel obstruction secondary to scar tissue or kink

BOWEL INFARCTION

Etiology

NOTE

The superior mesenteric artery provides arterial perfusion to the small intestine.

- Thrombus
- Hypercoagulability
- Arteriosclerosis
- Surgical procedure (aortic clamping)
- Vasopressors (endogenous or exogenous)
- Intra-abdominal infection

Pathophysiology

↓ Blood flow to the mesenteric vessels → prolonged ischemia → edema of the intestinal wall → full-thickness necrosis → perforation, peritonitis

Clinical Presentation

- Abdominal pain (periumbilical or diffuse), severe cramping
- Abdominal distension, vomiting
- Hypoactive or absent bowel sounds
- Fever, tachycardia, hypotension

Treatment

- Airway, breathing, circulation (ABCs)
- Fluids
- Gastric decompression (nasogastric tube)
- Treat pain
- Bowel resection with debridement of necrotic tissue
- Monitor for sepsis

BOWEL OBSTRUCTION

Tables 9-3 and 9-4 describe the types, etiologies, and clinical presentations of bowel obstructions.

Table 9-3. Types and Etiologies of Bowel Obstructions

Paralytic Ileus	Small Bowel	Large Bowel
Hypokalemia Abdominal surgery Peritonitis Intestinal distension Pneumonia Pancreatitis Opiates Sepsis (Paralytic ileus is usually transient)	Adhesions Hernia Volvulus Neoplasm (May be partial or complete, simple or strangulated)	Neoplasm Stricture Diverticulitis Fecal or barium impaction

Table 9-4. Clinical Presentation of Bowel Obstructions

Small Bowel	Large Bowel
Sharp, episodic pain Vomiting **early** (projectile and/or fecal) Hypokalemia High-pitched bowel sounds ($\uparrow$ early, $\downarrow$ late) KUB, dilated loops of gas-filled bowel	Dull pain Change in bowel habits Vomiting **late** Abdominal distension Low-pitched bowel sounds ($\uparrow$ early, $\downarrow$ late) KUB, dilated loops of gas-filled bowel

Treatment for Bowel Obstructions

- ABCs
- Prevent perforation (NG tube).
- Fluids/electrolytes
- Treat pain.
- Monitor for an infection or complications.
- Appropriate nutritional support (intravenous hyperalimentation or gut nutritional support via a feeding tube). If the gut is used, a feeding tube needs to be distal to the obstruction.
- Surgery
  - May or may not be needed
  - For a complete or strangulated small bowel obstruction (SBO), surgery will be done; if perforation has occurred, surgery will be done.
    - Lysis of adhesion, herniorrhaphy, reduction of volvulus
    - Bowel resection with debridement of necrotic tissue

BOWEL PERFORATION

Table 9-5 lists the etiology, clinical presentation, and pathophysiology of bowel perforations.

Table 9-5. Bowel Perforations

Etiology	Clinical Presentation
Peptic ulcer Bowel obstruction Appendicitis Penetrating wound Ulcerative colitis	Nausea Vomiting Fever, tachypnea, tachycardia Abdominal pain, tenderness that increases with coughing or with hip flexion Rigid abdomen, "boardlike" Rebound tenderness Bowel sounds are diminished or absent KUB, free air in the peritoneum may be seen
Pathophysiology	
Leakage of GI content into the peritoneal cavity → leakage of bacteria causes an infection, and chemical irritation causes inflammation of the peritoneum (peritonitis)	

Treatment for Bowel Perforation

- ABCs
- Gastric decompression (NG tube)
- Fluids/electrolytes
- Treat pain.
- Antibiotics, blood cultures

- Monitor for an infection and complications.
- Appropriate nutritional support
- **Surgery**
  - Repair of perforation; the patient may require temporary bowel diversion to allow anastomosis to heal.
  - Antibiotic lavage during surgery

See Table 9-6 for the differentiation of abdominal pain of select disorders.

Table 9-6. Differentiation of Abdominal Pain

Condition	Location of Pain	Quality of Pain	Associated Symptoms
Gastritis	Epigastric or slightly left	Indigestion	Nausea, vomiting May have hematemesis Abdominal tenderness
Peptic ulcer	Epigastric or RUQ	Gnawing, burning	Abdominal tenderness Hematemesis (gastric) or melena (duodenal)
Pancreatitis	Epigastric or LUQ May radiate to the back, flanks, left shoulder	Boring Worsened by lying down	Nausea, vomiting Mild fever Abdominal tenderness
Cholecystitis	Epigastric or RUQ May be referred to below the right scapula	Cramping	Nausea, vomiting Abdominal tenderness in RUQ
Appendicitis	Epigastric or periumbilical pain, later localizes to the RUQ	Dull to sharp	Anorexia, nausea, vomiting Fever, leukocytosis Diarrhea Rebound tenderness
Small bowel obstruction	Across the abdomen, in waves, tender to palpation	Cramping, severe, sharp	Distension, vomiting, hypokalemia, hyperactive to hypoactive bowel sounds
Ruptured spleen	Left shoulder (Kehr's sign)	Sharp	Abdominal distension, no bowel sounds
Peritonitis "acute abdomen"	Generalized, may become localized later	Dull initially; then intensifies and becomes worse with movement	Rigid abdomen, "boardlike" Rebound tenderness Bowel sounds are diminished or absent

Overview of Enteral Nutrition

- Use enteral nutrition (EN) for a critically ill patient who is unable to maintain volitional intake.
- EN is the preferred route of feeding over parenteral nutrition (PN).
- EN should be started early, within the first 24–48 hours following admission.
- Feeding should be advanced toward a goal over the next 48–72 hours.
- If a patient is hemodynamically unstable, EN should be withheld until the patient is fully resuscitated.
- In the ICU patient population, neither the presence or absence of bowel sounds nor the passage of flatus/stool is required for the initiation of enteral feeding.
- In the ICU setting, evidence of the resolution of clinical ileus is not required to initiate EN.
- Avoid bolus tube feedings in patients who are at a high risk for aspiration.
- Maintain an endotracheal tube cuff pressure > 20 cm H_2O and < 30 cm H_2O to prevent aspiration.

Advantages of Using Enteral Nutrition Rather than Parenteral Nutrition

- EN provides adequate metabolic support.
- EN maintains gut structure and function.
- EN prevents translocation of bacteria and gut toxins.
- EN is associated with fewer complications (infections, problems with catheter placement).
- EN is less costly and requires less monitoring.

Complications of Enteral Nutritional Therapy

- Inappropriate tube placement during insertion or maintenance
  - Esophageal placement: increased aspiration
  - Lung placement: pneumothorax, pneumonia
- Pulmonary aspiration despite appropriate tube placement (e.g., due to emesis or a loss of reflexes for airway protection)
- Digestive intolerance
  - High gastric residual volume—the definition of "high" has increased (see the gastric residual volume information later in this section).
  - Diarrhea
  - Constipation
- Tube obstruction

Enteral Nutritional Therapy Nursing Considerations

- Maintain a head of bed elevation of 30–45°.
- Use a variety of bedside methods to predict tube location **during** the insertion procedure:
  - Observe for signs of respiratory distress or misplacement into the lung.
  - Use capnography if available.
  - Measure the pH of aspirate from the tube if pH strips are available.
  - Observe visual characteristics of aspirate from the tube.
  - Recognize that auscultatory (air bolus) and water bubbling methods are unreliable.
- Obtain radiographic confirmation of correct placement of any blindly inserted tube prior to its initial use for feedings or medication administration.
  - The radiograph should visualize the entire course of the feeding tube in the gastrointestinal tract.
  - Mark the tube's exit site from the nose or mouth with an indelible marker immediately after radiographic confirmation of correct tube placement. Document the level of the tube exit site in the medical record after confirmation of correct placement.
- Check the tube location at 4-hour intervals after feedings are started.
  - Observe for a change in the length of the external portion of the feeding tube (as determined by movement of the marked portion of the tube).
  - Review routine chest and abdominal X-ray reports to look for notations about tube location.
  - Obtain an X-ray to confirm the tube position if there is doubt about the tube's location.
- Measure the gastric residual volume (GRV) every 4 hours.
  - If the GRV is greater than 250 mL after a second gastric residual check, consider a promotility agent.
  - A GRV greater than 500 mL should result in holding the feeding and reassessing the patient tolerance by using an established algorithm including a physical assessment, a GI assessment, an evaluation of glycemic control, minimization of sedation, and consideration of the use of a promotility agent if one has not already been prescribed.
  - Assess for abdominal distension/discomfort and/or nausea/vomiting.
- Use promotility agents to assist in timely gastric emptying; withhold for diarrhea.
- Dye should **not** be added to enteral feeding as a method for identifying aspiration of gastric contents.
- Provide free water as ordered in order to prevent dehydration.

Indications for Parenteral Nutrition (PN)

- If EN is not feasible or available over the first 7 days following admission to the ICU, no nutritional support therapy should be provided.
- For a patient who was previously healthy before a critical illness with no evidence of protein calorie malnutrition, the use of PN should be reserved and initiated only after the first 7 days.

NOTE

PN meets total nutritional needs but does not enhance anabolism as well as enteral nutritional support does.

- If there is protein calorie malnutrition at admission and EN is not feasible, initiate PN ASAP after adequate resuscitation.

> Now that you have reviewed the key gastrointestinal concepts, go to the Gastrointestinal Practice Questions. Answer the questions, and then check your answers. Continue to review the information until you answer 80% of the practice questions correctly.

GASTROINTESTINAL PRACTICE QUESTIONS

1. A patient is admitted after an assault with a tire iron. The nurse notices that the patient has a bluish discoloration to her left flank when turned to the side. This patient most likely has:

   (A) retroperitoneal bleeding.
   (B) hemorrhagic pancreatitis.
   (C) a ruptured spleen.
   (D) hypocalcemia.

2. A patient is admitted with acute epigastric pain that radiates to his back. He says he has been continuously vomiting for 12 hours, and his pain has been worsening. He reports drinking 2 six packs of beer a night. His lips are cracked, he has poor skin turgor, and his abdomen is distended and tender. He is restless and agitated. His vitals are as follows: his B/P is 90/50, his heart rate is 135 beats/minute, and his respiratory rate is 28 breaths/minute. When assessing the B/P, the nurse notices spasms of the patient's hand. This is indicative of:

   (A) hyponatremia due to overhydration.
   (B) metabolic acidosis due to hypoperfusion.
   (C) hypoalbuminemia due to protein loss.
   (D) hypocalcemia due to fat necrosis and calcium precipitation.

3. What is the most critical concern during the acute phase of care of a patient with an intestinal obstruction?

   (A) aspiration
   (B) hyperkalemia
   (C) hypovolemia
   (D) metabolic alkalosis

4. The following are complications related to the pathophysiological changes in acute pancreatitis EXCEPT:

   (A) hyperglycemia related to a beta cell injury.
   (B) hypercalcemia due to pancreatic auto-digestion.
   (C) ARDS related to a Type II alveolar cell injury.
   (D) left-sided atelectasis related to a left-sided diaphragm lift.

5. A patient with abdominal trauma and hypovolemic shock was stabilized. However, now hypotension has recurred, the patient's urine output has dropped, and the BUN and creatinine have increased. The nurse suspects intra-abdominal hypertension. Which of the following interventions would the nurse anticipate?

(A) Elevate the head of the bed to 45°.
(B) Remove the nasogastric tube.
(C) Measure the bladder pressure.
(D) Withhold opiates.

6. Which of the following is an appropriate intervention for a patient who is receiving enteral nutrition via a small-bore feeding tube?

(A) Maintain the head of bed elevation at less than 20°.
(B) Hold feeding if diarrhea develops.
(C) Assess the placement of the feeding tube with air insufflation.
(D) Mark the tube exit site with an indelible marker.

7. The following statements regarding hepatic failure are true EXCEPT:

(A) Alcohol abuse is the leading cause of acute hepatic failure.
(B) Pancytopenia may be a manifestation of the disease.
(C) A GI hemorrhage will increase the serum NH_3.
(D) The development of hepatorenal syndrome leads to high mortality.

8. A patient was admitted with generalized abdominal pain (that is dull in quality), diminished bowel sounds, and a low-grade fever. The patient now complains of more severe pain that is worse with movement. Upon examination, bowel sounds are absent, her abdomen is rigid to palpation, and her pain is less with palpation down than when released. Which of the following is a priority for the patient at this time?

(A) increasing the opiate dose
(B) surgery
(C) inserting a nasogastric tube
(D) antibiotic therapy

9. A patient with esophageal varices was admitted with hypovolemic shock secondary to upper GI bleeding. The following interventions related to the care of this patient are appropriate EXCEPT:

(A) preparing the patient for emergent surgery.
(B) ensuring that scissors are at the bedside if the patient has an esophageal balloon (Sengstaken-Blakemore tube) in place.
(C) administering lactulose if the patient has a history of cirrhosis.
(D) closely monitoring the patient's respiratory status and neurological status.

ANSWER KEY

1. **A**	3. **C**	5. **C**	7. **A**	9. **A**
2. **D**	4. **B**	6. **D**	8. **B**	

ANSWERS AND EXPLANATION

1. **(A)** The flank discoloration is indicative of Grey Turner's sign. The patient's history of trauma may lead to retroperitoneal bleeding. Although Grey Turner's sign may be due to acute hemorrhagic pancreatitis, choice (B), the patient's history indicates a traumatic etiology rather than pancreatitis. Grey Turner's sign is not a sign for choices (C) or (D).

2. **(D)** This clinical picture is one of acute pancreatitis. Hand spasms seen in this patient population indicate low calcium due to the precipitation of calcium secondary to auto-digestion. The other 3 choices would not result in hand spasms in the setting of acute pancreatitis.

3. **(C)** Sequestration of fluid from the vasculature to third spaces is a life-threatening phenomenon of bowel obstruction and is generally worse with small bowel obstruction. Although aspiration may occur if there is secondary abdominal distension, hyperkalemia and metabolic alkalosis are not associated with bowel obstructions.

4. **(B)** Hypocalcemia (not hypercalcemia) is a complication of acute pancreatitis. The other 3 choices are often a result of acute pancreatitis.

5. **(C)** The patient's history of trauma and his fluid resuscitation requirement, along with his cardiovascular and renal organ dysfunction, points to intra-abdominal pressure elevation. Measuring the bladder pressure, and comparing that pressure to the MAP, will help determine the appropriate therapy. The other 3 choices are not appropriate interventions for increased intra-abdominal pressure.

6. **(D)** The marking can be used as a reference for correct placement. Choices (A), (B), and (C) are not evidence-based practices related to enteral nutritional support.

7. **(A)** The leading cause of acute hepatic failure is acetaminophen overdose; alcohol abuse is the leading cause of chronic hepatic failure. Choices (B), (C), and (D) are all signs of hepatic failure.

8. **(B)** This clinical picture is one of peritonitis. Addressing the problem surgically will prevent increased morbidity. Although the patient may need the other 3 interventions, these will not definitively treat the urgent problem.

9. **(A)** Surgery is not indicated for esophageal varices. Rather, endoscopic procedures (banding, sclerosing) will address the cause more effectively. Esophageal balloon therapy may be used. If so, scissors should be at the bedside in order to cut the esophageal balloon in the event that it displaces upward and occludes the airway. Lactulose may be needed to move blood quickly through the bowel and decrease ammonia absorption. Choice (D) is indicated since aspiration and encephalopathy are possible complications.

Renal/Genitourinary Concepts

10

A dream doesn't become reality through magic; it takes sweat, determination, and hard work.

—Colin Powell

RENAL/GENITOURINARY TEST BLUEPRINT

Renal/Genitourinary 5% of total test   **7 questions***

→ Acute genitourinary trauma
→ Acute kidney injury (AKI)
→ Chronic kidney disease (CKD)
→ Infections (e.g., kidney, urosepsis)
→ Life-threatening electrolyte imbalances

*The number of questions and percentages in this category may vary slightly from test to test.

RENAL/GENITOURINARY TESTABLE NURSING ACTIONS

☐ Identify nephrotoxic agents
☐ Monitor patients and follow protocols pre-, intra-, and post-procedure (e.g., renal biopsy, ultrasound)
☐ Recognize indications for, and manage, patients requiring renal therapeutic intervention (e.g., hemodialysis, CRRT, peritoneal dialysis)

> Renal/genitourinary concepts comprise approximately 5% of the Adult CCRN test blueprint with approximately 7 questions. Therefore, you will need to study these concepts for approximately 7 hours.

RENAL ANATOMIC CONCEPTS

- The nephron is the functional unit of the kidneys, whose structure is complex.
- Each kidney has approximately 1 million nephrons, and each nephron has a vascular system and a tubular system (Table 10-1).

Table 10-1. Vascular System and Tubular System of a Nephron

Vascular System	Tubular System
Artery	Bowman's capsule
Afferent arteriole	Proximal tubule
Capillary (glomerulus)	Loop of Henle
Efferent arteriole	Distal tubule
Vein	Collecting duct

- If the blood pressure falls and renal perfusion is decreased, the compensatory response at the level of the nephron occurs (Figure 10-1).

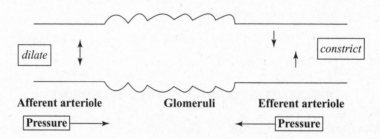

Figure 10-1. Renal arterioles

- The afferent arteriole DILATES, increasing flow to the glomerular capillaries, AND the efferent arteriole CONSTRICTS, decreasing flow from the glomerular capillaries.
  - These two mechanisms above result in an increased pressure gradient within the capillary bed.

- Any condition that prevents afferent arteriolar dilation or efferent arteriolar constriction interferes with this compensatory response.

PREVENTION OF ACUTE KIDNEY INJURY (AKI)

Prevention of AKI is of vital importance for the critically ill!

- Identify patient comorbidities that put the patient at an increased risk for developing AKI.

  - Diabetes
  - Heart failure
  - Hypertension

- Avoid potentially nephrotoxic substances as able, or monitor renal function more closely if nephrotoxic substances must be administered.

  - Antibiotics
  - NSAIDs
  - ACE inhibitors, ARBs
  - Antineoplastics
  - Contrast media
  - Diuretics, if overused, may result in vascular volume depletion.

- Carefully assess and monitor:
  - Fluid balance (especially in patients who present with signs of hypovolemia or who are being treated with diuretics)
  - Hemodynamics, hypotension
  - Renal function, labs
  - Urine output (decreased urine OP and the use of appropriate types and doses of medications)

Assessment of Fluid, Electrolyte, and Renal Function

LAB VALUES

- Serum blood urea nitrogen (BUN)
  - Measures the amount of nitrogen in the blood that comes from the waste product urea (formed in the liver)
  - Dehydration and shock may elevate BUN; therefore, BUN is not the best parameter for monitoring renal function or the glomerular filtration rate (GFR).
  - Normal BUN: 10–23 mg/dL
- Serum creatinine
  - Creatinine is a nonprotein waste product of creatine phosphate metabolism by skeletal muscle tissue. Most creatinine is removed by the kidneys.
  - Serum creatinine is a better indicator of renal function (GFR) than BUN.
  - Normal serum creatinine: males 0.8–1.4 mg/dL; females 0.6–1.1 mg/dL
- A 24-hour urine collection test for creatinine clearance (Cr. Cl.) is **the best indicator of the glomerular filtration rate (GFR)**.
  - The variables needed to calculate the 24-hour urine collection test for creatinine clearance include the urine creatinine, the serum creatinine, and the volume of the urine.

Glomerular Filtration Rate (GFR)

- GFR is the **volume** of plasma (filtered from the glomerular capillaries into Bowman's capsule) per minute.
  - Normal GFR is 125 mL/minute; this is the total blood volume filtered $\sim$ 60 times per day!
  - Normal urine volume is $\sim$ 1,000 mL/day, > 99% reabsorption of filtrate.
  - **Cr.Cl.** $= \dfrac{(140 - \text{age}) \times (\text{IBW}) \times (0.85 \text{ if female})}{72 \times \text{serum creatinine}}$
    - Note that IBW = ideal body weight in kg
  - The GFR is inversely related to the **serum creatinine** (NOT the BUN).
  - Only small molecules are filtered; the presence of large molecules (protein) in urine indicates glomerular damage.

NOTE

Do not memorize the creatinine clearance formula for this exam. However, be aware of the importance of the patient's age, sex, size, and serum creatinine when calculating the GFR.

- The urinalysis, spot urine test for electrolytes, and urine culture are also tests that are used to assess renal function.
  - Visual exam
  - Proteinuria: may be an early indication of renal disease
    - Normoalbuminuria = less than 30 mg/day albumin
    - Microalbuminuria = persistent excretion of albumin (30–300 mg/day)
    - Proteinuria = excretion of > 300 mg of albumin per day
    - Routinely assessing patients with diabetes for proteinuria is important in detecting **EARLY** diabetic nephropathy.
  - Normal specific gravity (SG) = 1.010–1.020
  - Spot urine Na^+: normal = 20 mEq/L
  - Urine culture/sensitivities are collected for select patients.
- Electrolytes: see Table 10-6 later in this chapter.
- Serum albumin: if it is low, there may be a decrease in oncotic pressure, increased third-spacing, and/or decreased vascular volume.
- Serum CK: extremely high CK is indicative of rhabdomyolysis (which is discussed in more depth in the Musculoskeletal Concepts chapter).
- ABGs: metabolic acidosis may be present if the patient is in intrarenal failure and has acute kidney injury due to an abnormal excretion of acids.

NOTE

A patient may have edema yet have intravascular dehydration.

Clinical Renal Assessment

- Flank pain: possible infection
- Bladder distension: obstruction
- Ultrasound: assesses the kidney size; checks for kidney stones and/or urine retention

Definitions Related to Types of Kidney Injury

NOTE

Do not memorize the RIFLE criteria for this exam. However, familiarize yourself with the categories.

- Acute renal failure, which is now often referred to as acute kidney injury (AKI), is an increase in serum creatinine by ≥ 1.5 times the baseline within 7 days.
- The stages of kidney injury are defined according to serum creatinine and urine output (Table 10-2).

Table 10-2. RIFLE Criteria for Kidney Injury

Stage	Serum Creatinine Criteria	Urine Output Criteria
Risk	Increase in serum creatinine (SCr) by 1.5 to > 2 times the baseline	UO < 0.5 mL/kg/h × 6 hours
Injury	Increase in SCr by 2 to > 3 times the baseline	UO < 0.5 mL/kg/h × 12 hours
Failure	Increase in SCr by ≥ 3 times the baseline	UO < 0.5 mL/kg/h × 12 hours or anuria × 12 hours
Loss	Persistent acute kidney injury for > 4 weeks	
End-stage kidney disease	Persistent acute kidney injury for > 3 months	

- In addition to the stages of the RIFLE criteria, acute kidney injury can be categorized as prerenal, intrarenal, and postrenal.

PRERENAL FAILURE

- Prerenal failure: perfusion to the kidneys is reduced (Figure 10-2 and Table 10-3), but there is no destruction of the tubular basement membranes.
- Prerenal failure is the most common type of acute renal failure and seldom requires hemodialysis.

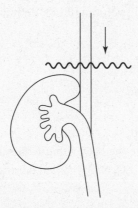

Figure 10-2. Illustration of prerenal failure

Table 10-3. Etiologies of Prerenal Failure

Impaired Cardiac Performance	Vasodilation	Intravascular Volume Depletion
Heart failure Myocardial infarction Cardiogenic shock Pericardial tamponade Dysrhythmias with low CO Acute pulmonary embolism	Sepsis Anaphylaxis Drugs (such as ACE inhibitors)	Volume depletion • Hemorrhage • GI losses Renal losses • Osmotic diuresis • Diuretic drugs
	Vasoconstriction	Volume shifts
	Pressors Compensatory response	• Burns • Pancreatitis • Ileus Inadequate volume replacement

Drugs That May Contribute to Prerenal Failure

- NSAIDs
  - ○ Block production of prostaglandins in the afferent arteriole → results in afferent arteriole constriction, ↓ inflow of blood into the glomerulus → GFR is ↓
  - ○ Prerenal failure can result with normal doses of NSAIDs, especially when associated with other renal risks (e.g., heart failure, sepsis, preexisting renal insufficiency).

NOTE

**Prerenal failure
can progress
to intrarenal
failure if it is not
corrected!**

- ACE inhibitors

  ○ Prevent the production of angiotensin II; the efferent arteriole will remain in a **dilated** state
  ○ Prevent the maintenance of adequate glomeruli pressure
  ○ May cause problems (such as heart failure and hypovolemia) for patients who are dependent upon efferent arteriole constriction to maintain adequate pressure within the glomeruli

Management of Prerenal Failure

- Correct the underlying problem, as able.
- Restore effective arterial blood volume (fluids) to maintain a MAP > 70 mmHg in order to improve renal perfusion.
- Wean pressors, as able.
- Improve cardiac performance.

  ○ Optimize preload/afterload.
  ○ Improve contractility.

- Control vasodilation: treat sepsis.
- Monitor the I&O and correlate the I&O with the daily weight for accuracy.
- Avoid nephrotoxic agents (ACEIs, NSAIDs) and contrast dyes; adjust drug doses in high-risk populations.

INTRARENAL FAILURE

- Intrarenal failure: destruction of the tubular basement membrane occurs (Figure 10-3 and Table 10-4).

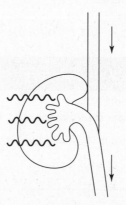

Figure 10-3. Illustration of intrarenal failure

Table 10-4. Etiologies of Intrarenal Failure

| Cortical | Medullary (ATN) | |
	Nephrotoxic (Often Nonoliguric, Better Prognosis)	Ischemic (Often Oliguric, Worse Prognosis)
Post-infectious (strep, hepatitis, varicella) Systemic lupus erythematosus (SLE) Vasculitis	Contrast dye Drugs (antibiotics, NSAIDs) Rhabdomyolysis Organic solvents	All causes of prerenal failure, postrenal failure Surgery (CABG, vascular, valve) Cardiopulmonary bypass Hypotension (sepsis, hypovolemia)

Contrast Medium Nephropathy

RISKS

- Pre-existing renal insufficiency
- Diabetes
- Dehydration
- Heart failure
- Older age
- Large doses of contrast material
- Use of NSAIDs
- Use of ACEIs
- Use of metformin

SIGNS

- Anuria
- Elevated BUN
- Elevated creatinine
- Fluid overload

INITIAL TREATMENT

- Diuretics; if there is no response, treat as intrarenal failure.

Prevention of Contrast Medium Nephropathy

- Evaluate the risks, and weigh the risks/benefits.
- Hydrate (with 0.9 NS) the patient before the procedure (1 mL/kg/hr) and after the procedure.
  - ○ Hydration is more important before the procedure than after the procedure.
  - ○ Hydration ↑ renal prostaglandins → improves renal medullary blood flow.
- Avoid drugs that may cause kidney injury.
- Decrease the volume of contrast media given.
- The use of acetylcysteine (before or after the procedure) is not shown to be effective in studies; this will most likely not be seen on the exam.

Rhabdomyolysis

Rhabdomyolysis may lead to intrarenal failure. Refer to the Musculoskeletal Concepts chapter (Chapter 15) of this book for more information on rhabdomyolysis.

Management of Acute Intrarenal Failure

- Maintain the fluid volume: monitor for fluid overload.
  - Administer loop diuretics; furosemide acts on the ascending limb of the loop of Henle to decrease sodium reabsorption and water reabsorption and to increase urine output.
  - The administration of furosemide may be able to "convert" nonoliguric renal failure to oliguric renal failure; however, furosemide will not resolve renal failure.
- Maintain a normal electrolyte balance: treat life-threatening electrolyte imbalances, especially hyperkalemia.
- Maintain a normal acid-base status: dialyze for extreme metabolic acidosis.
- Prevent uremia: dialyze early.
- Prevent infections: renal failure leads to weaker immune function (Note: Infections are the **HIGHEST CAUSE OF MORTALITY** in the population of patients who have renal failure).
- Address anemia: use packed red blood cells for extreme anemia; epoetin alfa (Epogen) is used for patients with chronic anemia.
- Prevent bleeding: platelet counts are normal, but platelet function is affected by renal failure.
- For drugs that may be nephrotoxic, use lower drug doses.
- Prevent malnutrition: do not restrict protein.
- Initiate dialysis as needed.

Who is most likely a candidate for dialysis? A patient who has any of the "AEIOU" criteria:

Acidemia
Electrolyte disorders (hyperkalemia)
Intoxication (methanol, ethylene glycol, aspirin*, lithium, theophylline)
Overload (heart failure)
Uremia (elevated BUN with associated mental status changes)

*Even if the admission GFR is normal, a salicylate (aspirin) overdose requires dialysis to PREVENT renal tubular damage.

Types of Dialysis Therapy

- Hemodialysis
  - Double-lumen central line access (temporary or permanent catheter)
  - Fistula access
  - AV graft access

- Peritoneal dialysis is not often used for the acutely/critically ill, but a patient may be admitted with peritoneal dialysis access.
- Continuous renal replacement therapy (CRRT)
  - Considered for certain patients with AKI
    - Hemodynamically unstable patients who cannot tolerate rapid fluid shifts that occur with intermittent hemodialysis are potential candidates for CRRT.
  - During CRRT, after the insertion of a double-lumen central venous line, the blood is continually passed through a filtration circuit via a machine to a filter where waste products and water are removed; replacement fluid is added, and the filtered blood is returned to the patient.

Differentiation of Prerenal Failure and Intrarenal Failure

- Occasionally, the patient history, clinical presentation, and labs do not clearly put the patient in either the prerenal (risk) category or the intrarenal (injury) category, and additional labs will need to be examined (Table 10-5).

☆ **Table 10-5. Differentiation of Prerenal (Risk) and Intrarenal (Injury)**

Laboratory Values	Prerenal	Intrarenal
BUN:creatinine ratio	20–40:1	10–15:1
Urine sodium	< 20 mEq/L	> 20 mEq/L
Urine concentration	Concentrated	Dilute
Urine osmolality	High (> 500 mOsm/kg)	Low (< 300 mOsm/kg)
Specific gravity	High (> 1.020)	Low (< 1.010)
Urinary sediment	Normal (Hyaline casts)	Abnormal (Cellular casts and debris)
Fractional excretion of sodium	≤ 1%	> 1%
Response to furosemide (Lasix)	> 40 mL/hr	No response

- When the BUN is elevated, look at the BUN:creatinine ratio.
  - A wide ratio (20–40:1) is usually associated with prerenal failure.
  - A narrower ratio (10–15:1) is usually associated with intrarenal failure.
- BUN:creatinine ratio examples:
  - BUN 90:creatinine 2.8 (prerenal)
  - BUN 50:creatinine 11 (intrarenal)
  - BUN 90:creatinine 9.5 (intrarenal)
  - BUN 70:creatinine 3.1 (prerenal)
  - BUN 108:creatinine 4.8 (prerenal)
- In general, when the renal tubules are still able to function, the urine sodium may be low (the renal tubules are able to hold onto sodium), and the urine osmolality is high (the renal tubules are able to concentrate urine).

- Postrenal failure accounts for 5–10% of the cases of AKI and is caused by any obstruction in the flow of urine from the collecting duct in the kidney to the external urethral orifice (Figure 10-4).
  - Examples: ureteral blockage (bilateral renal stones), urethral blockage (prostate stricture or benign prostatic hypertrophy), neurogenic bladder, or extrinsic source (tumor)

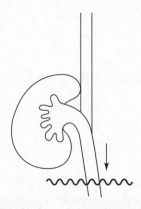

Figure 10-4. Illustration of postrenal failure

Treatment for Postrenal Failure

- Identify and correct the obstruction.
- Recovery of renal function is directly proportional to the duration of the obstruction.
- Generally, postrenal failure is the easiest renal failure to treat.

LIFE-THREATENING ELECTROLYTE ABNORMALITIES

The Adult CCRN test blueprint includes life-threatening electrolyte abnormalities. If you become familiar with the information in Table 10-6, you will be ready for these questions!

Table 10-6. Electrolyte Abnormalities

Electrolyte Problem	Signs/Symptoms	Causes	Treatment
Calcium (Ca^{++}): Normal is 8.5–10.5 mg/dL			

Hypocalcemia	Anxiety, irritability
	Twitching around the mouth
	Laryngospasm
	Seizures
	Chvostek sign (see below)
	Trousseau sign (see below)
	Torsades VT
		Acute pancreatitis
		Hyperkalemia
		Hypoparathyroidism
		Vitamin D deficiency
		Hypoalbuminemia
		Chronic renal failure
		Alkalotic states:
		  hyperventilation,
		  prolonged vomiting
		Massive infection of
		  subcutaneous tissues
			IV fluids, normal saline
			Calcium gluconate or calcium
			  chloride Vitamin D
			Correct the respiratory
			  alkalosis

Positive Chvostek sign (spasm of the lip and cheek)		Positive Trousseau sign (carpopedal spasm)	

Hypercalcemia	Lethargy, fatigue, altered
	  mental status
	DTRs decreased to absent
	Abdominal pain, constipation
	Muscle weakness
	Nausea/vomiting, "metallic"
	  taste
	Anorexia, weight loss
	Kidney stones
		Renal disease
		Hypokalemia
		Hyperparathyroidism
		Prolonged immobilization,
		  bed rest
		Malignancies
			IV 0.9 NS to promote diuresis
			Promote renal excretion with
			  furosemide; note: first rule
			  out hypokalemia
			Glucocorticoids, decrease GI
			  absorption of Ca^{++}
			Mithracin IV, calcitonin, or
			  etidronate; decrease Ca^{++}
			  release from bones

Potassium (K^{+}): Normal is 3.5–5.0 mEq/L			

Hyperkalemia	Muscle weakness; irritability
	Nausea, diarrhea
	Muscle cramps, pain
	ECG changes
	• Peaked T-waves
	• Widening of the QRS
	• Loss of P-waves
	• Bradycardia
	• PEA
		Renal failure
		Burns (early)
		Massive crush injuries
		Excessive potassium intake
		Metabolic acidosis
		Adrenocortical insufficiency
			Calcium chloride (or
			  gluconate), sodium
			  bicarbonate, insulin/
			  glucose, albuterol
			Elimination of potassium
			  intake
			Correct the acidosis
			Kayexalate
			Dialysis

Hypokalemia	Muscle weakness, ↓ reflexes
	Nausea, vomiting
	Paralytic ileus or abdominal
	  distension/gas
	Shallow respirations
	Mental depression
	ECG changes: ventricular
	  tachycardia, ventricular
	  fibrillation
		Diuretics
		Hypochloremic metabolic
		  alkalosis
		Acute alcoholism
		Uncontrolled diabetes
		Excessive perspiration
		Excess production of
		  aldosterone
		Cirrhosis
			KCl
			Correct the alkalosis by
			  replacing chloride
			IV lactated Ringer's
			Correct the hypomagnesemia

Table 10-6. Electrolyte Abnormalities (continued)

Electrolyte Problem	Signs/Symptoms	Causes	Treatment
Sodium (Na⁺): Normal is 135–145 mEq/L			
Hypernatremia	Classic signs of hypovolemic hypernatremia (thirst, tachycardia, orthostasis, and hypotension) may be present; dry, sticky mucous membranes may also be present Restlessness and irritability, later obtundation, stupor, coma	Insensible losses, dehydration Osmotic diuresis, mannitol Diabetic ketoacidosis (DKA) Hyperosmolar hyperglycemic state (HHS) Diabetes insipidus (DI)	Identify the cause, and evaluate the urine Na⁺ (the urine Na⁺ will be > 20 mEq/L if the patient is hypervolemic; the urine Na⁺ will vary with the other causes of hypernatremia) Correct slowly to prevent cerebral edema D_5W, 0.45 NS Sodium restriction Vasopressin for DI
Hyponatremia	Edema Fatigue, muscle cramps, weakness Abdominal cramps, diarrhea Lethargy, confusion, ↓DTRs Seizures, coma, brain herniation	Fluid overload: heart failure, cirrhosis Excessive water ingestion Excessive infusion of D_5W SIADH	If the patient is hypervolemic or euvolemic, water restriction Loop diuretics Treat dehydration with 0.9 NS Water intoxication: water restriction, avoid hypotonic fluids If acute, severe: 3% saline, small amounts
Magnesium (Mg⁺⁺): Normal is 1.5–2.5 mEq/L			
Hypermagnesemia	Decreased deep tendon re-flexes (DTRs), respiratory depression, respiratory arrest Bradyarrhythmias, hypotension Lethargy, coma Nausea/vomiting Flushing	Renal failure Magnesium-containing laxative abuse Magnesium-containing antacid abuse Iatrogenic OD	Stop magnesium substances Give calcium as for hyperkalemia Give furosemide as for hypercalcemia if renal function is OK The patient may need dialysis
Hypomagnesemia	Hyperreflexia (Chvostek sign, Trousseau sign) Ventricular arrhythmias, PSVT Sensitivity to digoxin Insulin resistance, hypokalemia, hypocalcemia, hypophospha-temia Agitation, confusion Impedes the correction of low K⁺	Chronic alcoholism (most common cause!) Vomiting, diarrhea, NG suction Malabsorption Post-CABG or acute MI DKA, HHS, hyperthyroidism Nephrotic syndrome Drugs: aminoglycosides, diuretics, ETOH, digoxin, cisplatin Malnutrition, enteral or parenteral feedings	$MgSO_4$, generally max of 1 gram/minute
Phosphate (PO₄³): Normal is 3.0–4.5 mg/dL			
Hypophosphatemia	Similar to hypercalcemia Lethargy, fatigue, altered mental status DTRs are decreased to absent Abdominal pain, peptic ulcers, constipation Muscle weakness, hypoventilation	Due to ↑ cellular uptake of phosphate with TPN administration ↑ glucose administration (TPN) Alcoholism	Oral or IV phosphate supplement
Hyperphosphatemia	Similar to hypocalcemia Anxiety, irritability Twitching around the mouth Laryngospasm Seizures	Due to ↓ renal excretion and/or renal failure	Phosphate binders: aluminum hydroxide (Amphojel, Basagel); calcium carbonate (Caltrate)

RENAL/GENITOURINARY PRACTICE QUESTIONS

1. A patient with acute kidney injury (AKI) has the following arterial blood gas: pH 7.32, $PaCO_2$ 35, and HCO_3 18. This acid-base abnormality is the result of the kidneys' inability to:

    (A) excrete the acid by-products of metabolism.
    (B) excrete carbon dioxide.
    (C) excrete bicarbonate ions.
    (D) excrete calcium ions.

2. Which of the following statements correctly describes a function of furosemide (Lasix)?

    (A) It acts as an osmotic agent, pulling fluid into the renal tubule.
    (B) It acts on the ascending limb of the loop of Henle to decrease sodium and water reabsorption.
    (C) It acts as an ADH antagonist.
    (D) It acts as an aldosterone antagonist.

3. What is the best lab test to evaluate a patient's glomerular filtration rate?

    (A) blood urea nitrogen (BUN)
    (B) serum creatinine
    (C) urine creatinine clearance
    (D) serum amylase

4. After a CT scan with contrast media, which of the following nursing interventions is most important?

    (A) ensuring adequate fluid intake
    (B) maintaining fluid restriction
    (C) providing extra doses of sodium
    (D) administering antibiotics

5. A 35-year-old man developed AKI after upper GI bleeding secondary to esophageal varices, in which he lost a great deal of blood. Which of the following lab results would he be expected to have?

    (A) low urine osmolality, high urine sodium concentration
    (B) high urine osmolality, high urine sodium concentration
    (C) low urine osmolality, low urine sodium concentration
    (D) high urine osmolality, low urine sodium concentration

6. A patient has a serum K⁺ of 8.8 mEq/L and has slowing of the heart rate with widening of the QRS. Which of the following would be an appropriate treatment for this patient?

   (A) Kayexalate enema
   (B) calcium gluconate, glucose, and insulin intravenously
   (C) lactulose by mouth
   (D) hemodialysis

7. A 17-year-old male patient, who sustained multiple traumas and subsequent multiple organ dysfunction syndrome, has a BUN of 60 mEq/L, a serum creatinine of 6.1 mEq/L, fluid overload, and blood pressure of 98/50 mmHg. Which of the following is the most appropriate treatment for this patient?

   (A) loop diuretics
   (B) hemodialysis
   (C) peritoneal dialysis
   (D) continuous renal replacement therapy (CRRT)

ANSWER KEY

1. **A**   3. **C**   5. **D**   7. **D**
2. **B**   4. **A**   6. **B**

ANSWERS AND EXPLANATIONS

1. **(A)** When the body accumulates H^+, the bicarbonate drops (HCO_3 18) in an attempt to neutralize the acid. The excretion of carbon dioxide is not the problem as evidenced by the normal $PaCO_2$. The excretion of bicarbonate ions is not the problem; this would be evidenced by an elevated bicarbonate level. The scenario described does not address calcium ions.

2. **(B)** Furosemide (Lasix) acts on the ascending limb of the loop of Henle (remember **L**asix, **l**oop). A decrease in sodium and water reabsorption leads to diuresis. Furosemide is not an osmotic agent. Instead, mannitol acts in this manner. Furosemide does not act as an ADH antagonist or as an aldosterone antagonist.

3. **(C)** Urine creatinine clearance best reflects the glomerular filtration rate (GFR) or tubular function. BUN may be altered by volume depletion, and serum amylase does not reflect renal function. Although serum creatinine is needed to calculate the GFR and is a better reflection of tubular function than BUN, it does not take into account the variables that urine creatinine clearance includes.

4. **(A)** Exposure to the contrast media that is used for this test can cause contrast media nephropathy in patients who have risk factors for the development of contrast media nephropathy. An increase in fluid (especially prior to the CT scan) has been shown to prevent renal damage. The other three choices either increase the chance of nephropathy or do not prevent it.

5. **(D)** This patient had volume depletion secondary to upper GI bleeding and most likely is experiencing prerenal failure. Initially, volume depletion will result in acute prerenal failure, yet the basement membranes of the renal tubules are not affected (intrarenal failure). In the presence of prerenal failure, the renal tubules can still concentrate urine and hold onto sodium. Choice (A) is seen in intrarenal failure. The other 2 choices are not typical of any renal problem.

6. **(B)** Calcium will stabilize the cell membranes. Insulin will drive potassium into the intracellular space, thereby decreasing the serum potassium. Kayexalate (choice (A)) and hemodialysis (choice (D)) will decrease the total body potassium but will take hours. Lactulose (choice (C)) does not decrease serum potassium; it decreases NH_3.

7. **(D)** This patient has acute renal failure with hemodynamic instability. CRRT is less likely than hemodialysis to worsen the patient's hemodynamic status. The other 2 choices have not been shown to improve the outcome of acute renal failure.

Endocrine Concepts

11

You've got to do your own growing no matter how tall your grandfather was.

—Irish saying

ENDOCRINE TEST BLUEPRINT

Endocrine 5% of total test   7 questions*

→ Adrenal insufficiency
→ Diabetes insipidus (DI)
→ Diabetes mellitus, types 1 and 2
→ Diabetic ketoacidosis (DKA)
→ Hyperglycemia
→ Hyperosmolar hyperglycemic state (HHS)**
→ Hyperthyroidism
→ Hypoglycemia (acute)
→ Hypothyroidism
→ SIADH

*The number of questions and percentages in this category may vary slightly from test to test.

**Also referred to as hyperglycemic hyperosmolar nonketotic (HHNK) syndrome

---

ENDOCRINE TESTABLE NURSING ACTIONS

☐ Identify and monitor normal and abnormal diagnostic test results
☐ Implement treatment modalities for acute hypoglycemia/hyperglycemia (e.g., insulin therapy)
☐ Manage patients who are receiving medications and monitor response
☐ Recognize normal and abnormal physical assessment findings
☐ Recognize the signs and symptoms of endocrine emergencies, initiate interventions, and seek assistance as needed

Endocrine concepts comprise approximately 5% of the Adult CCRN test blueprint with approximately 7 questions. Therefore, you will need to study these concepts for approximately 7 hours.

Serum Osmolality

- Endocrine problems often result in serum osmolality (osmo) abnormalities; therefore, a general knowledge of the regulation of serum osmolality is needed for this exam.
- Osmolality of body fluids: the measure of the number of particles in a solution
    - Expressed as milliosmoles.
    - Normal osmolality of body fluids is 275–295 mOsm/kg.
    - Hypo-osmolar is < 275 mOsm/kg.
    - Hyperosmolar is > 295 mOsm/kg.
- Cell membranes are permeable to water; therefore, serum osmo will affect the intracellular fluid (ICF) osmo.
- Upon examination of the equation for calculating the serum osmolality, note that serum sodium, BUN, and glucose each play a role:

$$2(Na^+) + \frac{BUN}{5} + \frac{Glucose}{20} = 275-295 \text{ mOsm/kg}$$

- According to this formula, an increase in the serum sodium, BUN, and/or glucose will **increase** the serum osmolality.

TIP

Do not memorize this equation for the exam, but be aware of the variables that affect osmolality.

Hypothalamus

- The hypothalamus (via the pituitary gland) is the endocrine "monitoring center" and regulates:
    - Temperature
    - Intake drives
    - Autonomic nervous system (sympathetic/parasympathetic)
- Only the pancreas and the parathyroid gland release hormones that are not controlled by the hypothalamus.

Antidiuretic Hormone (ADH) Imbalances

- ADH is formed in the hypothalamus.
- ADH is stored in the posterior pituitary.
- ADH works on the distal convoluted tubules and the collecting tubules of the kidneys to reabsorb water (which prevents diuresis).
- ADH concentrates urine.

    - Normal urine specific gravity (SG) is 1.010–1.020.
    - Urine SG that is 1.005 or less is considered dilute urine/a low SG.
    - Urine SG that is 1.030 or greater is considered concentrated urine/an elevated SG.

SYNDROME OF INAPPROPRIATE ADH (SIADH)

The pathophysiology of SIADH is shown in Figure 11-1.

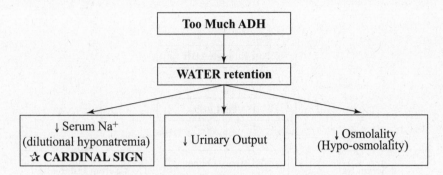

Figure 11-1. Pathophysiology of SIADH

Etiology of SIADH

- Oat cell carcinoma
- Viral pneumonia ⟩ Most Common
- Head problems
- Increased osmolality, anesthesia, analgesia, stress
- Thiazide diuretics (especially for the elderly)
- ☆ What is the biggest danger of hyponatremia? **SEIZURE!**

Treatment for SIADH

- Address the etiology:
  - ○ Oat cell carcinoma
  - ○ Viral pneumonia
  - ○ Head problems
- Fluid restriction
- 3% saline (generally reserved for a serum Na$^+$ less than 120 mEq/L)
- Administer phenytoin (Dilantin) → inhibits ADH secretion
- NO hypotonic solutions or free water

The pathophysiology of diabetes insipidus (DI) is described in Figure 11-2.

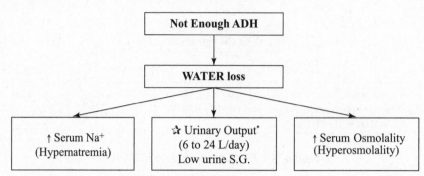

Figure 11-2. Pathophysiology of DI

☆ *DILUTE** urine with a specific gravity (SG) of 1.001–1.005.

Etiology of DI

- Head problems (surgery, trauma)
- Phenytoin (Dilantin)

Complication of DI

- Hypovolemia, hypovolemic shock

Treatment of DI

- Give ADH (Pitressin, DDAVP); use cautiously in those with heart disease, since ADH may cause coronary artery ischemia.
- Give fluids to replenish the intravascular volume.
- Monitor the urinary output/specific gravity.

DIABETIC KETOACIDOSIS (DKA) AND HYPEROSMOLAR HYPERGLYCEMIC STATE (HHS)

- Diabetic ketoacidosis (DKA) and hyperosmolar hyperglycemic state (HHS) are included in the Adult CCRN test blueprint. The best way to prepare for questions related to these 2 problems is to compare and contrast them (Table 11-1).

☆ Table 11-1. Comparison of DKA and HHS

	DKA	HHS
Etiologies	Younger age History of type 1 diabetes New onset of type 1 diabetes Infection Stress Noncompliance	Older age Type 2 diabetes Pancreatitis Total parenteral nutrition (TPN) Medications (steroids, thiazide diuretics, phenytoin, atypical antipsychotics)
Blood sugar	> 250 mg/dL	> 600 mg/dL
Develops	Rapidly over 1–2 days (no insulin production)	Slowly over 5–7 days (still making some insulin)
Fluid loss	4–6 L	6–9 L
Insulin production	No	Yes, but inadequate
Acidosis	Yes	No
Serum ketones	Positive, with high levels	Negative or positive, with low levels
Serum osmolality	Normal or high	> 320 mOsm/kg
Breathing pattern	Kussmaul	Rapid, shallow
Treatment	Insulin, fluids 0.9 saline, or, if the sodium is high and the B/P is normal or high, use 0.45 saline Decrease the blood sugar by 50–100 mg/dL/hour Add dextrose to the IV fluids after the serum glucose reaches ~ 250 mg/dL Continue the insulin infusion until the acidosis is resolved	Fluids, insulin 0.9 saline Decrease the blood sugar by 50–100 mg/dL/hour Add dextrose to the IV fluids after the serum glucose reaches ~ 300 mg/dL
Serum K^+	Elevated K^+ in the presence of acidosis, although the total body potassium is low (see Table 11-2); serum K^+ decreases as the acidosis is corrected	Often elevated due to insulin deficiency

- In a state of metabolic acidosis, hydrogen ions (H^+) move into the intracellular space. In exchange, potassium leaves the intracellular space. The movement of K^+ into the extracellular space results in hyperkalemia, yet the total body K^+ has not increased.

- For every 0.1 decrease in pH, the serum K^+ will increase by 0.6 mEq/L (Table 11-2).

**Table 11-2. Arterial pH and K^+ Relationship
in the Presence of Acidosis**

pH	K^+
7.4	4.0
7.3	4.6
7.2	5.2
7.1	5.8
7.0	6.4

- If the pH is 7.2 and the serum K^+ is 4.0, the total body K^+ (intracellular K^+ and serum K^+) is too low, resulting in total body relative hypokalemia!
- For a patient with DKA, there may be total body hypokalemia due to diuresis, which occurred as a result of elevated blood sugar.

ACUTE HYPOGLYCEMIA

Etiology of Acute Hypoglycemia

- Insulin (if the dose of insulin was more than what is necessary for body requirements)
- Oral hypoglycemic agents (if the dose of the oral agent was more than what is necessary for body requirements or if the dose was not adjusted as renal insufficiency developed)
- Increase in physical activity for diabetics, which may ↑ the utilization of glucose
- Sepsis (the process by which sepsis causes acute hypoglycemia is not well understood)
- Beta blockers mask the early signs of hypoglycemia (for Type 1 diabetics).

Table 11-3. Signs/Symptoms of Hypoglycemia

Initial Signs/Symptoms (Due to the sympathetic effects of adrenaline release in an attempt to raise the level of glucose)	Later Signs/Symptoms (Due to a lack of glucose in the brain)
Tachycardia	Confusion
Palpitations	Lethargy
Diaphoresis	Slurred speech
Irritability	Seizure
Restlessness	Coma

☆ **Note:** If a diabetic patient becomes hypoglycemic and is receiving beta-adrenergic blocking agents, the initial signs of hypoglycemia may be masked. The patient's first signs of hypoglycemia will be the later signs. You need to be aware of this, especially for patients with Type 1 diabetes.

Treatment for Hypoglycemia

- Complex carbohydrates by mouth
- 50% dextrose if the patient is unable to take oral carbohydrates (intravenous 50% dextrose may irritate the vein)
- 10% dextrose infusion for refractory hypoglycemia

- Glucagon 1 mg IM

  - Decreases GI motility
  - Monitor for nausea/vomiting: position the patient on his or her side in order to prevent aspiration.

ACUTE ADRENAL INSUFFICIENCY/CRISIS

Overview

- The adrenal glands produce cortisol (both glucocorticoid and mineralocorticoid). Adrenal crisis may develop due to acute insufficiency of these adrenal hormones.
- Acute adrenal insufficiency may be life-threatening.
- Chronic adrenal insufficiency may be seen in the presence of Addison's disease.
- Etiology of adrenal insufficiency/crisis—sepsis, trauma, head injury, medications (ketoconazole, phenytoin, rifampin, mitotane, the abrupt withdrawal of corticosteroids), acute physical stress, and/or inadequate medical treatment for someone with known Addison's disease
- Clinical presentation of adrenal insufficiency/crisis—altered mental status, weakness, severe hypotension, nausea/vomiting, fever, and/or abdominal pain
- Lab findings for adrenal insufficiency/crisis—hypoglycemia, hyponatremia, hyperkalemia, hypercalcemia, and/or low blood ACTH and cortisol (drawn PRIOR to treatment with steroids)
- A patient with suspected adrenal insufficiency/crisis will need a CT scan of the abdomen to rule out adrenal hemorrhage or calcification of the adrenal glands; the patient may also require a head CT to assess the pituitary gland.

Treatment for Adrenal Crisis

Rapid identification of the condition and treatment are the keys to a positive outcome.

- Fluids and glucocorticoid replacement

  - Normal saline or 5% dextrose in normal saline (if the patient is hypoglycemic), using the volume status and urine output to guide resuscitation
- Steroids

  - If the patient does not have a history of adrenal insufficiency, give dexamethasone (4 mg IV bolus); do not use hydrocortisone until testing (to rule out underlying adrenal insufficiency) is completed.

    - The patient will also need an ACTH stimulation test after he or she is stabilized.
  - If the patient has known adrenal insufficiency, give hydrocortisone (100 mg IV bolus).
  - Administer vasopressors if the patient's blood pressure is not responsive to fluids.

Hyperthyroidism and hypothyroidism are included in the most recent Adult CCRN test blueprint. There are 2 thyroid emergencies related to thyroid dysfunction: thyroid crisis (storm) and myxedema coma (severe hypothyroidism).

- **Thyroid crisis (storm)** occurs in patients with known hyperthyroid disease, in which there is increased action of the T3 and T4 hormones, resulting in a life-threatening emergency.
  - Etiologies include an infection, DKA, complications during labor and delivery, seizure disorder, radioactive iodine treatment or iodinated contrast dyes, multinodular goiter, poor compliance with antithyroid therapy, and/or thyroxine overdose.
  - Medications that may precipitate a thyroid storm include amiodarone, an ASA overdose, cytotoxic chemotherapy, insulin, lithium, thiazide diuretics, and/or tricyclic antidepressants.

- **Myxedema coma (severe hypothyroidism)** occurs in patients with known hypothyroid disease and results from a severe deficiency of thyroid hormones, creating a life-threatening emergency.
  - Etiologies include sepsis, stroke, heart failure, trauma or other physical stress, and/or a discontinuation of or inadequate dose of thyroid medication.
  - Medications that may precipitate myxedema coma include amiodarone, anesthetics, depressants, diuretics, lithium, narcotics, and/or phenytoin.

- The signs/symptoms and treatment of thyroid storm and myxedema coma are summarized in Table 11-4 and Table 11-5, respectively.

Table 11-4. Differentiation of the Signs/Symptoms of Thyroid Storm and Myxedema Coma

Thyroid Storm	Myxedema Coma

■ Altered mental status: confusion, psychosis, paranoia, coma
■ Hyperkinesis, tremor, agitation
■ Fever; warm, moist, flushed skin
■ Tachycardia
■ Tachypnea
■ Enlarged neck, goiter
■ Lab abnormalities
 	
  ○ ↑ total T3, T4 and ↑ free T3, T4; ↓ TSH
  ○ ↑ LDH, ↑ bilirubin
	■ Altered LOC, disorientation, poor memory, depression, coma
	■ Delayed deep tendon reflexes
	■ Hypothermia
	■ Bradycardia
	■ Slow, shallow respirations
	■ Macroglossia, vocal cord edema
	■ Lab abnormalities
	
	  ○ ↑ TSH; ↓ T3 and T4
	  ○ ↑ LDH, ↑ CK
	  ○ Anemia
	  ○ Respiratory acidosis, hypoxemia

Table 11-5. Treatment for Thyroid Storm and Myxedema Coma

Thyroid Storm	Myxedema Coma
<ul><li>Begin cooling, prevent shivering</li><li>IV fluids/electrolytes</li><li>Plasmapheresis, therapeutic plasma exchange</li><li>Medications<ul><li>Propylthiouracil (stops thyroid hormone synthesis)</li><li>Iodine or lithium (block thyroid hormone release)</li><li>Propranolol</li><li>Acetaminophen for a fever (do not administer ASA, which inhibits the binding of T3 and T4, thereby increasing T3 and T4)</li><li>Glucocorticoids</li></ul></li></ul>	<ul><li>Begin rewarming</li><li>Support the airway and provide ventilation as needed</li><li>Prevent infections</li><li>Administer (slowly) 3% saline for severe hyponatremia</li><li>Medications<ul><li>Levothyroxine (Synthroid) IV</li><li>Glucocorticoids if the patient is hypotensive despite adequate fluid resuscitation</li></ul></li><li>Rule out adrenal crisis (which may be masked by hypothyroidism)</li></ul>

Now that you have reviewed the key endocrine concepts, go to the Endocrine Practice Questions. Answer the questions, and then check your answers. Continue to review the information until you answer 80% of the practice questions correctly.

ENDOCRINE PRACTICE QUESTIONS

1. A patient was admitted with a blood sugar level of 450 mg/dL, a potassium level of 4.5 mEq/L, and an initial pH of 7.15. She received an insulin loading dose and an infusion of 2 L of normal saline. Now her blood sugar level is 215 mg/dL, and the pH is 7.32. Which of the following actions would be appropriate at this time?

(A) Change the IV solution to lactated Ringer's.
(B) Add potassium to the IV solution.
(C) Administer sodium bicarbonate.
(D) Increase the insulin infusion.

For questions 2 and 3

A post-op craniotomy patient began having an hourly urine output of 400–500 mL/hour, a serum glucose level of 100 mg/dL, a B/P of 100/68, a heart rate of 102 beats/minute, and a respiratory rate of 22 breaths/minute.

2. Which of the following lab results would you expect for this patient?

   (A) a serum osmolality of 265 mOsm/kg
   (B) a specific gravity of 1.030 and an Na$^+$ of 120 mEq/L
   (C) a serum osmolality of 280 mOsm/kg
   (D) a specific gravity of 1.001 and an Na$^+$ of 151 mEq/L

3. The IV solution that is most appropriate at this time for the patient described is:

   (A) lactated Ringer's.
   (B) 5% dextrose in water.
   (C) normal saline.
   (D) 10% dextrose in water.

_____

4. A 64-year-old female patient was admitted with a new-onset seizure that she had at home. She has a history of oat cell carcinoma of the lung, for which she had treatment over the past 6 months. A CT scan of the head was negative; additional findings included an Na$^+$ level of 116 mEq/L, a K$^+$ level of 3.9 mEq/L, a urine output of 25 mL/hour, a serum osmolality of 260 mOsm/kg, and a urine specific gravity of 1.030. Which of the following interventions is indicated for this patient?

   (A) Restrict free water.
   (B) Administer NSAIDs.
   (C) Administer 0.45 normal saline fluid boluses.
   (D) Administer Pitressin.

5. A 25-year-old male with Type 1 diabetes developed generalized weakness, palpitations, diaphoresis, and confusion after completing a 10K race. His wife stated that his diabetes had been controlled on the same dose of insulin for more than 1 year. This patient will most likely need:

   (A) insulin.
   (B) phenytoin (Dilantin).
   (C) 50% dextrose.
   (D) a beta blocker.

6. Which of the following findings would be expected for a patient with HHS?

   (A) a pH of 7.15
   (B) a urine specific gravity of 1.030
   (C) a K$^+$ level of 6.1 mEq/L
   (D) a serum osmolality of 270 mOsm/kg

7. A diabetic patient with hypoglycemia is most likely to present with a coma if the patient is also receiving which of the following?

(A) glipizide (Glucotrol)
(B) phenytoin (Dilantin)
(C) hydrochlorothiazide
(D) metoprolol (Lopressor)

8. A female patient with a history of heart failure and thyroid disease was admitted with acute exacerbation of heart failure. Three days after she was admitted, she developed a decreased level of consciousness, bradycardia, and hypothermia secondary to a thyroid emergency. Based on this situation, the nurse should anticipate initiating:

(A) propylthiouracil.
(B) iodine.
(C) levothyroxine (Synthroid) IV.
(D) a diuretic.

9. A patient was treated for septic shock secondary to necrotizing fasciitis. He initially responded well to therapy with fluids and a norepinephrine (Levophed) infusion, but he is now hypotensive despite appropriate antibiotic therapy, fluid resuscitation, and high-dose vasopressors. The physician suspects adrenal insufficiency, although the patient has no known history of this problem. Which of the following is the first priority for treating this patient?

(A) correction of hypernatremia
(B) administration of dexamethasone
(C) an ACTH stimulation test
(D) administration of hydrocortisone

ANSWER KEY

1. **B**	3. **A**	5. **C**	7. **D**	9. **B**
2. **D**	4. **A**	6. **B**	8. **C**	

ANSWERS AND EXPLANATIONS

1. **(B)** If the potassium was normal (4.5 mEq/L) when the pH was 7.15, it would have decreased as the pH was corrected, unmasking a deficit in the total body potassium. The intravenous solution should be changed to include dextrose, not lactated Ringer's. The pH is now close to normal, so there is no need for the administration of sodium bicarbonate. The insulin infusion needs to be decreased, not increased.

2. **(D)** This clinical scenario describes diabetes insipidus (DI) secondary to a head injury. Insufficient ADH is produced (low ADH), resulting in a large-volume diuresis of dilute urine. The serum osmolality due to the large volume loss would be expected to be high, not low or normal. The serum sodium would be expected to increase due to volume loss and resultant dehydration.

3. **(A)** This patient requires an isotonic crystalloid, one with lower amounts of sodium (normal saline has higher levels of sodium). A hypotonic solution, a solution that is high in sodium, or one that is high in dextrose will not prevent hypovolemic shock.

4. **(A)** This patient scenario describes SIADH with dilutional hyponatremia secondary to oat cell carcinoma. Free water will further decrease the serum sodium. Therefore, restriction of free water is crucial. No evidence is provided to indicate that the administration of NSAIDs will be useful. A solution containing 0.45 normal saline is a hypotonic solution. Therefore, administering this solution will worsen the hypotonicity that is already present. The administration of Pitressin will further increase the ADH and worsen the SIADH.

5. **(C)** These symptoms describe hypoglycemia. Therefore, the administration of 50% dextrose is appropriate. The other 3 choices will either worsen the hypoglycemia or not be of any benefit.

6. **(B)** A person with HHS has extremely high blood sugar that progresses over several days. During this time, the patient has extreme diuresis with fluid loss. Of the 4 available choices, only an elevated urine specific gravity would be the result of this hypovolemia. Acidosis and hyperkalemia are seen with DKA. A low serum osmolality is seen with fluid overload, not volume loss.

7. **(D)** Metoprolol, a beta-adrenergic blocker, will prevent the early signs of hypoglycemia (irritability, shakiness, increased heart rate) that are due to sympathetic nervous system activation precipitated by the low blood sugar. Therefore, for this patient, the first signs of hypoglycemia may be lethargy and a coma. The other 3 choices will not result in sudden lethargy and a coma.

8. **(C)** The clinical signs are those of myxedema coma, and treatment with a levothyroxine (Synthroid) IV is needed. Propylthiouracil (choice (A)) and iodine (choice (B)) are treatments for thyroid storm and are not indicated for this patient. This scenario does not include signs/symptoms that necessitate the use of a diuretic (choice (D)).

9. **(B)** A patient with adrenal insufficiency/crisis requires emergent administration of cortisol to prevent cardiovascular collapse. Dexamethasone is preferred in this situation because if hydrocortisone (choice (D)) is given, it will interfere with the diagnosis of underlying adrenal insufficiency, which may be corroborated with an ACTH stimulation test. Hypernatremia (choice (A)) is not a feature of adrenal crisis; hyponatremia is more common. An ACTH stimulation test (choice (C)) is completed after the patient is stabilized.

Hematology/Immunology Concepts

12

Believe you can and you're halfway there.

—Theodore Roosevelt

HEMATOLOGY/IMMUNOLOGY TEST BLUEPRINT

Hematology/Immunology 2% of total test   **3–4 questions***

→ Anemia
→ Coagulopathies (e.g., ITP, DIC, HIT)
→ Immune deficiencies
→ Leukopenia
→ Oncologic complications (e.g., tumor lysis syndrome, pericardial effusion)
→ Thrombocytopenia
→ Transfusion reactions

*The number of questions and percentages in this category may vary slightly from test to test.

HEMATOLOGY/IMMUNOLOGY TESTABLE NURSING ACTIONS

☐ Manage patients receiving transfusion of blood products
☐ Monitor patients and follow protocols:

  ○ Pre-, intra-, post-intervention (e.g., plasmapheresis, exchange transfusion, leukocyte depletion)
  ○ Related to blood conservation

> This exam includes only 3–4 questions on hematology/immunology concepts. Therefore, 3–4 hours of studying these topics is generally adequate in order to do well. Most test versions include DIC and HIT questions.

- Blood is a river of living tissue and needs to know when to be liquid and when to be solid (clot).
- Blood has several "jobs," one of which is to clot in the presence of an injury.

Platelet Phase of Clot Formation

- Platelets are the smallest type of blood cell and are made in bone marrow.
- 200 billion platelets are produced per day, with more than 1 trillion platelets circulating at all times.
- Platelets are white blood cells that live 7–10 days.
- A platelet plug (white clot) is effective for small injuries.
- Ordinarily, platelets do not react with endothelium, **but** in the presence of an injury, platelets become activated and actually change shape and appearance.

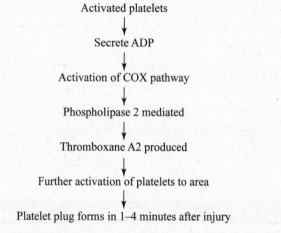

Activated platelets

↓

Secrete ADP

↓

Activation of COX pathway

↓

Phospholipase 2 mediated

↓

Thromboxane A2 produced

↓

Further activation of platelets to area

↓

Platelet plug forms in 1–4 minutes after injury

Figure 12-1. Physiology of platelet "white" clot formation

- **Platelet count** measures platelet quantity.
- **Bleeding time** measures platelet function/how well platelets work.

Coagulation Pathway Phase of Clot Formation

- Various pathophysiological problems may trigger either the intrinsic or the extrinsic coagulation pathways, followed by clotting (Figure 12-2).

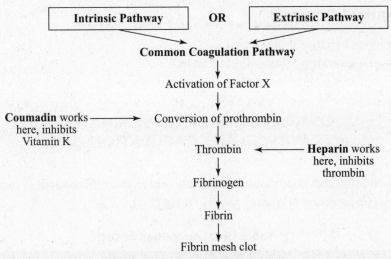

Figure 12-2. Coagulation pathways

- The **intrinsic coagulation pathway** is stimulated by a vascular endothelial injury.

  - Cell trauma (valve, IABP)
  - Sepsis
  - Shock
  - ARDS
  - Hypoxemia, acidemia
  - Cardiopulmonary arrest

- The **extrinsic coagulation pathway** is stimulated by tissue injury and releases "tissue thromboplastin."

  - Extensive trauma
  - OB emergencies
  - Malignancies
  - Dissecting aortic aneurysm
  - Extensive MI

Inhibition of Clot Formation

- As we are making clots, we are also dissolving clots (Figure 12-3).

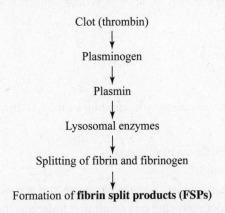

Figure 12-3. Inhibition of clot formation

Anticoagulant Reversal

- What reverses heparin? Protamine
- What reverses warfarin (Coumadin)? Vitamin K

COAGULOPATHIES: DISSEMINATED INTRAVASCULAR COAGULATION (DIC)

- DIC is a complex condition caused by activation of clotting (fibrinolytic system) with the resultant consumption of clotting factors (Table 12-1).

☆ Table 12-1. Lab Values of DIC

Primary	Secondary
↓ Platelets	↑ **D-dimer** assesses the presence of clotting
↓ Fibrinogen	↑ Antithrombin III
↓ Hematocrit	
↑ **FSP (due to ↑ fibrinolysis)**	
↑ PT, PTT, INR, bleeding time	

- DIC results in the deposition of thrombi in the microvasculature (**microembolism**) and the consumption of clotting factors (**hemorrhage**).
- DIC is primarily a clotting problem, **not** a bleeding problem.
- DIC is **always** secondary to another problem.
- Fortunately, massive bleeding from multiple sites is now rare since there is a better understanding of the etiology; massive bleeding is screened for DIC in its early stages, and treatment occurs earlier in most cases.

Etiology

- **Endothelial damage**
    - Sepsis, hypoxemia, shock, ARDS, AAA, acidemia, cardiopulmonary arrest
- **Release of tissue thromboplastin**
    - Extensive trauma, malignancies, OB emergencies, dissecting aortic aneurysm
- **Factor X activation**
    - Acute pancreatitis
    - Liver disease
- **Miscellaneous**
    - Massive transfusions, PE, hemolytic anemia, fresh H_2O drowning, ASA poisoning

Normals:

- Fibrin split products (FSP) is < 10 mcg/mL.
- Fibrinogen is 200–400 mg/dL.
- The normal D-dimer value depends upon the assay that is used by each institution.
    - ☆ Elevated FSP is the definitive lab test result that indicates the presence of DIC.
    - ☆ D-dimer must be elevated; however, it is not a definitive test for DIC.

Treatment for DIC

- Identify and eliminate the underlying cause, as able.
- Administer vitamin K.
- Administer blood component therapy.
    - Fresh frozen plasma (FFP)
    - Cryoprecipitate
    - Platelets
- Heparin (low-dose) is controversial but may be used for patients with chronic, low-grade DIC who have predominantly thrombotic manifestations.
- Maintain hemodynamic stability.

COAGULOPATHIES: HEPARIN-INDUCED THROMBOCYTOPENIA (HIT)

- ~ 50% of patients who are exposed to heparin are positive for heparin antibodies.
    - Most of those who are positive for heparin antibodies are asymptomatic.
    - ~ 5% of those who are positive for heparin antibodies develop HIT or "white clot syndrome."

Etiology of HIT

- Due to an immune (IgG) response
- Results in thrombosis (white clots) that consumes platelets

Signs/Symptoms of HIT

- Platelets decrease to < 150,000 **or** precipitously drop by 30–50% from the baseline.
- Early sign—petechiae
- Clots may lead to PE, MI, stroke, and/or amputation.
- Many signs/symptoms of HIT are frequently unrecognized.

Treatment for HIT

- Stop heparin (fractionated as well as unfractionated).
- Test for the presence of heparin antibodies by obtaining an enzyme-linked immuno-sorbent assay (ELISA) test, but do not wait for the test results to stop heparin and start treatment.
- Start a direct thrombin inhibitor and continue until the platelets stabilize; monitor PTTs.
    - Argatroban
- Start warfarin (Coumadin).
- If the platelet count is less than 10,000 platelets, monitor for changes in the LOC (intracranial bleed).

COAGULOPATHIES: IMMUNE (IDIOPATHIC) THROMBOCYTOPENIC PURPURA (ITP)

☆ This coagulopathy is seldom covered on the Adult CCRN exam but is included in the current test blueprint.

ITP is a chronic, **autoimmune** disorder that affects adults and has 2 criteria for a diagnosis:

1. Only a decrease in platelets is present. The rest of the complete blood count is normal.
2. ITP is NOT associated with any other systemic disease (e.g., lupus, chronic lymphocytic leukemia) or drugs.

Signs/Symptoms of ITP

- Patients with ITP are often asymptomatic, with the only sign being a low platelet count; if symptoms do develop, expect: petechiae, purpura, easy bruising, epistaxis, gingival bleeding, and/or menorrhagia.
- The spleen is normal in size unless there is a coexistent viral infection.
- Rare symptoms include: GI bleeding, hematuria, and/or intracranial hemorrhage.
- Numerous differential diagnoses need to be ruled out.
- Life-threatening bleeding is rarely seen.
- As with other types of thrombocytopenia, thrombosis is a possibility.

Treatment for ITP

- Corticosteroids
- If life-threatening bleeding develops, administer a platelet transfusion, IV steroids, or IV immunoglobulin.

PLASMAPHERESIS

- Plasmapheresis is the filtering and separation of plasma from whole blood via semipermeable membranes; this process is done via a central line that is similar to the catheters that are used for hemodialysis.
- Therapeutic plasmapheresis is indicated for disorders that are thought to be caused by an abnormal immunologic response:
  - Guillain-Barré syndrome
  - Myasthenia gravis
  - Thrombotic thrombocytopenic purpura
- Contraindications include:
  - Patients who cannot tolerate central line placement
  - Patients who are actively septic or are hemodynamically unstable
  - Patients who have allergies to fresh frozen plasma or albumin, depending upon the type of plasma exchange

- ○ Patients with heparin allergies should not receive heparin as an anticoagulant during plasmapheresis.
- ○ Patients with hypocalcemia are at risk for worsening of their condition because citrate is commonly used to prevent clotting and can potentiate hypocalcemia.

RECOGNITION AND MANAGEMENT OF TRANSFUSION REACTIONS

- Although included in the Adult CCRN test blueprint, transfusion reactions are less likely to be covered on the exam than DIC or HIT.

Signs of Transfusion Reactions

- **Acute transfusion reaction:** occurs within 24 hours of the administration of a blood product (Table 12-2)
- **Delayed transfusion reaction:** occurs 24 hours after the administration of a blood product (Table 12-2)

Table 12-2. Transfusion Reactions to Blood Products

Body System	Acute Reaction: Signs and Symptoms
Respiratory	Tachypnea, dyspnea, wheezing, rales, stridor, hypoxia
Cardiovascular	Tachycardia, bradycardia, hypertension, hypotension, jugular venous distention, arrhythmia
Immune	Fever (temperature increase > 1°C), chills, rigors
Cutaneous	Pruritus, urticaria, erythema, flushing, petechiae, cyanosis
Gastrointestinal	Nausea, vomiting
Pain	Headache, chest pain, abdominal pain, back/flank pain, pain at the infusion site
Renal	Red-colored urine (hemolytic, non-antibody mediated)

Management of Transfusion Reactions

- General interventions for ALL suspected reactions
  - ○ Stop the transfusion.
  - ○ Disconnect the blood tubing at the intravenous catheter hub and administer normal saline, using new tubing to keep the vein open.
  - ○ Assess the patient.
  - ○ Monitor the patient's vital signs until the patient is stable.
  - ○ Perform a clerical check on the blood product and the patient's identification.
- Acute hemolytic reactions (antibody mediated)
  - ○ Anticipate hypotension, renal failure, and DIC.
  - ○ Prophylactic measures to reduce the risk of renal failure may include vigorous hydration with crystalloid solutions (3,000 mL/m^2/24 hour) and osmotic diuresis with 20% mannitol (100 mL/m^2/bolus, followed by 30 mL/m^2/hour for 12 hours).

- If DIC is documented and bleeding requires treatment, transfusions of fresh frozen plasma, pooled cryoprecipitate, and/or platelet concentrates may be indicated.

■ Acute hemolytic reactions (non-antibody mediated)

- The transfusion of serologically compatible, although damaged, RBCs usually does not require rigorous management.
- Infuse 500 mL of 0.9% sodium chloride per hour, or as tolerated by the patient, until the intense red color of the urine subsides.

■ Febrile, non-hemolytic reactions

- Acetaminophen

■ Allergic reactions

- Diphenhydramine (Benadryl) is usually effective for relieving the pruritus that is associated with hives or a rash.

■ Anaphylactic reactions

- A subcutaneous injection of epinephrine (0.3–0.5 mL of a 1:1,000 aqueous solution) is standard treatment.
- IV steroids

■ Transfusion-related acute lung injury (TRALI)

- Oxygen, mechanical ventilation if necessary
- Diuretics (only if there is also volume overload or cardiogenic pulmonary edema)

■ Circulatory (volume) overload

- Oxygen
- If practical, the unit of blood component being transfused may be lowered.
- Diuretics

■ Bacterial contamination (sepsis)

- Blood cultures
- Antibiotics

ALTERED IMMUNE RESPONSE, NEUTROPENIA

Acute and critical care nurses care for a variety of patient populations with immune deficiencies. These populations include patients with acute leukemia, hematopoietic stem cell transplantation, organ transplantation, and HIV infection, among others. Additionally, critical illnesses and invasive therapies themselves also alter the immune response.

■ The **immune response** is the body's ability to recognize and defend itself against bacteria, viruses, and substances that appear foreign and harmful. At times, antigens, antibodies, and other cells produced by the immune response result in allergies and abnormal autoimmune responses.

■ Neutrophils are the white blood cells that are responsible for the immune response.

■ Segmented neutrophils (segs) are mature neutrophils; bands are immature neutrophils. Segs + bands = absolute neutrophil count (ANC).

■ Neutropenia is defined as an absolute neutrophil count (ANC) of less than 1,000 cells/mcL; severe neutropenia is an ANC of less than 500 cells/mcL.

- The etiology of neutropenia may be either decreased neutrophil production (e.g., bone marrow malignancy, radiation, medications, or autoimmune disorders) or increased neutrophil use (e.g., an overwhelming bacterial or viral infection).

Management of Neutropenia

- Monitor patients (especially high-risk populations) for signs of an infection, such as neutropenia, a fever (although some patients have a normal or even low temperature due to an inability to mount a normal inflammatory response), malaise, dyspnea, purulent drainage/sputum, chest infiltrates, pain, and/or confusion.
- Prevent an infection.
    - Neutropenic precautions if the ANC is less than 500 cells/mcL
    - Close assessment for the signs and symptoms of an infection, including a neutropenic fever
    - Note that a neutropenic fever is a single oral temperature of 38.3°C (101°F) or a temperature greater than 38.0°C (100.4°F) sustained for more than 1 hour in a patient with **neutropenia**; in the event of a neutropenic fever, administer prophylactic, empiric, or therapeutic antibiotics or antifungals, as ordered.
- Assess the daily WBC count, the WBC differential, and the ANC.
- Monitor fluid/nutritional intake.
- Administer granulocyte colony-stimulating factor (G-CSF or GM-CSF), which enhances bone marrow production of neutrophils and monocytes (e.g., filgrastim (Neupogen), pegfilgrastim (Neulasta)).
- Address infections to prevent sepsis.
    - Perform prompt cultures, as indicated.
    - Administer antibiotics/antifungals/antivirals as soon as possible to decrease mortality.
    - Provide system support.

ONCOLOGIC COMPLICATION—PERICARDIAL EFFUSION

- Pericardial effusion is seen in 5–20% of patients with cancer and is most commonly associated with breast cancer, lung cancer, or Hodgkin's lymphoma.
    - Rapid development results in cardiac tamponade.
    - Slow progression results in progressively worsening dyspnea.
    - A diagnosis is confirmed with an ECHO; fluid that is collected via pericardiocentesis may be examined to determine whether the etiology of the pericardial effusion is due to the malignancy or the treatment (chemotherapy, radiation).
- Treatment
    - Medical (chemotherapy, steroids)
    - A pericardiocentesis may be scheduled to provide symptom relief and to examine the fluid; note that pericardial effusion secondary to cancer has a high recurrence rate.
    - Emergent pericardiocentesis for signs of cardiac tamponade
    - Insertion of a pericardial catheter to provide prolonged drainage
    - A pericardial window, with surgical removal of a section of the pericardium to prevent a recurrence of pericardial effusion

Overview

- Studies that involve similar populations have demonstrated that there is a relationship between the number of blood products that are administered to a patient and increased levels of morbidity/mortality.
- Frequent lab draws have been shown to result in nosocomial anemia.
- Blood conservation reduces costs.
- Transfusion practices may vary from clinician to clinician.

Strategies to Conserve Blood

- Develop evidence-based, standard order sets; set the default unit ordered from multiple units to one.
- Develop massive transfusion protocols.
- Add a device to invasive monitoring lines to reduce the volume of blood obtained for lab draws.
- Include tools and information in the electronic health record (EHR) order sets, such as recent lab values and patient vital signs, that can be used to enhance decision making during order entry.
- Add the requirement for an in-person evaluation of the patient's condition, basing the decision to transfuse on the patient's symptoms and lab results.
- Update the cardiac bypass protocols to specify that the patient's blood, rather than donated blood, should be used to prime the heart-lung machine.
- Discontinue platelet inhibitors pre-op.
- Administer erythropoietin (EPO) plus iron pre-op to select patients (e.g., those who are anemic, those who are Jehovah's Witnesses).
- Use blood derivatives for select patients under certain circumstances.
- Use blood salvage techniques as able.
- Implement autotransfusion protocols (a process in which patients receive their own blood, which is collected from surgical sites and is then filtered for reinfusion) for surgical cardiac and orthopedic patients.
- Use small tubes, and draw only the volume necessary for laboratory testing.
- Provide clinician education.
- Monitor transfusion practices, and provide feedback to clinicians.

> Now that you have reviewed the key hematology/immunology concepts, go to the Hematology/Immunology Practice Questions. Answer the questions, and then check your answers. Continue to review the information until you answer 80% of the practice questions correctly.

HEMATOLOGY/IMMUNOLOGY PRACTICE QUESTIONS

For questions 1 and 2

A 54-year-old woman was admitted with deep vein thrombosis and pulmonary emboli. She received a heparin bolus and a continuous heparin infusion. The next day, heparin-induced thrombocytopenia (HIT) was suspected, and the heparin infusion was discontinued.

1. Which of the following would be most indicative of HIT?

   (A) surface bleeding from IV sites, a PTT of 50 seconds
   (B) loss of pulse, an INR of 5
   (C) petechiae, a platelet count of 50,000/mm^3
   (D) a change in the level of consciousness

2. Two days later, this patient is scheduled for insertion of a Greenfield filter to protect her lungs from future emboli. The preoperative laboratory results show a platelet count of 20,000/mm^3. Which nursing action is most appropriate?

   (A) Notify the surgeon.
   (B) Start an extra IV line with a large-gauge catheter.
   (C) Monitor the patient's neurological status carefully.
   (D) Discontinue argatroban.

   ----

3. A patient with septic shock is thought to be developing DIC. Which of the following lab results would be most indicative of DIC?

   (A) prolonged PT, PTT, and bleeding time
   (B) decreased platelet count
   (C) positive ELISA
   (D) elevated fibrin split products and D-dimer

4. A patient who has been receiving chemotherapy was admitted with a pulmonary embolism. Lab results indicated an absolute neutrophil count (ANC) of 450 cells/mcL. Neutropenic precautions were initiated, and filgrastim (Neupogen) was ordered. The latest vital sign assessment revealed: a temperature of 38.1°C (100.6°F), a B/P of 102/72, a heart rate of 96 beats/minute, and a respiratory rate of 18 breaths/minute. Which of the following interventions would be indicated in this situation?

   (A) Provide/encourage fluids.
   (B) Administer acetaminophen (Tylenol).
   (C) Assess oxygenation.
   (D) Recheck the patient's vital signs in an hour.

ANSWER KEY

1. **C**　　　2. **A**　　　3. **D**　　　4. **D**

ANSWERS AND EXPLANATIONS

1. **(C)** Petechiae are a sign of HIT (although they are not present in all cases). A platelet count of 50,000/mm^3 would meet the criteria for HIT (a decrease to < 150,000 platelets **or** a precipitous drop in the platelet count by 30–50% from the baseline platelet count). Surface bleeding from IV sites and/or a prolonged PTT are not indications of HIT. Although loss of pulse may be seen, a prolonged INR is not a sign of HIT. Even though a change in the level of consciousness may be due to a stroke secondary to HIT, petechiae and a drop in the platelet count are more specific signs of HIT.

2. **(A)** The surgeon needs to know of the extreme drop in platelet count as he or she may want to transfuse platelets prior to the procedure. The other interventions are not a priority. (An intracranial bleed would be more likely with a platelet count less than 20,000/mm^3.)

3. **(D)** Elevated fibrin split products (FSP) is due to the breakdown of the massive amount of clots that occur with DIC. The other lab values are not specific to DIC.

4. **(D)** A single oral temperature of 38.3°C (101°F) or a temperature greater than 38.0°C (100.4°F) sustained **for more than 1 hour** in a patient with neutropenia is a sign of a neutropenic fever. The patient's temperature needs to be rechecked, and if it is still 38.1°C (100.6°F) an hour later, the physician needs to be notified for possible prophylactic antibiotic therapy. The patient did not have evidence of dehydration; therefore, the provision and encouragement of fluids (choice (A)) are not priorities. The administration of Tylenol (choice (B)) may mask the neutropenic fever. There are no signs that the patient had a problem with oxygenation, so choice (C) is also incorrect.

Behavioral/Psychosocial Concepts

13

A year from now, you may have wished that you started today.

—Karen Lamb

BEHAVIORAL/PSYCHOSOCIAL TEST BLUEPRINT

Behavioral/Psychosocial 2% of total test — **3–4 questions***

➜ Abuse/neglect
➜ Aggression
➜ Agitation
➜ Anxiety
➜ Suicidal ideation and/or behaviors
➜ Depression
➜ Medical nonadherence
➜ PTSD
➜ Risk-taking behavior
➜ Substance use disorders (e.g., withdrawal, chronic alcohol or drug dependence)

*The number of questions and percentages in this category may vary slightly from test to test.

Note: Although *delirium* and *dementia* are included in the Neurological section of the Adult CCRN test blueprint, these topics are covered in this chapter. Delirium and dementia are brain disorders, but they are manifested in behavioral signs/symptoms.

BEHAVIORAL/PSYCHOSOCIAL TESTABLE NURSING ACTIONS

☐ Respond to behavioral emergencies (e.g., nonviolent crisis intervention, de-escalation techniques)
☐ Use behavioral assessment tools (e.g., delirium, alcohol withdrawal, cognitive impairment)
☐ Recognize indications for, and manage, patients requiring:

○ Behavioral therapeutic interventions
○ Medication management for agitation
○ Physical restraints

This exam includes only 3–4 questions on behavioral/psychosocial concepts. Therefore, 3–4 hours of studying these topics is generally adequate in order to do well.

- Delirium may cause agitation. However, not all delirious patients are agitated and not all agitated patients are delirious!
- Delirium is an acute organic mental syndrome with potentially reversible impairment of consciousness and cognitive function that fluctuates in severity.
- Types of delirium:
  - **Mixed** delirium (hyperactive and hypoactive type in the same patient) is the most common and is seen in approximately 55% of patients with delirium.
  - **Hypoactive** delirium is the second most common type and is seen in approximately 43% of patients with delirium.
  - Purely **hyperactive** delirium is the least common type and is seen in approximately 2% of patients with delirium.
- Note that a patient with dementia may develop delirium **superimposed on dementia**.
- The risk factors for delirium are listed in Table 13-1.
- Studies have shown that delirium is associated with a worse cognitive outcome, increased ICU and hospital length of stay (LOS), increased costs, and patient/family distress.

Table 13-1. Risk Factors for Delirium

Non-Modifiable Risk Factors	Modifiable Risk Factors*
History of dementia	Benzodiazepines
Recent history of substance abuse	Blood transfusions
Greater age	Immobility
Increasing APACHE score	Restraints
Prior coma	Pain
Pre-ICU emergency surgery or trauma	Sensory deprivation or overload
	Sleep disruption/deprivation

*Alternatives are available or strategies exist to reduce these risk factors

Assessment of Delirium—Overview

- Identifying delirium is important because delirium has an effect on morbidity and mortality; using an assessment tool to determine whether or not any type of delirium is present increases the identification of patients with delirium.
- Two valid/reliable tools can be used to assess for delirium in a critically ill patient:
  - The Confusion Assessment Method for the ICU (CAM-ICU)
  - The Intensive Care Delirium Screening Checklist (ICDSC)
- Studies have shown that, even when assessment tools are available, nurses have a difficult time recognizing delirium, especially identifying hypoactive delirium.

STEPS TO ASSESS DELIRIUM

☆ **Do not assess for delirium if the patient is not responsive or is heavily sedated.**

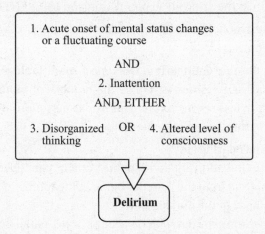

1. Acute onset of mental status changes or a fluctuating course

AND

2. Inattention

AND, EITHER

3. Disorganized thinking   OR   4. Altered level of consciousness

Delirium

Figure 13-1. Summary of the assessment of delirium

1. The patient must have an **acute onset of mental status changes or a fluctuating course**.

   ■ Is the patient different now than at his or her baseline mental status?

   ■ Alternatively, has the patient had any fluctuation in his or her mental status in the past 24 hours, as evidenced by fluctuation on the sedation scale (MAAS or RASS) or on the Glasgow Coma Scale (GCS)?

   If the patient is negative for either an acute onset of mental status changes or a fluctuating course, then the patient is negative for delirium. In that case, STOP the assessment. If the patient is positive for either, continue the assessment.

AND

2. The patient must also exhibit **inattention** (i.e., administer the "Letters Attention Test").

   ■ Say to the patient, "I am going to read you a series of 10 letters. Whenever you hear the letter A, indicate that by squeezing my hand." Read the letters from the following letter list in a normal tone and 3 seconds apart:

   ### SAVEAHAART or CASABLANCA

   ○ Errors are counted when the patient fails to squeeze on the letter A and when the patient squeezes on any letter other than A.

   ■ The patient is positive for inattention if more than 2 errors are made.

If the patient is negative for inattention, then the patient is negative for delirium. In that case, STOP the assessment. If the patient is positive for inattention, continue the assessment.

In addition to the first 2 criteria, for the patient to be diagnosed with delirium, he or she also needs to exhibit **EITHER feature 3 or feature 4:**

3. Disorganized thinking—assess for this by either asking a question or by testing the patient's ability to follow a specific command.

OR

4. Altered level of consciousness—anything other than calm and cooperative (RASS score of 0 or MAAS score of +3) could suggest delirium.

Prevention of Delirium

- Measures to prevent delirium should be utilized for ALL critically ill patients since delirium is common in the critically ill population and **PREVENTION** is key!

  - Remember that hypoactive delirium (which is often not diagnosed) also adversely affects the outcome.

- Interventions may not prevent delirium when **non-modifiable risk factors** are present, but taking preventative measures to reduce the number of **modifiable risk factors** for delirium may result in less severe delirium and/or a shorter duration of delirium.

- Utilize strategies to promote patient orientation.

  - Provide visual and hearing aids.
  - Encourage communication and reorient the patient repetitively.
  - Place familiar objects from the patient's home in the room.
  - Attempt consistency in the nursing staff.
  - Allow television during the day with daily news or per patient preference.
  - Play music (instrumental, without words).

- Assess/manage the environment.

  - Promote sleep hygiene: lights off at night and on during the day.
  - Control excess noise (staff, equipment, visitors) at night.
  - Avoid restraints, as able.
  - Remove/camouflage tubes.

- Control clinical parameters, as able.

  - Maintain a systolic blood pressure > 90 mmHg.
  - Maintain oxygen saturation > 90%.
  - Treat underlying metabolic derangements and infections.

- Prevent delirium secondary to substance abuse (alcohol, opiates, benzodiazepines, nicotine).

  - Assess for chronic substance abuse and adjust medication doses accordingly, keeping in mind that the patient may have developed a tolerance to select medications and thus may require higher doses.
  - Provide benzodiazepines to prevent/minimize alcohol or benzodiazepine withdrawal; provide opiates to a patient with known chronic opiate use.
  - Consider the use of a nicotine patch, as indicated.

- Ensure that processes are in place to implement the evidence-based strategies of the **ABCDEF bundle** for critically ill adults:

  A: <u>A</u>ssess, prevent, and manage pain
  B: <u>B</u>oth spontaneous awakening and breathing trials
  C: <u>C</u>hoice of analgesia and sedation
  D: <u>D</u>elirium—assess, prevent, and manage
  E: <u>E</u>arly mobility and exercise
  F: <u>F</u>amily engagement/empowerment

- Do NOT use pharmacological agents to **prevent** delirium (except for select patients with a substance abuse history).

Pharmacological Management of Delirium

The use of drugs to treat delirium is generally reserved for **hyperactive** delirium that is not responsive to non-pharmacological measures. As mentioned earlier, there is no pharmacological "magic bullet" for the treatment of delirium. Paradoxically, sedation agents can cause delirium in some patients. The following are general recommendations for the pharmacological management of delirium:

- Address pain with analgesics.
- For delirium that is related to alcohol or benzodiazepine withdrawal, use benzodiazepines.
- For delirium that is unrelated to alcohol or benzodiazepine withdrawal, when treating a patient who is receiving mechanical ventilation, use dexmedetomidine rather than benzodiazepine infusions.
- The use of haloperidol (Haldol) or a statin is not recommended for the treatment of delirium; studies have not demonstrated that the use of either of these agents is associated with a shorter duration of delirium, a shorter duration of mechanical ventilation, a shorter ICU LOS, or decreased mortality.
  - Short-term use of haloperidol (Haldol) may be utilized for patients with significant distress secondary to the symptoms of delirium (e.g., hallucinations and/or delusion-associated fearfulness) or for those who are delirious and have agitation that could be physically harmful to themselves or others.

☆ Haloperidol may prolong the QT interval and cause torsades de pointes ventricular tachycardia.
  - Obtain a baseline QTc interval measurement, and monitor the QTc regularly throughout therapy.
  - Monitor for the addition of other drugs that may prolong the QT interval.

DEMENTIA

- Dementia (a neurocognitive disorder) affects the brain's ability to think, reason, and remember clearly.
- The most commonly affected areas include memory, visual-spatial, language, attention, and problem solving.
- Unlike delirium, which is acute and temporary, most types of dementia are slow and progressive in onset and are permanent. Refer to Table 13-2 for a comparison of delirium and dementia.

☆ **Table 13-2. Comparison of Delirium and Dementia**

Delirium	Dementia
Acute, fluctuating	Chronic
Rapid progression	Slow progression
Reversible	Irreversible
Strategies are available for prevention	No known prevention
Organic brain changes	Organic brain changes
May include agitation, but not in all cases	May include agitation, but not always

- The most common cause of dementia is Alzheimer's disease (75% of all cases of dementia); vascular brain disease/stroke is another cause, among others.
- Symptoms vary depending upon whether the dementia is in early, mid, or late stages.
- If a patient with dementia requires care in an ICU, there is a higher likelihood of delirium.
- Patient safety is a priority, and inclusion of the family/significant others in the plan of care is required.

AGGRESSIVE/VIOLENT BEHAVIOR

- Be aware and alert.
- Maintain a calm, quiet manner.
- Maintain a quiet environment.
- Stand at a slight angle to the patient.
- Do not provide care alone.
- Activate an emergency response, as needed.

DEPRESSION

- Depression affects all age groups and all social classes.
- Depression is twice as frequent in women.
- 17.3 million adults in the U.S. (7.1% of all adults in the U.S.) have had at least 1 major depressive episode.

Cause of Depression

- There is no single known cause, although researchers have noted some hereditary, environmental, physiological, and psychological factors that may contribute to depression.
  - MRIs of the brains of depressed individuals have shown changes.
  - Depression has been associated with an imbalance of brain neurotransmitters.

Diagnosis of Depression

1. Depressed mood (feeling sad or low) **or**
2. Loss of interest or pleasure in nearly all activities

Plus 4 additional signs/symptoms from the following:
- Significant loss of appetite or weight loss or gain
- Insomnia or hypersomnia
- Psychomotor agitation or retardation
- Fatigue or loss of energy
- Feelings of worthlessness or guilt
- Impaired thinking or concentration; indecisiveness
- Suicidal thoughts/thoughts of death

Therapeutic Interventions for Depression

- Do NOT isolate the patient.
- Provide safety.
- Avoid excessive environmental stimulation.
- Do not force decision-making.
- Encourage expressions of feelings.
- Explore sources of emotional support.
- Involve family members/a personal support system.
- Ensure the continuation of home medications, as the condition permits.
- Assess the suicide risk.
- Obtain a psychiatric referral.

Pharmacological Management of Depression

TRICYCLIC ANTIDEPRESSANTS

- Use has declined with the availability of SSRIs.
- Examples of tricyclic antidepressants that are used include:

  - Amitriptyline
  - Nortriptyline
  - Imipramine
  - Clomipramine
  - Desipramine

- Adverse effects of tricyclic antidepressants

  - Highly lethal in an overdose (tachycardia, hypotension, fatal arrhythmias)
  - Vertigo
  - Dry mouth, dental caries
  - Urinary retention
  - Constipation
  - Orthostatic hypotension
  - Prolonged QT

SELECTIVE SEROTONIN REUPTAKE INHIBITORS (SSRIs)

- SSRIs are the first-line pharmacological therapy for depression. Table 13-3 outlines the types of SSRIs.
- Abnormalities in brain serotonin activity have been implicated in many emotional and behavioral disorders, including mood disorders, obsessive-compulsive disorder, and aggressive behaviors.
- SSRIs block the action of the presynaptic serotonin reuptake pump, thereby increasing the amount of serotonin available in the synapse and increasing postsynaptic serotonin receptor occupancy.
- SSRIs are usually well tolerated and can be administered once a day. They also usually have fewer adverse effects than tricyclic antidepressants.

Table 13-3. Types of SSRIs (New-Generation Antidepressants)

Generic Name	Brand Name
Fluoxetine	Prozac
Citalopram	Celexa
Escitalopram	Lexapro
Sertraline	Zoloft
Paroxetine	Paxil
Fluvoxamine	Luvox
Bupropion	Wellbutrin
Mirtazapine	Remeron
Venlafaxine	Effexor
Duloxetine	Cymbalta
Desvenlafaxine	Pristiq

Adverse Effects of SSRIs

- SSRIs are generally well-tolerated, and any adverse effects are dose-dependent. Most subside after 1–2 weeks or after a dose reduction.
- More common adverse effects—headache, abdominal pain, nausea, diarrhea, sleep changes, jitteriness, agitation
- Less common adverse effects—diaphoresis, akathisia (restlessness and an inability to sit still), bruising, changes in sexual functioning
- SSRIs can induce a manic or hypomanic episode.
- SSRIs have the potential for increased suicidality.
- SSRIs can inhibit the metabolism of some medications, such as antiarrhythmics, benzodiazepines, warfarin, tricyclics, and neuroleptics.

SUICIDE

- Over 500,000 patients per year are admitted for suicide-related injuries.
- There are over 47,000 suicides annually.
- Suicide is the 10th leading cause of death in the U.S.
- By gender:
  - Four men succeed for every woman who succeeds.
  - Women attempt **twice** as often as men.
  - Men over 65 years of age are at a greater risk.
- Suicide behavior continuum:
  - Ideation—contemplation without action
  - Gesture—nonlethal action
  - Attempt—potentially lethal
  - Suicide—30% of people are successful on their first attempt.

Assessment for Suicide Intent

Evaluate the patient's **intent**, determine whether there is or was a **plan**, and assess the patient's **ability** to follow through with the plan.

- Are you feeling depressed, sad, or discouraged?
- How long have you felt like this?
- Do you feel that your life is no longer worth living?
- Are you thinking of acting on that feeling by hurting yourself or taking your own life?
- Do you have a suicide plan?
- Can you tell me about your plan?

Nursing Interventions for a Patient with Suicide Intent/Attempt

- Establish a **safe** environment.
- Provide one-on-one observation.
- Explain the precautions to the patient.
- Document comprehensive assessments, interventions, and the patient's response to those interventions.

Safety Measures

- Remove hazards from the room.
  - Sharp or hazardous objects (plastic bags, cords, metal coat hangers)
  - Personal items (shoelaces, belts, lighters)
- Conduct a contraband check on the patient's personal belongings.
- Provide only paper or plastic food utensils.
- Do not allow visitors to leave anything with the patient unless the nurse approves of it.
- Make sure the patient swallows his or her medications.
- Move the patient near the nurses' station.

SUBSTANCE USE DISORDERS

- Some patients who are admitted to the critical care unit for acute physiological problems may find that their treatment is complicated if they have a chronic dependence on opiates, benzodiazepines, nicotine, alcohol, and/or other substances.
- The chronic dependence will need to be identified, the withdrawal symptoms will need to be differentiated from any acute physiological problems, and the withdrawal symptoms will need to be controlled as part of the overall plan of care.

Signs of Alcohol Withdrawal Syndrome (AWS)

- AWS is evidenced by 2 or more symptoms of autonomic hyperactivity: insomnia, agitation, sweating, tremulousness, a heart rate > 100 beats/minute.
- Seizures may occur during the first 48 hours.
- "Alcoholic hallucinosis" may occur after 12–48 hours without alcohol; visual, auditory, and/or tactile hallucinations may occur; patient orientation and vital signs are normal.

- Delirium tremens (DTs) may occur after 48–96 hours without alcohol; delirium, agitation, tachycardia, hypertension, fever, and/or diaphoresis may be present.
    - With early treatment, the mortality rate of DTs is ~ 5%; without early treatment, the mortality rate is even higher.

☆ Treatment for Alcohol Withdrawal Syndrome (AWS)

- For patients with known heavy alcohol intake or a previous history of DTs, preventative therapy with oral benzodiazepines, such as lorazepam (Ativan), is recommended.
    - Benzodiazepines enhance the effect of the neurotransmitter gamma-aminobutyric acid (GABA) at the $GABA_A$ receptor, resulting in sedative, hypnotic (sleep-inducing), anxiolytic (anti-anxiety), anticonvulsant, and muscle relaxant properties.
- Provide symptom-triggered treatment with benzodiazepines, using a valid tool.
    - The Clinical Institute Withdrawal Assessment for Alcohol—Revised (CIWA-Ar) is a valid tool to measure the severity of alcohol withdrawal. This tool relies on the patient being capable of answering. This tool is **not** valid if the patient cannot answer questions (e.g., if the patient is receiving mechanical ventilation and/or is disoriented).
    - The Richmond Agitation-Sedation Scale (RASS) is appropriate for the critical care setting, with a goal score of 0 to –2.
- Correct volume deficits that are the result of diaphoresis, a lack of oral intake, or insensible loss.
- ☆ Administer glucose and thiamine to prevent Wernicke encephalopathy (gait disturbances, nystagmus, eye muscle paralysis) and Korsakoff syndrome (decreased spontaneity, amnesia, denial of memory loss by making up facts).
- Administer multivitamins with folate.
- Correct potassium, magnesium, and/or phosphate deficiencies.
- Provide as quiet of an environment as possible.
- Evaluate the need for restraints for patient safety, especially until agitation is controlled.
- Remove the restraints once sedation is achieved, since resistance against restraints may lead to a temperature increase or rhabdomyolysis and may cause a physical injury.
- Following acute treatment, follow-up treatment should be planned.
    - Encourage and support abstinence.
    - Involve the patient's family and social services.

Benzodiazepine Withdrawal

- Identify a history of chronic benzodiazepine use by a patient or family report.
- The onset of signs and symptoms may occur 2–21 days after the last dose of benzodiazepines, depending upon the half-life of and the amount of the benzodiazepine that was taken chronically.
- The signs and symptoms include tremors, anxiety, perceptual disturbances, psychosis, and seizures.

MANAGEMENT OF BENZODIAZEPINE WITHDRAWAL

- The goal is to prevent or eliminate symptoms without causing respiratory depression or moderate to deep sedation.
- Administer a benzodiazepine (the same agent that the patient was taking chronically) or a long-acting agent, such as chlordiazepoxide (Librium), as the patient's condition warrants.

Signs of Opioid Withdrawal

- In the first 24 hours, the patient may experience a fear of withdrawal, anxiety, and/or drug craving.
- Insomnia, restlessness, yawning, lacrimation, rhinorrhea, and/or diaphoresis may follow after the first 24 hours.
- Severe signs include vomiting, diarrhea, fever, chills, muscle spasm, tremor, tachycardia, and hypertension.

MANAGEMENT OF OPIOID WITHDRAWAL

- Controlling the signs/symptoms of opioid withdrawal may be done with the use of one or more of the following agents:
  - Opioid agonists (morphine, methadone)
    - Often used initially, then gradually tapered
  - Partial opioid agonists (buprenorphine)
  - Alpha-2 agonists (clonidine)
  - Anti-nausea agents (ondansetron (Zofran))
  - Dicyclomine (Bentyl) for abdominal cramping
  - Ibuprofen for pain

POST-TRAUMATIC STRESS DISORDER (PTSD)

Studies have demonstrated that patients who have been critically ill in an ICU have significant rates of post-traumatic stress disorder (PTSD) after discharge; additionally, some patients have PTSD upon admission due to past traumatic events.

- Definition
  - A mental health condition that is triggered by a traumatic event; symptoms last longer than 1 month.
- Symptoms
  - Flashbacks
  - Nightmares
  - Anxiety
  - Difficulty coping
  - Uncontrollable thoughts of the event
- Management of PTSD in the ICU
  - Consider a psych consult.
  - Provide emotional support and allow time for the expression of emotions.

- Administer medications, which may include antidepressants (paroxetine, sertraline, venlafaxine) or alpha blockers (prazosin).
  - AVOID benzodiazepines!
- Risks for developing PTSD post-ICU stay
  - History of anxiety or depression prior to a critical illness
  - Deep level of sedation during a critical illness
  - Frightening memories of the ICU stay post-discharge
  - Increased severity of a critical illness during the ICU stay
  - Use of benzodiazepines for sedation while in critical care
- Prevention of PTSD post-ICU stay
  - Initiate strategies to prevent delirium.
  - Involve the patient's family/significant others in the plan of care.
  - Encourage the patient to express his or her emotions.
  - Utilize an ICU notebook or diary—clinicians and family write daily messages about what is happening to the patient, which assists the patient in filling in memory gaps.

USE OF RESTRAINTS

- The use of restraints has been associated with increased incidences of delirium and with the endangerment of patient safety.
- The reduction of the use of restraints is a team effort and is dependent upon many factors, including unit leadership and unit culture.
- Physical restraints should only be used to prevent a patient from harming himself/herself or others after alternatives have been attempted.
- Rule out physiological causes for the patient's behavior (e.g., hypoxemia, hypotension, pain, withdrawal), and address them as able.
- Frequently assess the patient, and remove the restraints as soon as the behavior that had necessitated the use of restraints has been resolved.
  - Restraints that are applied as a result of violent behavior require a face-to-face evaluation by a provider or a specially trained practitioner within 1 hour of application, more frequent monitoring, and more frequent orders than restraints that are used for nonviolent behavior.
- Explain the plan of care for restraint use to the patient and the patient's family.
- Restraint use is closely monitored by regulatory agencies.

ABUSE/NEGLECT

Unfortunately, various types of abuse occur. Table 13-4 compares and contrasts domestic abuse with elder abuse.

Table 13-4. Domestic Abuse and Elder Abuse

Domestic Abuse	Elder Abuse

■ 85% of victims are female
■ Individuals who are at risk include children younger than 12 years old, those who are 16–25 years old, those who are recently separated, those who are homeless, and those who are pregnant
■ Signs include
  ○ Evasiveness, hesitancy
  ○ Inconsistent explanations
  ○ Frequent visits to the Emergency Department
  ○ Injuries to the trunk and/or extremities
	■ Includes physical abuse, emotional abuse, sexual abuse, financial abuse, abandonment, and/or a violation of personal rights
	■ Signs include
	  ○ Soft-tissue injuries
	  ○ Untreated medical problems
	  ○ Withdrawal
	  ○ Lack of personal hygiene

Nursing Interventions for an Abused Patient

- Interview the patient privately.
- Utilize therapeutic communication.
  - This involves exploring how the person actually feels while interpreting spoken words, gestures, and facial expressions. Do they match?
  - In a case where the patient's words do not match his or her gestures or facial expressions, further explore how the person actually feels.
  - For therapeutic communication to be effective, the nurse needs to be aware of how he or she appears to the patient and be able to assess the overall message that is communicated by the patient, such as fear, pain, sadness, anxiety, or apathy.
- Provide support.
- Do not judge.
- Document the assessment and any referrals.
- Refer the patient to social services.
- It is the law to report elder abuse to Adult Protective Services.

Now that you have reviewed the key behavioral/psychosocial concepts, go to the Behavioral/Psychosocial Practice Questions. Answer the questions, and then check your answers. Continue to review the information until you answer 80% of the practice questions correctly.

BEHAVIORAL/PSYCHOSOCIAL PRACTICE QUESTIONS

1. A patient who is in the critical care unit with sepsis has a known history of PTSD secondary to a physical assault, including a rape 6 months prior to admission. Which of the following is a recommended strategy for the nurse to utilize in the care of this patient?

   (A) Administer benzodiazepines for anxiety.
   (B) Limit family visitation.
   (C) Insist on having a discussion about the assault.
   (D) Provide the opportunity for the patient to record her daily activities while critically ill.

2. The development of delirium has been shown to have a negative effect on the patient's outcome. Therefore, it is important to PREVENT delirium. Which of the following is an effective strategy to prevent delirium?

   (A) Restrain the patient's wrists loosely to provide safety.
   (B) Maintain a target of deep sedation for most patients.
   (C) Encourage communication and reorient the patient repetitively.
   (D) Keep the patient on bed rest until he or she is weaned off a ventilator and pressors.

3. A 69-year-old female is admitted for a suicide attempt after being found unresponsive at home by her husband with an open bottle of zolpidem (Ambien). As soon as the nurse enters the room, the patient greets the nurse cheerfully and claims it was all a "big mistake," stating that she would never want to end her life. Which of the following should be included in this patient's plan of care?

   (A) Stay with the patient until she swallows her scheduled medications.
   (B) Update the patient's husband that the patient is not depressed.
   (C) Advise the patient that she will need to be honest in order to improve.
   (D) Provide privacy in order to increase the patient's self-esteem.

4. A 45-year-old male is admitted with acute respiratory failure secondary to pneumonia. The nurse notices that he appears increasingly restless and suspects delirium. Which of the following must be present for the patient to be delirious?

   (A) agitation
   (B) disorganized thinking
   (C) acute onset of mental status changes or a fluctuating course
   (D) withdrawal

5. A patient with a long history of alcohol abuse may develop gait disturbances due to a thiamine deficiency that, in turn, affects glucose metabolism. Gait disturbances are a sign of which of the following problems?

(A) Grey Turner's sign
(B) Wernicke encephalopathy
(C) alcohol poisoning
(D) Korsakoff syndrome

6. A patient has suddenly become verbally aggressive and loud. Which of the following is the best strategy for the nurse to use at this time?

(A) Speak loudly to the patient.
(B) Restrain the patient.
(C) Stand directly in front of the patient.
(D) Provide direct care with a colleague.

ANSWER KEY

1. **D**   2. **C**   3. **A**   4. **C**   5. **B**   6. **D**

ANSWERS AND EXPLANATIONS

1. **(D)** Providing a process that encourages the patient/her family to record daily activities prevents the anxiety that is associated with memory gaps during a critical illness. Benzodiazepines (choice (A)) have been shown to lead to PTSD. Family visitation should be encouraged, not limited (as choice (B)) suggests, because family presence may prevent anxiety and PTSD symptoms. Choice (C) is incorrect because the traumatic event should only be discussed if the patient brings it up.

2. **(C)** Studies have shown that engaging patients in communication and frequent reorientation will help prevent delirium. Restraining patients, using deep sedation, and limiting mobility will all increase the likelihood of developing delirium.

3. **(A)** Patients who have attempted suicide have been known to either hoard medications to use in a future suicide attempt or be suspicious of medications that are ordered by health care providers. This patient is most likely depressed, as evidenced by her actions. Her statement otherwise is not to be entirely believed. Confrontation is most likely not therapeutic. Patients who have attempted suicide should not be left alone.

4. **(C)** Delirium always has an acute onset of mental status changes or a fluctuating course (as opposed to dementia, which is chronic). Additionally, the patient needs to manifest inattention in order for delirium to be present. Not all patients with delirium are agitated (as choice (A) suggests) since some have symptoms of hypoactivity. Disorganized thinking (choice (B)) may be present, but it is not required since an altered LOC may be present instead of disorganized thinking. Withdrawal (choice (D)) may be present, but the change in baseline may be agitation, not withdrawal. Note that the use of a valid assessment tool, such as the CAM-ICU or the ICDSC, increases the chance of accurately detecting all types of delirium.

5. **(B)** Gait disturbances are one of several signs of Wernicke encephalopathy, which is due to a severe lack of thiamine. The remaining 3 choices do not result in gait changes and/or are not due to alcohol abuse.

6. **(D)** When more than one caregiver is in the room, the patient is less likely to be aggressive. The remaining 3 choices may provoke aggression or put the nurse in an unsafe position.

Integumentary Concepts

14

Spectacular achievement is always preceded by unspectacular preparation.

—Robert H. Schuller

INTEGUMENTARY TEST BLUEPRINT

Integumentary 2% of total test   **3-4 questions***

→ Cellulitis
→ IV infiltration
→ Necrotizing fasciitis
→ Pressure injury
→ Wounds
  ○ Infectious
  ○ Surgical
  ○ Trauma

*The number of questions and percentages in this category may vary slightly from test to test.

INTEGUMENTARY TESTABLE NURSING ACTIONS

☐ Recognize indications for and manage patients requiring therapeutic interventions (e.g., wound VACs, pressure reduction surfaces, fecal management devices, IV infiltrate treatment)

This exam includes only 3–4 questions on integumentary concepts. Therefore, 3–4 hours of studying these topics is generally adequate in order to do well.

Overview

- **Complex wounds** are usually accompanied by comorbidities that complicate healing (e.g., diabetes, peripheral vascular disease, infections, immune deficiency, poor nutritional status, and burns).
  - Surgical intervention and/or wound care consults are often required.
- A **pressure injury (PI)** is localized damage to the skin and underlying soft tissue. It usually occurs over a bony prominence and/or is related to improper use of a medical device, such as a tube securement device or SCD tubing. A pressure injury may be present with either intact skin or an open ulcer; pain may or may not be present.
  - Pressure injuries are preventable in most cases, depending upon the quality of care provided.

Prevention of a Pressure Injury

- Look for the presence of a PI upon admission and assess the skin surfaces each shift.
  - Note that not all wounds are due to pressure; it is important to differentiate.
- Identify high-risk patients with the use of a valid risk assessment tool (Braden Scale or Norton Scale), and those with known risk factors for developing a PI (low body weight, poor nutritional status, inadequate hydration, decreased perfusion, immobility, and/or hypoxemia).
- Utilize strategies to prevent pressure injuries and to maintain intact skin integrity: reposition the patient, prevent shearing/friction when moving, moisturize the skin, maintain clean/dry skin, protect the skin from incontinence, use skin barrier products, off-load bony prominences and lines/tubes, use paper tape for those with fragile skin, provide nutritional support if needed, and/or provide special pressure-redistributing surfaces (including mattresses, mattress overlays, and seat cushions).
  - Avoid the use of diapers, which cause dermatitis in adult patients; use absorbent bed padding.

Assessment of a Pressure Injury

- When a patient is admitted, and during each shift, assess the skin. If a PI is identified, determine the stage of the pressure injury, document the stage, and determine and evaluate the plan of care.
  - Stage 1
    - Characterized by intact skin with redness of a localized area
  - Stage 2
    - Characterized by partial thickness skin loss with exposed dermis
    - The wound bed is pink or red and moist and may appear as a blister
  - Stage 3
    - Characterized by full thickness skin loss
    - Subcutaneous fat is visible.

- ○ Stage 4
  - – Characterized by full thickness skin loss with exposed or directly palpable fascia, bone, tendon, ligament, or muscle
  - – Slough or eschar may be present.
- ○ Unstageable
  - – A PI may be classified as "unstageable" if there is full thickness skin loss and tissue loss in which the extent of the tissue damage within the ulcer cannot be confirmed because it is obscured by slough or eschar. If the slough or eschar is removed, the wound may then be classified as Stage 1, 2, 3, or 4 based on an assessment of it.

Treatment for a Pressure Injury

- As soon as a PI is identified, notify the provider to discuss a detailed treatment plan. Request a wound care consult, if available. Treatment is based upon an assessment of the patient and the PI.
- Keep the affected area clean and dry.
- Provide pressure relief over bony prominences by utilizing pressure-reducing surfaces, repositioning the patient at least every 2 hours (even when using pressure-reducing surfaces), and keeping the head of the bed at 30° while the patient is side-lying.
- Perform wound debridement to support healing. Examples of wound debridement include:
  - ○ Enzymatic debridement using proteolytic enzymes
  - ○ Nonselective mechanical debridement (whirlpool treatments, forceful irrigation, or wet-to-dry dressings)
  - ○ Surgical debridement
- Apply dressings as indicated (the type of dressing depends upon the wound assessment).
- Ensure adequate nutrition.
- Apply antibiotic ointment as indicated.
- Initiate and care for a wound VAC system, if one is ordered by the provider.

NEGATIVE-PRESSURE WOUND THERAPY (WOUND VAC THERAPY)

Overview

- Negative-pressure wound therapy, also known as wound VAC therapy, is used for acute or chronic complex wounds (e.g., diabetic ulcers, surgical wounds, or burns).
- A sealed wound dressing is placed over the wound and connected to a vacuum pump, which provides continuous or intermittent negative pressure (–75 mmHg to –125 mmHg).
  - ○ The continued application of negative pressure promotes healing by increasing blood flow to the area.
- This type of therapy is usually applied by a provider or a wound care nurse and is maintained by an acute/critical care nurse.

Management of Wound VAC Therapy

- Address alarms that may be caused by a full canister, an air leak in the system, a low battery, or blocked or dislodged tubing.
- Change the evacuation canister when it is full, if there are signs of damage, and according to manufacturer recommendations (generally once per week).
- Do not allow the therapy to be interrupted for longer than 2 hours; a longer interruption puts the patient at a greater risk for infection.
  - If the therapy needs to be interrupted for longer than 2 hours, replace the dressing with a wet-to-damp dressing until the therapy can be resumed.
- Report any bleeding to the provider.

NECROTIZING FASCIITIS

Necrotizing fasciitis is a rapidly progressive inflammatory infection of the fascia, with secondary necrosis of the subcutaneous tissues. Early identification of and treatment for this infection are the keys to decreasing morbidity and mortality.

- Causative organisms: group A *Streptococcus*, *Clostridial myonecrosis* (gas gangrene), salt water that contains a *Vibrio* species, or multiple organisms may be the cause; at times, the cause of necrotizing fasciitis may be unknown.
- Risk factors: the presence of open skin (e.g., the site of an injection, abrasion, insect bite, or surgical procedure), more often seen in those who are immunocompromised, such as those with diabetes, cancer, alcoholism, vascular insufficiency, organ transplants, HIV infection, or neutropenia
- Signs and symptoms: intense pain over the involved skin and underlying muscle, minor redness, the infection quickly spreading out onto normal skin, developing dusky or purplish discoloration, and necrosis; subsequent systemic signs of an infection (such as a fever and malaise) will occur.
  - Necrotizing fasciitis may progress to septic shock, MODS, and/or limb loss.
- Treatment: this is a surgical emergency! An early and aggressive implementation of a regimen of surgical debridement (until the spread of necrosis is resolved) is associated with a decrease in morbidity and mortality; however, the patient may require surgical reconstruction.
  - Treat hemodynamic instability with fluids/pressors.
  - Provide antibiotic therapy (that will initially be empiric, but will subsequently be guided by the blood culture results).
  - Provide nutritional support to address the catabolism that is caused by large necrotic wounds.
  - Consider using hyperbaric oxygen and intravenous immunoglobulin for select cases.

FECAL MANAGEMENT SYSTEM (FMS)

- A fecal management system (FMS) is used for a patient with involuntary, liquid diarrhea in order to prevent skin excoriation and breakdown and to prevent contamination of a surgical site, wounds, or invasive lines.
- An internal device is inserted into the rectum and is held in place by a balloon catheter; the balloon is then inflated, and the device is flushed as directed by the manufacturer.
  - A provider order is needed to use an internal device.
  - An internal FMS is contraindicated for patients with a rectal injury, patients who have recently had lower large bowel surgery, patients with fecal impaction, and patients who have severe hemorrhoids or formed stool.
- An external device is applied externally around the anus.
  - An external device is indicated when an internal device cannot be used.
  - Do not apply over excoriated skin.
- Provide frequent monitoring of device patency, stool quality/amount, and the condition of the skin.

MANAGEMENT OF INTRAVENOUS THERAPY (INFILTRATION, PHLEBITIS, EXTRAVASATION)

Infiltration

- Infiltration is the inadvertent infusion of a medication or solution into the surrounding tissue rather than into the intended vascular system; the medication or solution may or may not be a vesicant.
- If infiltration occurs, stop the infusion.
- Assess and document the infiltration using an infiltration scale:

  0 = No symptoms
  1 = Blanched skin, edema < 1 inch in any direction
  2 = Blanched skin, edema 1–6 inches in any direction
  3 = Blanched and translucent skin, edema > 6 inches in any direction, possible numbness
  4 = Blanched and translucent skin, tight skin that's leaking fluid, deep pitting edema, moderate to severe pain; an extravasation of blood product, irritant, or vesicant is a grade 4 infiltration, regardless of whether the site assessment is normal or abnormal

- If infiltration occurs, elevate the extremity and apply a warm, moist compress, or provide whatever treatment is indicated for that specific type of irritant/vesicant.
- Reinsert the IV using the opposite extremity (if able).

Phlebitis

- Phlebitis is a venous inflammatory reaction that is caused by an irritant drug or mechanical device and results in a local inflammatory reaction such as redness, red streaks, pain, burning, or swelling.

- Utilize strategies to prevent phlebitis (e.g., use the smallest gauge catheter indicated, avoid placing the catheter near joints or vein valves, use more diluted agent if indicated, use a central line for medications that are known to have a high osmolality or a low pH).
- Stop the infusion, and elevate the extremity.
- Attempt to identify the cause of the reaction and address it as able; restart the IV.

Extravasation

- Extravasation is an infiltration of a vesicant drug that may cause severe and/or irreversible tissue injury and necrosis. This may result in blisters, pain, tissue sloughing, a loss of mobility, and/or an infection.
- More serious cases may require surgical intervention.
- Consult a pharmacist or hospital procedures to determine which drugs are vesicants, since there are many agents used that are non-cytotoxic agents that will cause tissue damage, and determine:
  - Whether an antidote is available
  - Whether warm or cold compresses are indicated and the frequency/duration of application
    - Most vesicant agents are treated with cold compresses, although warm compresses are indicated when the antidote **hyaluronidase** is used or when **phentolamine** (Regitine) is used; always double-check!
- Provide an antidote, as indicated, **as soon as possible**.
- Examples of antidotes include:
  - Hyaluronidase (used for non-cytotoxic agent extravasations [e.g., amiodarone, calcium gluconate, mannitol] **or** for cytotoxic extravasations [e.g., teniposide])
  - Phentolamine (Regitine), terbutaline, or 2% nitroglycerin ointment (used for vasopressor extravasations [e.g., norepinephrine, dopamine])

> Now that you have reviewed the key integumentary concepts, go to the Integumentary Practice Questions. Answer the questions, and then check your answers. Continue to review the information until you answer 80% of the practice questions correctly.

INTEGUMENTARY PRACTICE QUESTIONS

1. A patient has copious involuntary diarrhea secondary to a *C. difficile* infection and has developed red, excoriated skin with blisters on the coccyx/buttocks area. Which of the following is the most appropriate intervention for this patient?

   (A) Keep the area clean and dry, and apply a diaper and barrier cream.
   (B) Obtain an order for the insertion of a fecal management system (FMS).
   (C) Keep the area clean and dry, and apply an external fecal collection device.
   (D) Contact the provider for an anti-diarrheal medication and order a wound care consult.

2. A patient has a norepinephrine infusion running via a left antecubital IV. The skin appears puffy about a half inch above the IV insertion site and is also reddened and tender. What is a priority intervention for this patient?

(A) Apply cool compresses.

(B) Administer hyaluronidase, and apply cold compresses.

(C) Restart the IV with a smaller gauge catheter in the opposite arm.

(D) Administer phentolamine (Regitine), and apply warm compresses.

3. Which of the following is the priority treatment for a patient with necrotizing fasciitis?

(A) surgical debridement of the necrotic tissue

(B) nutritional support

(C) hyperbaric oxygen therapy

(D) antibiotic ointment

ANSWER KEY

1. **B**   2. **D**   3. **A**

ANSWERS AND EXPLANATIONS

1. **(B)** The skin damage is over a bony prominence with blisters. Therefore, it is a Stage 2 PI, and an internal fecal management system (FMS) will help prevent further skin irritation. Pressure relief measures are also needed. The use of diapers (choice (A)) is not recommended as a skin protection strategy. External fecal collection devices (choice (C)) are not indicated for excoriated skin. An anti-diarrheal medication (choice (D)) is not indicated for a *C. difficile* infection, and generally, wound care consults are not required for a partial thickness PI.

2. **(D)** This patient has a Grade 1 infiltration of a vesicant; therefore, this is an extravasation. The antidote for a vasopressor extravasation is phentolamine (Regitine), which should be given as soon as possible after the extravasation is identified. Then, warm compresses should be applied. The remaining three choices are not appropriate interventions for this scenario.

3. **(A)** Early debridement of the necrotic tissue and repeating debridement as the necrotic tissue spreads leads to decreased morbidity and mortality. Nutritional support (choice (B)) is important, although without the removal of necrotic tissue, nutritional support alone will not improve the outcome. Hyperbaric oxygen therapy (choice (C)) may be helpful (when available), but evidence has not supported that it decreases morbidity and mortality. Antibiotic ointment (choice (D)) is not a therapy for necrotizing fasciitis.

Musculoskeletal Concepts

15

Optimism is the faith that leads to achievement. Nothing can be done without hope and confidence.

—Helen Keller

MUSCULOSKELETAL TEST BLUEPRINT

Musculoskeletal 2% of total test　　　　　　**3–4 questions***

→ Compartment syndrome
→ Fractures (e.g., femur, pelvic)
→ Functional issues (e.g., immobility, falls, gait disorders)
→ Osteomyelitis
→ Rhabdomyolysis

*The number of questions and percentages in this category may vary slightly from test to test.

MUSCULOSKELETAL TESTABLE NURSING ACTIONS

☐ Manage patients requiring progressive mobility
☐ Recognize indications for, and manage patients requiring, compartment syndrome monitoring

This exam includes only 3–4 questions on musculoskeletal concepts. Therefore, 3–4 hours of studying these topics is generally adequate in order to do well.

PROGRESSIVE MOBILITY

Overview

■ Immobility is a consequence of all types of critical illnesses, and studies have demonstrated its deleterious effects on all body systems. The goal is to progress patients to the highest level of mobility that they are safely capable of achieving each day during their acute care stay.

Negative Outcomes of Immobility

- Physiological changes such as increased heart rate, decreased vital capacity, atelectasis, pneumonia, muscular weakness, urinary retention, constipation, and pain
- Pressure injuries
- Sleep deprivation
- Delirium
- Prolonged ventilator days, ICU stay, and/or hospital stay

Contraindications for Mobility Progression

- **M**yocardial instability—chest pain, ischemia, an arrhythmia requiring an antiarrhythmic in the past 24 hours
- **O**xygenation issues—pulse oximetry $< 90\%$, respiratory rate < 10 breaths/minute or > 35 breaths/minute, extreme fatigue/dyspnea; if the patient is receiving mechanical ventilation, contraindications include any of the previously mentioned oxygenation issues OR FiO_2 60% or greater and/or PEEP > 10 cm H_2O.
- **V**asopressor—increase in dose needed in the past 2 hours or the patient has 2 or more vasopressors infusing.
- **E**ngagement issues—the patient does not respond to verbal stimulation or follow commands.

Strategies to Address the Challenges of Early Progressive Mobility for the Acute/Critically Ill

- Develop and utilize a nurse-driven protocol for the progression of patient mobility.
- Minimize sedation.
- Provide effective, safe patient handling equipment.
- Maintain the safety of lines and tubes.
- Schedule and coordinate mobilization with the interdisciplinary team; that MUST be a team effort with the physician and nursing leadership.
- Address any patient discomfort and explain the rationale for and importance of moving to the patient and his or her family.
- Assess for hemodynamic stability.
  - If the patient is unstable, attempt position changes and/or continuous lateral rotation therapy and provide passive range of motion.
- Provide education on the rationale for mobility, the protocol involved, and the equipment used.
- Consult the physical therapy team for more complex mobility challenges.

Overview

- Studies have shown that patients suffer harm in approximately 25% of cases that involve sustaining a fall while hospitalized.
- Patient falls lead to negative clinical outcomes, including an increased length of stay, increased costs, increased 30-day readmission rate, and higher mortality.
- Almost all critically ill patients are at a high risk for a fall at some point during their hospital stay.

Risk Factors for Falls

- Age > 65 years old
- History of a fall in the past year
- Orthostatic hypotension
- Impaired mobility or gait
- Altered mental status
- Incontinence
- Need for assistive devices
- Medications, especially those that were recently ordered (e.g., benzodiazepines, diuretics, antihypertensives)
- Medical devices that limit mobility (e.g., urinary catheters, monitor leads, IV lines)
- Restraints

Fall Prevention Strategies

- Routinely assess the patient's risk for falls using a validated fall risk assessment tool (e.g., Morse Fall Scale).
- Communicate the patient's fall risk status (document this in the patient's medical record, in signage, on the patient's wristband, on whiteboards, and verbally) to all members of the health care team.
- Provide ongoing education about the patient's high-risk status and the rationale for fall prevention strategies to the patient and his or her family.
- Adhere to hospital procedures and protocols regarding the assessments, interventions, and documentation related to fall risk factors and the utilization of preventive measures.
- Provide orientations and ongoing staff education.
- Ensure adequate staffing.
- Assess the physical environment for safety issues and orient the patient to the environment.
- Accompany the patient during mobilization in and out of bed and to the commode.
- Study and learn from past patient falls; perform a root cause analysis of each fall.
- Ensure that unit managers are engaged in and communicate about fall prevention in each hospital unit.

- Rhabdomyolysis is a potentially life-threatening syndrome due to the massive destruction of skeletal muscle cells.
- The etiologies of rhabdomyolysis include crush injuries, prolonged immobility, compartment syndrome, hyperthermia, and delirium tremens (DTs).
- Massive muscle injury results in the release of myoglobin, creatine kinase (CK), and potassium into the extracellular and intravascular spaces due to damaged muscles.
- Kidney injury occurs when creatine kinase and myoglobin obstruct the renal tubules.
- Clinical sequelae of rhabdomyolysis:
  - Hypovolemia
  - Hyperkalemia
  - Metabolic acidosis
  - Acute renal failure
- Refer to Table 15-1, which summarizes the signs/symptoms of and treatment for rhabdomyolysis.

Table 15-1. Signs/Symptoms of and Treatment for Rhabdomyolysis

Signs/Symptoms	Treatment
• Dark, tea-colored urine • Low urine output • Urine dipstick is positive for hemoglobin, but a urinalysis is negative for RBCs • Myoglobin in urine • Elevated CK > 10,000 U/L • Muscle cramping • Arrhythmias	• Administer fluids (0.9 NS) to maintain a urine flow of ~ 300 mL/hour; it may be necessary to infuse up to 500 mL/hour of 0.9 NS to maintain a urine output of 300 mL/hour • Initiate a sodium bicarbonate infusion to alkalinize the urine • Administer mannitol • Monitor for and treat hyperkalemia • Therapy should continue until the urine is cleared of any myoglobin

COMPARTMENT SYNDROME

Acute compartment syndrome is the development of elevated pressure within the muscle fascia, which may lead to decreased blood flow. This results in damage to the muscle tissue and nerves within the compartment.

- Causes: a crush injury to or surgery on a limb, a fracture, severe muscle hematoma or sprain, a constricting cast or bandage, and/or prolonged tourniquet or positioning during surgery that leads to a loss of blood supply to a limb
- Signs/symptoms: pain (worse than expected based on an assessment of the injury), numbness, a loss of movement, a firm, "wooden" feeling upon palpation, and/or elevated intracompartmental pressure
  - Loss of pulse and/or the development of pallor are not reliable clinical signs of compartment syndrome; they may occur late (after permanent damage has already been done).

- Management
  - Measure the intracompartmental pressure as soon as compartment syndrome is suspected and continue to monitor the intracompartmental pressure as indicated.
    - A normal compartment pressure = 0–8 mmHg
    - A compartment pressure > 30 mmHg = compartment syndrome; if that is the case, **emergent decompressive fasciotomy** is indicated to prevent permanent nerve and/or vascular injuries.
  - Maintain the level of the affected limb at the **level of the heart**; do NOT elevate the limb higher than the level of the heart because elevation decreases arterial blood flow to the tissues.
  - Remove any bandages or casts.
  - Provide pain control with opioids or NSAIDs.
  - Approximately 3 hours after decompression procedures, monitor for postischemic tissue swelling due to altered capillary permeability (mannitol may be considered).
  - Monitor for the development of rhabdomyolysis.

Now that you have reviewed the key musculoskeletal concepts, go to the Musculoskeletal Practice Questions. Answer the questions, and then check your answers. Continue to review the information until you answer 80% of the practice questions correctly

MUSCULOSKELETAL PRACTICE QUESTIONS

1. An ICU nurse feels that patients in the ICU where he currently works are not sufficiently mobilized. He plans to bring a proposal of strategies to use for the successful implementation of a progressive mobility program to the unit manager, and he plans to offer to assist with the program's implementation. Which of the following is an evidence-based strategy that can be used to help make a progressive mobility program successful?

   (A) discouraging the use of opioids for pain
   (B) developing a physician-driven protocol for mobility progression
   (C) proposing that physical therapists see all ICU patients
   (D) requesting the purchase of safe patient handling equipment

2. A patient has been in bed for 2 days and is scheduled to get up and sit in a chair today. The patient was admitted with heart failure and hypertension, and he has been started on 2 antihypertensive medications. Which of the following would most likely help prevent this patient from falling?

   (A) Assess the patient for orthostatic hypotension before he gets out of bed.
   (B) Hold the B/P medications until after the mobility session.
   (C) Stay with the patient while he gets out of bed.
   (D) Keep the patient on bed rest.

For questions 3 and 4

A female patient who was brought in after having fallen on the kitchen floor and was unable to move for approximately 48 hours has dark, tea-colored urine that is positive for myoglobin, a BUN of 52 mEq/L, a serum creatinine of 4.2 mEq/L, and a serum potassium of 5.6 mEq/L.

3. Which of the following is a priority treatment for this patient?

   (A) Administer a loop diuretic.
   (B) Administer an amp of sodium bicarbonate.
   (C) Administer 0.9 normal saline at a rate that will maintain a urine output of 300 mL/hour.
   (D) Dialyze the patient as soon as possible.

4. Which of the following lab values would be an expected finding for this patient?

   (A) CK 30,000 U/L
   (B) amylase 500 U/L
   (C) troponin 12 ng/mL
   (D) bilirubin 4.2 mg/dL

ANSWER KEY

1. **D**   2. **A**   3. **C**   4. **A**

ANSWERS AND EXPLANATIONS

1. **(D)** The availability of safe patient handling equipment assists with mobilization of the most dependent critically ill patients. Pain control, often with opioids, is important for the patient to move comfortably; as long as they are timed and dosed appropriately, opioid use would not be a barrier to patient mobility. Therefore, choice (A) is incorrect. A nurse-driven protocol, not a physician-driven protocol, has been demonstrated to be effective. Therefore, choice (B) is incorrect. Physical therapy resources are used to assist with the management of the more challenging patients, but physical therapists do not need to see all ICU patients. Therefore, choice (C) is also incorrect.

2. **(A)** The prolonged period of time in bed and the addition of antihypertensive medications puts the patient at risk for orthostatic hypotension. Therefore, an assessment for orthostatic hypotension needs to be done to keep the patient safe. Medications should not be held, since they are needed for controlling the patient's B/P, and it is important to know how the patient will do while taking these medications in the hospital. Therefore, choice (B) is incorrect. It goes without saying that someone needs to stay with the patient during first-time ambulation, but that alone may not prevent a patient or nurse injury if orthostatic hypotension is severe and if the patient stumbles or loses consciousness. Therefore, choice (C) is incorrect. The addition of 2 antihypertensive medications increases the patient's fall risk, but that is not a reason to keep the patient on bed rest and prolong immobility. Therefore, choice (D) is also incorrect.

3. **(C)** This clinical scenario describes rhabdomyolysis (tea-colored urine that is positive for myoglobin). Administering large volumes of fluid in order to maintain "flushing" of the kidneys is needed to prevent permanent renal tubular damage. Diuretics and hemodialysis have not been shown to prevent permanent renal tubular damage. Alkalinization of urine is beneficial. However, it is done by placing sodium bicarbonate into large-volume IV bags and infusing it over several hours. Alkalinization should not be done by giving the patient an amp of sodium bicarbonate through an IV.

4. **(A)** Rhabdomyolysis is the result of a crush injury of skeletal muscle cells, which releases myoglobin and CK into the blood. This release may "clog" the renal tubules. The other 3 lab values are not typical of rhabdomyolysis.

Professional Caring and Ethical Practice Concepts

16

Don't worry about failures, worry about the chances you miss when you don't even try.

—Jack Canfield

PROFESSIONAL CARING AND ETHICAL PRACTICE TEST BLUEPRINT

Professional Caring and Ethical Practice 20% of total test   **30 questions**

→ Advocacy/Moral Agency (3%)*
→ Caring Practices (4%)*
→ Collaboration (4%)*
→ Systems Thinking (2%)*
→ Response to Diversity (1%)*
→ Clinical Inquiry (4%)*
→ Facilitation of Learning (2%)*

*The number of questions and percentages in each of these categories may vary slightly from test to test.

OVERVIEW

The AACN places a great deal of importance on a nurse's ability to provide care to critically ill patients and their families beyond the physiological realm. A nurse's ability to assess the entire patient situation is expected. Novice critical care nurses tend to focus on learning the many clinical issues and management of symptoms. As a nurse progresses from novice to competent to expert level of nursing practice, he or she increases his/her ability to see the whole patient and consider patient characteristics beyond physiology. The competencies that will be discussed throughout this chapter are described in the AACN Synergy Model for Patient Care, which can be found at *www.aacn.org*. The Adult CCRN exam questions will require you to take into account all of the patient's characteristics, not just the physiological ones, when planning care.

TEST PREPARATION

- Read the AACN Synergy Model for Patient Care, but do not attempt to memorize it. Simply understand the AACN's philosophy on professional caring and ethical practice.
- Review the concepts presented in this chapter.

- Answer the practice questions and review the answer explanations to identify areas you may need to review further.
- Although the total number of Professional Caring and Ethical Practice questions is greater than the number of questions devoted to any one Clinical Judgment topic on the Adult CCRN exam, you will not need to study this chapter for as many hours as you will need to study the Cardiovascular Concepts chapter (the Clinical Judgment topic with the greatest number of questions); you'll probably only need half that time to review this chapter.
- Familiarize yourself with the AACN Practice Alerts that are related to Professional Caring and Ethical Practice. The Practice Alerts are available at *https://www.aacn.org/clinical-resources/practice-alerts* and can be saved as PDFs for your files. Two important Practice Alerts to review are:
  - "Family Presence During Resuscitation and Invasive Procedures"
  - "Family Presence: Visitation in the Adult ICU"

NURSE CHARACTERISTICS THAT ARE NECESSARY TO PROVIDE PROFESSIONAL CARING AND ETHICAL PRACTICE

Clinical Judgment

An expert nurse has the ability to synthesize and interpret multiple pieces of data and demonstrate critical thinking.

- At the expert level of practice, the nurse interprets multiple, sometimes conflicting, pieces of data and makes decisions based on a grasp of the whole picture. He or she can anticipate problems based on previous experiences.
- The nurse helps the patient and the patient's family see the "big picture."
- It takes time for a nurse to develop clinical judgment.
- For example, when caring for a patient with multiple organ dysfunction syndrome with comorbidities, a less-experienced nurse will focus solely on the patient's immediate physiological instability. This will be reflected in patient/family communication. An expert nurse who is demonstrating clinical judgment will address the patient's physiological instability, but he or she will also realize the impact of the comorbidities and will include this when communicating with the patient and the patient's family.

Advocacy and Moral Agency

An expert nurse works on the behalf of others, represents the concerns of others (including the patient/family and other nurses), and is able to identify and help resolve ethical issues.

- At the expert level of practice, the nurse advocates from the patient's/family's perspective, even when their views are different from the nurse's personal values.
- The nurse may work to adjust the rules (i.e., policies) to work for the benefit of the patient/family.
- The integrity of the family support system is crucial to the patient's long-term outcome (i.e., the patient's support system is always considered in the plan of care).
- The nurse will empower the patient/family to speak for themselves.
- For example, if the wife of an unresponsive patient on a ventilator requests to use an herbal remedy ointment that is known to be a cure in her culture, a less-experienced nurse might tactfully explain that using an herbal remedy ointment is not allowed, thereby supporting

the rules. An expert nurse, who is demonstrating advocacy and moral agency, would understand the importance of this ointment to the wife and would explain that he or she will consult a pharmacist to see if the ointment is safe. If the ointment is safe to use, the expert nurse will allow the wife to apply it on the patient under supervision.

Caring Practices

An expert nurse creates a compassionate, supportive, and therapeutic environment for the patients and their families. He or she prevents unnecessary suffering.

- At the expert level of practice, the nurse engages the patient/family, is aware of the patient's needs and the family's needs, and anticipates their needs.
- The nurse coordinates care to provide comfort for the patient/family, even at the time of death.
- The nurse ensures that **all** patients and their families understand that palliative options exist to relieve suffering at the end of life.
- For example, if a young athlete has an acute traumatic injury that may impact her future ability to play sports and she exhibits "difficult" behavior, a less-experienced nurse may sympathize and do what is necessary in an attempt to meet the patient's demands. An expert nurse who is demonstrating caring practices will understand that this behavior may be a symptom of grief and loss, and he or she will encourage the patient to express her feelings related to that loss. The expert nurse may also seek expert consultation and engage the rehab team early in the patient's treatment.

Collaboration

An expert nurse works with others in a manner that promotes and encourages each person's contributions toward achieving optimal, realistic goals.

- At the expert level of practice, the nurse initiates collaboration. He or she does not wait for others to reach out.
- The nurse seeks opportunities to teach, coach, and mentor.
- The nurse seeks opportunities to be taught, coached, and mentored.
- The nurse values consistent communication.
- For example, if a nephrologist explains to the wife of an 89-year-old unresponsive patient with metastatic cancer that hemodialysis is required and will provide a chance for improvement, and then the wife expresses doubt after the physician leaves the room, a less-experienced nurse may either comfort the wife or perhaps contradict what the physician explained. An expert nurse who is demonstrating collaboration will seek to collaborate with the wife and the physician by first discussing the prognosis with the wife, then listening to the wife's hesitancy, and finally working with the physician to determine a better solution.

Systems Thinking

An expert nurse manages the environmental and system resources to meet the patient's/family's needs. He or she considers factors outside of the immediate unit. He or she considers the hospital a community.

- At the expert level of practice, the nurse navigates the system on behalf of the patient/family.
- The nurse sees the patient/family in the "big picture," not only in terms of the immediate unit environment.

- The nurse understands that the processes and systems that are in place may cause human errors and inefficiencies.
- The nurse participates in a culture of patient safety:
    - When errors are made, the response is to analyze the system processes that led to the error (not punitive).
    - The number of incident reports or patient safety event reports generally increases in a culture of patient safety, since reports are made to assess and identify how processes can be improved to prevent future errors, not to target individuals.
- For example, a patient received 2 stents during a PCI procedure for acute coronary syndrome and will need to take clopidogrel (Plavix). The patient does not have health insurance. A less-experienced nurse may not realize the cost of the drug and may not be aware of resources that can be recommended to the patient. An expert nurse who is demonstrating systems thinking may be aware of a special program that is sponsored by a pharmaceutical company. The expert nurse may also consult social services or a case manager in an attempt to get financial assistance for the patient.

Response to Diversity

An expert nurse will recognize, appreciate, and incorporate differences into the plan of care. Differences include age, gender, race, cultural differences, ethnicity, lifestyle, educational level, socioeconomic status, values, and beliefs.

- At the expert level of practice, the nurse does not expect the patient/family to have the same characteristics or values as the health care providers, and the nurse is able to explore and identify differences.
- The nurse accepts the patient's/family's individualized responses to acute illnesses and modifies the plan of care to accommodate the patient/family.
- For example, a patient's family may have what seems like an unrealistic expectation for the patient's recovery, which is frustrating to health care providers. A less-experienced nurse may experience frustration and provide explanations in the same manner as for all other patients. An expert nurse who is demonstrating a response to diversity may attempt to identify where the family is "coming from," obtain background information, and then revise his or her explanations accordingly.

Clinical Inquiry

An expert nurse questions and evaluates practices, maintains familiarity with professional literature, and shares the best practices.

- At the expert level of practice, the nurse identifies circumstances when standards and guidelines may be improved upon or deviated from in order to address individualized patient situations or populations.
- The nurse stays current on new, updated, or revised evidence-based practices and and updates his or her own nursing practices accordingly.
- According to the AACN Synergy Model for Patient Care, the domains of clinical judgment and clinical inquiry converge at the expert level and cannot be separated.
- For example, if a patient requires feeding tube placement, a less-experienced nurse may continue to determine the correct placement of an enteral feeding tube by auscultation of air. He or she may continue this outdated practice since all other nurses use this technique.

An expert nurse who is demonstrating clinical inquiry will be aware that studies show that this practice is not an accurate method for determining feeding tube placement. He or she will bring in the literature, share the information with the staff, and engage in the process of updating hospital procedures.

Facilitation of Learning

An expert nurse promotes learning for patients, their families, the nursing staff, and members of the health care team, both formally and informally.

- At the expert level of practice, the nurse creatively finds opportunities to provide accurate information.
- The nurse adapts educational programs to the patient/family and the need/situation.
- The nurse obtains input from the patient/family when setting educational goals.
- The nurse collaborates with all members of the health care team and incorporates health care goals into the patient's educational plan.
- For example, a patient may have 3 major risk factors for coronary artery disease status post PCI with stent deployment. A less-experienced nurse might provide all available written resources on risk factor modification and advise the patient to attend cardiac rehab after being discharged. An expert nurse who is demonstrating the facilitation of learning will ask the patient to identify which risk factors he wants to target the most and provide advice based on the patient's motivation, as well as the seriousness of the risk factors.

PATIENT CHARACTERISTICS TO CONSIDER WHEN PROVIDING PROFESSIONAL CARING AND ETHICAL PRACTICE

In addition to the nurse characteristics that affect professional caring and ethical practice, the AACN has identified patient characteristics (other than physiological ones) that nurses need to consider when planning care. If only physiological problems are identified without consideration of nonclinical individual differences, the outcome will be negatively affected. The patient characteristics to consider include:

- Resiliency
  - The patient's ability to "bounce back"
- Vulnerability
  - The patient's susceptibility to actual or potential stressors
- Stability
  - The patient's ability to maintain equilibrium (not only physiological)
- Complexity
  - The patient's family interactions and environment
- Resource availability
  - Resources of the patient **and** the family (personal, fiscal, technical, social)
- Participation in care
  - The extent that the patient and the family are engaged in the patient's care

- Participation in decision making
  - The extent that the patient and the family are engaged in making decisions
- Predictability
  - The degree to which the outcome and events are expected

> Now that you have reviewed the key professional caring and ethical practice concepts, go to the Professional Caring and Ethical Practice Practice Questions. Answer the questions, and then check your answers. Continue to review the information until you answer 80% of the practice questions correctly.

PROFESSIONAL CARING AND ETHICAL PRACTICE PRACTICE QUESTIONS

1. A nurse is having difficulty with a patient's family and requests assistance from a more experienced nurse. The best approach for the experienced nurse would be to:

   (A) offer to speak with the family.
   (B) advise the nurse colleague to ignore the family's behavior.
   (C) suggest the use of active listening techniques.
   (D) suggest that the patient assignment be changed.

2. The health care team believes that a patient with multiple organ dysfunction syndrome will not survive and is dying. Which of the following is the most appropriate action at this time?

   (A) Avoid a discussion of death since it is upsetting to the patient's wife.
   (B) Ensure that the patient's wife understands the availability of palliative care at the end of life.
   (C) Refer the family's questions to the attending physician.
   (D) Portray the hopelessness of the situation so that the patient's wife accepts the reality of the situation.

3. Upon entering the room of a patient who is receiving mechanical ventilation, a nurse notices that the nursing assistant allowed the patient to remain supine and did not elevate the head of the bed to at least 30° before leaving the room. The best response would be to elevate the head of the bed and:

   (A) mention the nursing assistant's omission to the charge nurse.
   (B) point out the omission to the nursing assistant later in the shift.
   (C) advocate for a policy change related to nursing assistant responsibilities.
   (D) explain the rationale (for elevation of the head of the bed for patients on a ventilator) to the nursing assistant.

4. A nurse is approached by the patient's family during active resuscitation for full cardiopulmonary arrest and requests to be present. The nurse's best response would be to:

(A) call security.
(B) allow them to stay as long as they do not interfere.
(C) follow the current hospital policy.
(D) explain that the physician in charge does not permit family presence during CPR.

5. A 25-year-old male patient is recovering from septic shock. His mother has a homeopathic ointment and is applying it on the patient's hands and feet "for the swelling." The nurse should:

(A) take the ointment from the mother and explain it is not allowed.
(B) instruct the mother to hold off on ointment application until the pharmacist is consulted.
(C) allow the mother to continue to use the ointment since doing so is comforting her.
(D) explain that the ointment will not be of any help to the patient's edema.

6. A nurse reads a meta-analysis of a clinical intervention that supports its adoption in a nursing procedure. The most effective action to be taken by the nurse is to:

(A) bring a copy of the study to nursing and physician leadership with a request to consider revising the current nursing procedure.
(B) incorporate the clinical intervention into practice.
(C) discuss the clinical intervention with the charge nurse.
(D) assume that the nursing leadership will be adopting the new practice in the near future.

7. While receiving a report from the nurse who was working during the previous shift, a nurse notices that her colleague provided a sedative drug but no analgesic to a post-op patient. The best response would be to:

(A) point out to the nurse colleague that an omission of analgesia for a post-op patient is negligent.
(B) consider that the previous shift was busier than usual, and provide the analgesic as soon as possible.
(C) point out to the nurse colleague that it appears as if an analgesic was not given, inquire why, and then explain the importance of post-op analgesia.
(D) report the omission to the charge nurse.

8. Which of the following statements related to patient characteristics is TRUE?

(A) A quadriplegic patient who was admitted with septic shock has low resiliency.
(B) A patient with multiple comorbidities has low complexity.
(C) A patient who was admitted with multiple fractures and no other problems has low predictability.
(D) Restricted family visitation improves patient resource availability.

9. The family of a patient who is in critical, unstable condition is critical of the hospital and nursing staff and is highly distraught. What is the most appropriate response for the nurse?

(A) Explain all interventions in detail.
(B) Listen to the family's concerns and provide reassurance.
(C) Provide information on the hospital's clinical excellence.
(D) Call the nursing supervisor to meet with the family.

10. The wife of a 29-year-old critically ill trauma patient requests that she be able to bring in their 9-month-old daughter for the patient to see. The patient, who is lightly sedated, nods "yes" when asked if he wants to see his daughter. Which of the following would be the nurse's best response?

(A) Explain that children under the age of 12 cannot visit.
(B) Ignore the policy, and allow the wife to bring in their daughter.
(C) Explain to the wife that the patient will not remember the visit.
(D) Tell the wife that the physician and charge nurse will be consulted to request permission.

11. A nurse receives information from her colleague at 0700 that, during the previous shift, a 21-year-old female patient who was admitted with acute complications related to sickle cell crisis had not reported a pain score of less than 8 (on a 0–10 scale). The attending physician was contacted at 0500 for additional analgesia but stated, "The order is adequate; the patient is drug-seeking." During the initial day shift assessment, the patient rates her pain as a 9. The best response by the day shift nurse would be to:

(A) explain to the patient that the physician has been notified but no further orders were received.
(B) reassure the patient that the next dose of analgesia is due in an hour.
(C) call the physician, report the current assessment, and recommend the analgesia order that the nurse feels is most appropriate for the patient's pain.
(D) contact the nurse manager, and explain the situation.

12. A patient reported to the nurse that the physician told him he would be transferred to the step down unit later in the evening, but his wife was told that the patient would be transferred the next day. The nurse should:

(A) explain to them both that physicians often change their minds after getting more information.
(B) contact the physician to clarify the plan of care.
(C) tell the patient and his wife to wait and see what is decided.
(D) contact the charge nurse to discuss the matter.

13. A nurse has found out about an innovative IV tubing labeling system from a friend who is a nurse at another hospital. The nurse feels strongly that the innovative system would promote patient safety, and she would like to be able to use the system in her unit. The best approach to use to get the new system would be to:

    (A) obtain written information and samples of the system, and present those materials to nursing leadership.
    (B) advise the unit manager that the current IV tubing labeling system is not safe, citing examples.
    (C) complete an incident report each time a nurse forgets to label IV tubing.
    (D) point out the multiple problems with the unit's current IV tubing labeling system to colleagues.

14. The nursing staff is reacting negatively when assigned a patient with a large family that has been labeled "demanding." The best resolution would be to:

    (A) hold a team conference to discuss the issue.
    (B) rotate the patient assignment from day to day.
    (C) meet with the family, to explain that the demands need to cease.
    (D) request a psychiatric consult from the attending physician.

15. The nurse does not understand the physician's plan of care and the treatments ordered for a particular patient. It is the nurse's responsibility to:

    (A) plan to look up the patient diagnosis and treatment after work.
    (B) complete the orders as written.
    (C) tell the charge nurse to reassign the patient to another nurse.
    (D) approach the physician and seek to understand the plan of care.

16. One of the newer nurses continues to struggle when setting up the IV infusion pump despite several explanations and the provision of written material. The optimal strategy for the more experienced nurse would be to:

    (A) provide coaching while she sets up a pump.
    (B) obtain a video that shows how to set up the pump.
    (C) report the issue to the charge nurse.
    (D) demonstrate how the setup is done.

17. Which of the following statements is TRUE?

    (A) Speaking up when safety lapses are identified increases errors.
    (B) It is easier to assess system problems as the source of medication errors than to take a punitive approach.
    (C) Family presence benefits the family, not the patient.
    (D) The AACN expects nurses to consider nonphysiological patient characteristics as well as physiological data.

18. A nurse discovers that a medication error was made as the infusion pump was programmed incorrectly 30 minutes ago. The patient has not experienced any adverse reaction and is stable. The nurse should:

(A) continue to monitor the patient for adverse effects and notify the physician if any adverse effects occur.
(B) report the error to the physician, but not mention it to the patient.
(C) contact the pharmacist to determine the next steps.
(D) notify the physician, tell the patient of the error, and complete a safety event report.

19. A patient arrives on the critical care unit from the post-anesthesia care unit (PACU) with a chest tube drainage system that has never been seen before by the nurse who is receiving the patient. The nurse's best response would be to:

(A) request that the nurse from the PACU explain the system operation and answer questions as the system is reviewed.
(B) call the charge nurse into the room and explain the situation.
(C) call the surgeon and explain how disruptive and unsafe the use of the new system has been.
(D) assume the new drainage system is similar to those used in the past.

20. Several nurse colleagues of a nurse who has attained certification have asked what the value of certification is. The certified nurse's best response would be to explain that certification:

(A) validates clinical skills.
(B) is a process that leads to higher levels of professionalism.
(C) provides fiscal rewards.
(D) contributes to the professional reputation of the hospital.

21. A nurse is caring for a 71-year-old male with respiratory failure secondary to pneumonia who requires mechanical ventilation. The patient is married and has 9 children and 20 grandchildren. Many of them are either coming to see the patient or are calling to inquire about the patient. Which of the following is the best response to this situation?

(A) Ask security to intervene.
(B) Ask the family to leave the hospital, limiting the visits to 2 to 3 family members in the hospital at the same time.
(C) Answer questions succinctly as they arise, and take calls when not providing patient care.
(D) Ask the family to decide on 1 spokesperson, and communicate the plan of care to whomever the spokesperson is.

22. The critical care unit upgraded the patient beds, and the beds have many new features. All nurses received education on the new beds. On the first day at work with the new beds, a nurse realizes that he has forgotten most of the education. The nurse should:

    (A) complain to colleagues that the education took place too far in advance of actual use.
    (B) make a point to review the new bed at some point during the shift.
    (C) request that the unit educator or another nurse colleague (who worked with the beds during the previous shift) review essential operations.
    (D) look up the bed vendor on the Internet as soon as possible.

23. The unit education committee is developing written resources for patients with heart failure. An effective approach would include:

    (A) shrinking the information so that it fits on 1 page.
    (B) using more pictures than words.
    (C) developing an online program.
    (D) ensuring that the material is written at a fourth-grade reading level.

24. A nurse and her ICU colleagues have seen what they believe is an increase in lapses in care by the Emergency Department nurses. The most effective course of action would be to:

    (A) document all of the problems and send them to Risk Management.
    (B) ask the unit manager to set up a meeting between the leadership and staff representatives from each unit to plan a course of action.
    (C) request that the Emergency Department nurses receive more education.
    (D) arrange to have all ICU nurses ask more detailed questions of the Emergency Department nurses when getting a report on a patient's status prior to receiving the patient.

25. A nurse has reason to believe that one of her nurse colleagues is diverting controlled substances. The nurse should:

    (A) report her suspicions to the nurse manager.
    (B) approach the colleague to discuss her suspicions.
    (C) call security.
    (D) not take any action until more information is obtained.

26. Nurse staffing and patient assignments are best based on:

    (A) nurse/patient ratio.
    (B) patient acuity.
    (C) nurse seniority.
    (D) patient characteristics.

27. A physician orders a medication that is not considered compatible with another medication that the patient is already receiving. The nurse should:

(A) call the pharmacist to get more information.
(B) ask the physician to explain the order.
(C) ask a nurse colleague what he or she thinks of the order.
(D) administer the medication as ordered.

28. A 25-year-old female patient sustained a double amputation due to a traumatic injury. She seems withdrawn and appears to have poor self-esteem related to her body image, even though she has a strong family support system, good health insurance, and no previous health problems. An effective strategy for this patient would be to:

(A) ask for an order for an antidepressant.
(B) point out to the patient what she has in her life for which she can be grateful.
(C) encourage the patient to participate in her care, and provide options.
(D) ask for a psychiatric consult.

29. A 25-year-old non-English speaking trauma patient is unable to make decisions for himself. His wife seems to understand English and nods "yes" that she understands. However, she only speaks in short sentences and does not ask questions. The best course of action would be to:

(A) request an interpreter.
(B) attempt to contact another family member of the patient who speaks English.
(C) call a phlebotomist who speaks Spanish.
(D) continue to speak English with the wife as long as she does not object.

30. The attending physician of a patient with multisystem problems continues to express hope of a positive outcome to the patient's husband. However, the consultants have portrayed a more bleak outcome to the husband. The patient's husband has expressed his frustration to the nurse. The nurse's best response would be to:

(A) support the attending physician's opinions when speaking with the husband.
(B) support the consultants' opinions when speaking with the husband.
(C) contact the attending physician and express concern regarding the conflicting information that is being provided to the husband.
(D) empathize with the husband and explain that conflicting information often happens when multiple physicians are providing care.

ANSWER KEY

1. **C**	6. **A**	11. **C**	16. **A**	21. **D**	26. **D**
2. **B**	7. **C**	12. **B**	17. **D**	22. **C**	27. **B**
3. **D**	8. **A**	13. **A**	18. **D**	23. **D**	28. **C**
4. **C**	9. **B**	14. **A**	19. **A**	24. **B**	29. **A**
5. **B**	10. **D**	15. **D**	20. **B**	25. **A**	30. **C**

ANSWERS AND EXPLANATIONS

1. **(C)** Most difficult situations are related to gaps in communication, and listening is a major part of communication. This response demonstrates the nurse characteristic of facilitation of learning. Choices (A) and (D) do not provide an opportunity for the nurse colleague to develop professionally. Choice (B) is avoidance behavior.

2. **(B)** All critically ill patients and their families, even those in situations where the outcome is uncertain and may not be the "end of life," are entitled to palliative care, which provides a plan for the family. Choice (B) illustrates the nurse characteristics of advocacy and caring practices. Choice (A) is not a solution for the family and is not helpful. Choice (C) is not a strategy for a proactive, professional nurse. Although it may be honest, choice (D) is not helpful for the family.

3. **(D)** The nursing assistant must understand the importance of elevating the head of the bed for this patient population in order to prevent ventilator-associated complications. The correct choice also demonstrates the nurse's ability to teach. Choice (A) is passive. Choice (B) is not optimal since the ward may get too busy or the nurse may forget, and coaching should be done as close to the situation as possible. Choice (C) is not a solution. Elevation of the head of the bed is a responsibility that can be delegated to unlicensed assistants.

4. **(C)** Although choice (B) may be considered, this is not the time to allow the family's presence, since systems are not in place that would ensure a good experience. Choice (A) is an overreaction. Choice (D) is not a valid reason to prevent the family's presence.

5. **(B)** As long as homeopathic remedies are not harmful to the patient, allowing the family to practice within their culture is acceptable. Choices (A) and (D) do not acknowledge cultural diversity. Choice (C) is not correct because some homeopathic remedies may harm the patient, especially when used in conjunction with some medical therapies that are already in use.

6. **(A)** Choices (C) and (D) are not effective strategies. Choice (B) may contradict current policy that, despite being outdated, cannot be ignored without special physician approval.

7. **(C)** Choice (C) gives the nurse the chance to teach and provides an opportunity to hear the colleague's point of view. Choices (A) and (D) are not effective strategies. Choice (B) is passive behavior and ignores the opportunity for coaching.

8. **(A)** This patient has 2 major problems that will decrease his ability to "bounce back" and have a positive outcome. The plan of care should optimally take this into consideration. The remaining 3 choices are not accurate.

9. **(B)** This strategy allows the family to be heard and also allows the nurse to show a degree of empathy. The remaining 3 choices do not acknowledge the family's stress or provide support.

10. **(D)** Choices (A) and (C) do not attempt to provide patient-centered care. Although it acknowledges the patient's and wife's needs, choice (B) may send the wrong message regarding hospital policies in general. Plus, choice (B) shows a lack of ability to collaborate on the part of the nurse.

11. **(C)** This strategy, unlike the other choices, puts the patient's needs first. It has the potential to get a more appropriate order for the patient going forward.

12. **(B)** This choice is the most collaborative and direct approach.

13. **(A)** Although this choice requires the most effort, it is the one that is most likely to result in an improvement over the current process.

14. **(A)** The team needs to discuss strategies for handling this type of situation because a solution that everyone can support might be used in the future for similar situations. Choice (B) prevents continuity of care. Choice (C) does not consider the family's needs. Choice (D) implies that the issue is all the family's "fault." A social worker or psychiatric specialist may be consulted, but that alone would not be the solution.

15. **(D)** A professional nurse needs to actively collaborate to ensure his or her own understanding and to facilitate his or her own learning. The other choices are not effective strategies for ensuring the nurse understands the plan of care.

16. **(A)** This allows visual, auditory, and sensory learning. It also provides immediate feedback to the learner. All of these factors are principles of effective adult learning. The other choices do not provide multiple learning modalities.

17. **(D)** Choice (A) is not correct because speaking up decreases errors. Choice (B) is not correct because system assessments are more difficult. Choice (C) is incorrect because family presence benefits both the patient and the family.

18. **(D)** Transparency (notifying both the physician and the patient) is the appropriate response when a medication error is committed, even if the patient does not experience any adverse effects.

19. **(A)** The best immediate solution for the patient is for the nurse to get information about the new system and get his questions answered from a more knowledgeable source. Introducing new equipment without preparation will need to be addressed by unit leadership in order to prevent a repeat incident in the future.

20. **(B)** The "journey" of attaining certification results in the professional growth of the nurse. Certification does **not** validate clinical skills, and it does **not** guarantee fiscal rewards, although that may be the result. Certification is not directly associated with the hospital's reputation.

21. **(D)** This will help control the volume of family that the nurse will need to communicate with, allowing the nurse to care for the patient, yet it will also provide a means to include the family. The other 3 choices do not provide an organized approach for the nursing staff that also meets the family's needs.

22. **(C)** This is the best strategy. It will allow the nurse to care for the patients safely during the present shift. The remaining choices are not effective, safe strategies.

23. **(D)** In order for educational materials to meet the requirements for the majority of the population, information needs to be written at a fourth-grade reading level. The other 3 choices do not provide effective strategies for patient/family comprehension for the majority of the adult population.

24. **(B)** Collaboration between the units will provide the most effective solution.

25. **(A)** Diversion of controlled substances is not an issue that is dealt with collaboratively between 2 nurses. Suspicions need to be pursued for the safety of the patients and the nurse who may be diverting the drugs. Human resources has the knowledge and expertise for handling these situations.

26. **(D)** Basing resources on the individual needs and characteristics of the patient (which includes more than just patient acuity) is the best practice for providing quality care.

27. **(B)** The nurse is responsible for understanding the plan of care. The best strategy is to actively collaborate with the physician. If the nurse still has doubts after doing this, those doubts need to be taken up the chain of command.

28. **(C)** Active participation and providing choices may allow some patient control and decrease passivity, which may improve the patient's self-esteem.

29. **(A)** It is the nurse's responsibility to ensure that the family (and the patient) understands the information and that the nurse's communication is delivered accurately and objectively. The remaining 3 choices do not ensure accuracy and objectivity.

30. **(C)** The goal is to provide realistic, consistent information to the patient's husband. The best strategy to achieve this is for the nurse to express concerns directly to the attending physician and contribute feedback as well as possible recommendations about the situation.

Practice Tests

NOTE

Don't forget that, in addition to the pretest and the following 2 practice tests, there is also an additional full-length online practice test. Refer to the card at the beginning of this book, which provides instructions for accessing this online practice test.

*Be sure to have your copy of this book on hand to complete the registration process.

ANSWER SHEET
Practice Test 1

1. Ⓐ Ⓑ Ⓒ Ⓓ
2. Ⓐ Ⓑ Ⓒ Ⓓ
3. Ⓐ Ⓑ Ⓒ Ⓓ
4. Ⓐ Ⓑ Ⓒ Ⓓ
5. Ⓐ Ⓑ Ⓒ Ⓓ
6. Ⓐ Ⓑ Ⓒ Ⓓ
7. Ⓐ Ⓑ Ⓒ Ⓓ
8. Ⓐ Ⓑ Ⓒ Ⓓ
9. Ⓐ Ⓑ Ⓒ Ⓓ
10. Ⓐ Ⓑ Ⓒ Ⓓ
11. Ⓐ Ⓑ Ⓒ Ⓓ
12. Ⓐ Ⓑ Ⓒ Ⓓ
13. Ⓐ Ⓑ Ⓒ Ⓓ
14. Ⓐ Ⓑ Ⓒ Ⓓ
15. Ⓐ Ⓑ Ⓒ Ⓓ
16. Ⓐ Ⓑ Ⓒ Ⓓ
17. Ⓐ Ⓑ Ⓒ Ⓓ
18. Ⓐ Ⓑ Ⓒ Ⓓ
19. Ⓐ Ⓑ Ⓒ Ⓓ
20. Ⓐ Ⓑ Ⓒ Ⓓ
21. Ⓐ Ⓑ Ⓒ Ⓓ
22. Ⓐ Ⓑ Ⓒ Ⓓ
23. Ⓐ Ⓑ Ⓒ Ⓓ
24. Ⓐ Ⓑ Ⓒ Ⓓ
25. Ⓐ Ⓑ Ⓒ Ⓓ
26. Ⓐ Ⓑ Ⓒ Ⓓ
27. Ⓐ Ⓑ Ⓒ Ⓓ
28. Ⓐ Ⓑ Ⓒ Ⓓ
29. Ⓐ Ⓑ Ⓒ Ⓓ
30. Ⓐ Ⓑ Ⓒ Ⓓ
31. Ⓐ Ⓑ Ⓒ Ⓓ
32. Ⓐ Ⓑ Ⓒ Ⓓ
33. Ⓐ Ⓑ Ⓒ Ⓓ
34. Ⓐ Ⓑ Ⓒ Ⓓ
35. Ⓐ Ⓑ Ⓒ Ⓓ
36. Ⓐ Ⓑ Ⓒ Ⓓ
37. Ⓐ Ⓑ Ⓒ Ⓓ
38. Ⓐ Ⓑ Ⓒ Ⓓ

39. Ⓐ Ⓑ Ⓒ Ⓓ
40. Ⓐ Ⓑ Ⓒ Ⓓ
41. Ⓐ Ⓑ Ⓒ Ⓓ
42. Ⓐ Ⓑ Ⓒ Ⓓ
43. Ⓐ Ⓑ Ⓒ Ⓓ
44. Ⓐ Ⓑ Ⓒ Ⓓ
45. Ⓐ Ⓑ Ⓒ Ⓓ
46. Ⓐ Ⓑ Ⓒ Ⓓ
47. Ⓐ Ⓑ Ⓒ Ⓓ
48. Ⓐ Ⓑ Ⓒ Ⓓ
49. Ⓐ Ⓑ Ⓒ Ⓓ
50. Ⓐ Ⓑ Ⓒ Ⓓ
51. Ⓐ Ⓑ Ⓒ Ⓓ
52. Ⓐ Ⓑ Ⓒ Ⓓ
53. Ⓐ Ⓑ Ⓒ Ⓓ
54. Ⓐ Ⓑ Ⓒ Ⓓ
55. Ⓐ Ⓑ Ⓒ Ⓓ
56. Ⓐ Ⓑ Ⓒ Ⓓ
57. Ⓐ Ⓑ Ⓒ Ⓓ
58. Ⓐ Ⓑ Ⓒ Ⓓ
59. Ⓐ Ⓑ Ⓒ Ⓓ
60. Ⓐ Ⓑ Ⓒ Ⓓ
61. Ⓐ Ⓑ Ⓒ Ⓓ
62. Ⓐ Ⓑ Ⓒ Ⓓ
63. Ⓐ Ⓑ Ⓒ Ⓓ
64. Ⓐ Ⓑ Ⓒ Ⓓ
65. Ⓐ Ⓑ Ⓒ Ⓓ
66. Ⓐ Ⓑ Ⓒ Ⓓ
67. Ⓐ Ⓑ Ⓒ Ⓓ
68. Ⓐ Ⓑ Ⓒ Ⓓ
69. Ⓐ Ⓑ Ⓒ Ⓓ
70. Ⓐ Ⓑ Ⓒ Ⓓ
71. Ⓐ Ⓑ Ⓒ Ⓓ
72. Ⓐ Ⓑ Ⓒ Ⓓ
73. Ⓐ Ⓑ Ⓒ Ⓓ
74. Ⓐ Ⓑ Ⓒ Ⓓ
75. Ⓐ Ⓑ Ⓒ Ⓓ
76. Ⓐ Ⓑ Ⓒ Ⓓ

77. Ⓐ Ⓑ Ⓒ Ⓓ
78. Ⓐ Ⓑ Ⓒ Ⓓ
79. Ⓐ Ⓑ Ⓒ Ⓓ
80. Ⓐ Ⓑ Ⓒ Ⓓ
81. Ⓐ Ⓑ Ⓒ Ⓓ
82. Ⓐ Ⓑ Ⓒ Ⓓ
83. Ⓐ Ⓑ Ⓒ Ⓓ
84. Ⓐ Ⓑ Ⓒ Ⓓ
85. Ⓐ Ⓑ Ⓒ Ⓓ
86. Ⓐ Ⓑ Ⓒ Ⓓ
87. Ⓐ Ⓑ Ⓒ Ⓓ
88. Ⓐ Ⓑ Ⓒ Ⓓ
89. Ⓐ Ⓑ Ⓒ Ⓓ
90. Ⓐ Ⓑ Ⓒ Ⓓ
91. Ⓐ Ⓑ Ⓒ Ⓓ
92. Ⓐ Ⓑ Ⓒ Ⓓ
93. Ⓐ Ⓑ Ⓒ Ⓓ
94. Ⓐ Ⓑ Ⓒ Ⓓ
95. Ⓐ Ⓑ Ⓒ Ⓓ
96. Ⓐ Ⓑ Ⓒ Ⓓ
97. Ⓐ Ⓑ Ⓒ Ⓓ
98. Ⓐ Ⓑ Ⓒ Ⓓ
99. Ⓐ Ⓑ Ⓒ Ⓓ
100. Ⓐ Ⓑ Ⓒ Ⓓ
101. Ⓐ Ⓑ Ⓒ Ⓓ
102. Ⓐ Ⓑ Ⓒ Ⓓ
103. Ⓐ Ⓑ Ⓒ Ⓓ
104. Ⓐ Ⓑ Ⓒ Ⓓ
105. Ⓐ Ⓑ Ⓒ Ⓓ
106. Ⓐ Ⓑ Ⓒ Ⓓ
107. Ⓐ Ⓑ Ⓒ Ⓓ
108. Ⓐ Ⓑ Ⓒ Ⓓ
109. Ⓐ Ⓑ Ⓒ Ⓓ
110. Ⓐ Ⓑ Ⓒ Ⓓ
111. Ⓐ Ⓑ Ⓒ Ⓓ
112. Ⓐ Ⓑ Ⓒ Ⓓ
113. Ⓐ Ⓑ Ⓒ Ⓓ
114. Ⓐ Ⓑ Ⓒ Ⓓ

115. Ⓐ Ⓑ Ⓒ Ⓓ
116. Ⓐ Ⓑ Ⓒ Ⓓ
117. Ⓐ Ⓑ Ⓒ Ⓓ
118. Ⓐ Ⓑ Ⓒ Ⓓ
119. Ⓐ Ⓑ Ⓒ Ⓓ
120. Ⓐ Ⓑ Ⓒ Ⓓ
121. Ⓐ Ⓑ Ⓒ Ⓓ
122. Ⓐ Ⓑ Ⓒ Ⓓ
123. Ⓐ Ⓑ Ⓒ Ⓓ
124. Ⓐ Ⓑ Ⓒ Ⓓ
125. Ⓐ Ⓑ Ⓒ Ⓓ
126. Ⓐ Ⓑ Ⓒ Ⓓ
127. Ⓐ Ⓑ Ⓒ Ⓓ
128. Ⓐ Ⓑ Ⓒ Ⓓ
129. Ⓐ Ⓑ Ⓒ Ⓓ
130. Ⓐ Ⓑ Ⓒ Ⓓ
131. Ⓐ Ⓑ Ⓒ Ⓓ
132. Ⓐ Ⓑ Ⓒ Ⓓ
133. Ⓐ Ⓑ Ⓒ Ⓓ
134. Ⓐ Ⓑ Ⓒ Ⓓ
135. Ⓐ Ⓑ Ⓒ Ⓓ
136. Ⓐ Ⓑ Ⓒ Ⓓ
137. Ⓐ Ⓑ Ⓒ Ⓓ
138. Ⓐ Ⓑ Ⓒ Ⓓ
139. Ⓐ Ⓑ Ⓒ Ⓓ
140. Ⓐ Ⓑ Ⓒ Ⓓ
141. Ⓐ Ⓑ Ⓒ Ⓓ
142. Ⓐ Ⓑ Ⓒ Ⓓ
143. Ⓐ Ⓑ Ⓒ Ⓓ
144. Ⓐ Ⓑ Ⓒ Ⓓ
145. Ⓐ Ⓑ Ⓒ Ⓓ
146. Ⓐ Ⓑ Ⓒ Ⓓ
147. Ⓐ Ⓑ Ⓒ Ⓓ
148. Ⓐ Ⓑ Ⓒ Ⓓ
149. Ⓐ Ⓑ Ⓒ Ⓓ
150. Ⓐ Ⓑ Ⓒ Ⓓ

17

Practice Test 1

Directions: This is the first of two 150-question comprehensive practice tests at the end of this book. Do not attempt to complete these tests until you have reviewed each chapter in this book and completed the practice questions within each chapter. The pretest questions and the questions within each chapter focused more on "facts." The questions found on each final comprehensive practice test require application, evaluation, and analysis of knowledge. Master the book's contents until you can achieve a score of at least 80% on these comprehensive practice tests prior to taking the Adult CCRN exam.

1. After attending an educational session that reviewed drug dosing and provided a review of the literature, the nurse would like to start using the admission weight to calculate drug dosing during titration of vasoactive drugs rather than the current practice of using daily weights. What would be the most effective next step for the nurse to take to implement this change?

   (A) Begin the adaptation of the practice by using the admission weight for patients.
   (B) Identify the key stakeholders related to the proposed change in practice.
   (C) Ask the attending physician on rounds what her thoughts are about the practice.
   (D) Discuss the educational session with nurse colleagues.

2. A patient presents with a productive cough, hypoxemia, a fever, hypotension, tachycardia, and tachypnea. Hypoxemia was corrected with the administration of oxygen. Which of the following should be done next?

   (A) Administer antibiotics.
   (B) Start a vasopressor.
   (C) Collect a sputum culture.
   (D) Initiate 0.9 normal saline.

3. A patient with a urinary tract infection presented with a temperature of 39°C (102.2°F), a heart rate of 132 beats/minute, a respiratory rate of 24 breaths/minute, a B/P of 78/49 (a MAP of 59 mmHg), and a lactate of 2.8 mmol/L. The patient received 2 L of 0.9 NS within 1 hour. The B/P is now 100/52 (the MAP is 68 mmHg), the heart rate is 118 beats/minute, the respiratory rate is 20 breaths/minute, and the lactate is 2.1 mmol/L. The patient requires treatment for:

   (A) bacteremia.
   (B) sepsis.
   (C) SIRS.
   (D) septic shock.

4. A patient is 48 hours post aortic valve replacement. Which of the following would be a major goal for this patient?

   (A) diuretic therapy
   (B) stabilizing the blood pressure
   (C) prophylactic antibiotics
   (D) preventing a thrombus

5. A patient with hypoxic encephalopathy has been opening his eyes to touch for the past 24 hours. The patient now withdraws to painful stimuli, has developed unequal pupils, and has a positive Babinski's sign. Which of the following interventions should the nurse anticipate?

(A) ventriculostomy, oxygen, steroids
(B) sedation, vasopressin (Pitressin), thiazide diuretic
(C) osmotic diuretic, intubation, and monitor the pCO_2
(D) lumbar puncture and increase the FiO_2

6. A 19-year-old patient who was admitted with sickle cell crisis and acute kidney injury requests to use a phone to update her friends on her condition. The nurse's best response would be to:

(A) explain to the patient that calls can be made when she is transferred out of the critical care unit.
(B) allow the patient to make the calls in order to meet the patient's need for social support.
(C) explain to the patient that she needs to rest in order for the analgesic medication to take effect.
(D) allow the patient to make the calls in order to reduce the patient's anxiety.

7. The unit quality council wants to reduce the number of CAUTIs. Which of the following strategies has been demonstrated to reduce incidences of CAUTIs?

(A) Remove the indwelling urinary catheter on day 3 post-op.
(B) Place the drainage collection system on the patient's abdomen during transport.
(C) Assess the competency of the staff using a simulated environment.
(D) Avoid the use of intermittent straight catheterization.

8. A patient has cardiogenic shock and cardiogenic pulmonary edema. Which of the following therapies would be most effective for this patient?

(A) an intra-aortic balloon pump to increase coronary artery perfusion
(B) a beta blocker to increase cardiac contractility
(C) an alpha-adrenergic drug to increase coronary artery perfusion
(D) angiotensin-converting enzyme inhibitors to decrease afterload

9. The care team is considering whether a patient is a candidate for hospice care. Which of the following is a specific service provided by hospice care?

(A) advance care planning
(B) symptom management
(C) care for a terminal illness
(D) consideration of patient/family wishes

10. A patient has a history of chronic respiratory failure secondary to COPD and now has acute respiratory failure secondary to pneumonia. Upon arrival at the critical care unit, his ABGs were a pH of 7.29, a $PaCO_2$ of 77, a PaO_2 of 51, and an HCO_3 of 31. He is receiving noninvasive ventilation with settings that read as follows: FiO_2 0.40, IPAP 12 cm, and EPAP 5 cm. After 1 hour of therapy, the patient's ABG results are a pH of 7.20, a $PaCO_2$ of 89, a PaO_2 of 48, and an HCO_3 of 32.

What is the correct evaluation of this data?

(A) Alveolar hyperventilation is getting worse; the BiPAP settings need adjustment.
(B) Metabolic acidosis is worse; the FiO_2 needs to be increased.
(C) Alveolar hypoventilation is getting worse; the patient needs to be intubated.
(D) The pH is acceptable for a patient with COPD; continue the current therapy.

11. Which of the following is true regarding plateau pressure?

    (A) It is a pressure that is used to calculate static compliance and reflects pressure in the lungs.

    (B) It is a pressure that is used to calculate vital capacity and reflects pressure in the lungs.

    (C) It is a pressure that is used to calculate dynamic compliance and reflects pressure in the airways.

    (D) It is a pressure that is used to measure tidal volume and reflects pressure in the airways.

12. A patient is admitted with a salicylate overdose. Which of the following treatments is most effective for this patient?

    (A) N-acetylcysteine, support the airway, fluids

    (B) gastric lavage, an antidote, fluids

    (C) activated charcoal, urine alkalinization, dialysis

    (D) support the airway, gastric lavage, ethanol

13. Which of the following patients who have sustained multiple trauma is most likely to have a poor outcome based on patient characteristics?

    (A) the college graduate

    (B) the owner of a successful business

    (C) the married man

    (D) the homeless man

14. Which of the following may be a reason to use restraints for a patient?

    (A) The patient is screaming obscenities.

    (B) The patient is spitting.

    (C) The patient is pulling at his central venous catheter.

    (D) The patient has an endotracheal tube.

15. A patient has acute right ventricular infarct and RV failure. Which of the following is an indication that this patient's condition has improved?

    (A) The PAOP has decreased.

    (B) The RA pressure has decreased.

    (C) The RV pressure has increased.

    (D) The PA diastolic pressure has decreased.

16. At 1 day status post AAA repair with a Dacron graft, the patient's serum BUN and creatinine increase, and the urine output decreases. Which of the following is the most likely etiology of these new patient findings?

    (A) acute renal failure

    (B) graft rejection

    (C) septic shock

    (D) acute hemorrhage

17. A patient complains of chest pain with deep inspiration that is worse when lying supine. There is a friction rub upon auscultation and sinus tachycardia. Which of the following would you expect to find on the stat 12-lead ECG?

    (A) ST depression in V1–V4

    (B) ST elevation in II, III, aVF, and V2–V5

    (C) ST depression in rV2 and rV3

    (D) ST elevation in II, III, and aVF

18. A trauma patient's morning labs return with the following values:

Hemoglobin 8.2 g/dL; hematocrit 30%; platelets 50,000/mcL; PTT 50 seconds; INR 3.0 seconds; fibrinogen 150 mg/dL; fibrin split products 45 mcg/dL

What is most likely the cause of this patient's lab profile?

    (A) autoimmune reaction

    (B) consumption of clotting factors

    (C) occult blood loss

    (D) drug reaction

19. A patient has a temporary transvenous VVI pacemaker with a set rate of 72 beats/minute and an mA output of 5. The monitor shows 1:1 pacing at the set rate. The physician asks the nurse to determine the capture threshold. Which of the following should the nurse do?

    (A) Slowly increase the sensitivity until the heart rate increases.
    (B) Slowly decrease the sensitivity until the capture is lost.
    (C) Slowly increase the mA output until the native beats are seen.
    (D) Slowly decrease the mA output until the capture is lost.

20. A patient is alert and is receiving mechanical ventilation with the following settings: assist-control mode at 10 breaths/minute, FiO_2 0.40, and PEEP 5 cm H_2O pressure. Vital signs include a B/P of 104/58, a heart rate of 90 beats/minute, and a respiratory rate of 18 breaths/minute, with norepinephrine at 7 mcg/min for the past 4 hours. The patient has tolerated repositioning in bed and a head of bed elevation up to 90°. Which of the following would be an appropriate next step in terms of mobility for this patient?

    (A) Allow the patient to sit on the edge of the bed, with assistance.
    (B) Reduce the head of bed elevation to 45°.
    (C) Maintain the patient's current level of mobility.
    (D) Help the patient stand and pivot to a chair.

21. A 70 kg patient with ARDS is mechanically ventilated with the following settings: FiO_2 70%, tidal volume 450 mL, assist-control mode 10 breaths/minute, and PEEP 20 cm H_2O pressure. On these settings, the patient's PaO_2 is 76 mmHg and the $PaCO_2$ is 58 mmHg. The patient's core temperature is 37°C, his heart rate is 116 beats/minute, and his B/P is 78/58. Which of the following interventions should the nurse now anticipate?

    (A) Decrease PEEP to decrease the intrathoracic pressure.
    (B) Administer a 500 mL fluid bolus of normal saline.
    (C) Initiate a norepinephrine drip to maintain a SBP of 80 mmHg.
    (D) Increase the tidal volume to 750 mL.

22. Which of the following is accurate regarding nursing responsibilities related to brain death?

    (A) The nurse should report a loss of brain stem reflexes (gag, corneal) to the physician.
    (B) The nurse should obtain an order from the physician to call the organ procurement agency.
    (C) The nurse should request permission from the patient's family to remove the ventilator.
    (D) The nurse should ensure that the patient receives an EEG, a transcranial Doppler ultrasound, and a cerebral angiogram to make the diagnosis of brain death.

23. A 70 kg patient with ARDS is intubated and mechanically ventilated. The patient is on continuous infusions of an opiate, a sedative, and neuromuscular blocking drugs. The plateau pressure is 45 cm H_2O. The PaO_2 is 60 mmHg. The physician orders the following ventilator settings: SIMV mode, tidal volume 700 mL, rate 12 breaths/minute, FiO_2 1.00, and PEEP 15 cm H_2O pressure. Which of the following needs to be discussed with the physician?

(A) the ventilator mode
(B) the tidal volume
(C) the PEEP
(D) the FiO_2

24. Which of the following is an appropriate strategy to use when providing mechanical ventilation to a patient with status asthmaticus?

(A) Provide a long inspiratory time and a short expiratory time.
(B) Utilize a PEEP setting of 10–15 cm.
(C) Use a lower respiratory rate.
(D) Set the tidal volume to 10–12 mL/kg.

25. A large (32 mm) V-wave appears on the pulmonary artery occlusion pressure (PAOP) tracing of an unstable patient after an extensive inferior wall myocardial infarction. This finding is consistent with:

(A) cardiogenic shock.
(B) congestive heart failure.
(C) pericarditis.
(D) mitral regurgitation.

26. A patient is admitted with a serum calcium of 15.1 mEq/L. Which of the following interventions should the nurse anticipate?

(A) ruling out hypermagnesemia and administering vitamin D
(B) treating hypoalbuminemia
(C) emergent hemodialysis and ruling out hyperphosphatemia
(D) ruling out hypokalemia and then administering diuretics

27. Which of the following patients is most likely to experience heart block?

(A) a patient who has had a cardiac transplant
(B) a patient who has had CABG surgery
(C) a patient who has had mitral valve repair
(D) a patient who has had ventricular septal defect repair

28. A patient with a head injury was admitted last night. This morning, she is increasingly less responsive, and her right pupil has become unresponsive to light. Now, her systolic pressure has increased, her heart rate has slowed, and her respirations have also slowed. These vital sign changes are referred to as:

(A) Battle's sign.
(B) Cushing's triad.
(C) halo sign.
(D) Chvostek sign.

29. A 68-year-old patient is admitted with syndrome of inappropriate antidiuretic hormone (SIADH). Which of the following lab findings and interventions would the nurse anticipate for this patient?

(A) serum sodium low, serum osmolality low, urine output low; order for phenytoin (Dilantin)
(B) serum sodium elevated, serum osmolality elevated, urine output low; order for Pitressin
(C) serum sodium low, urine specific gravity low, urine output elevated; order for 3% saline
(D) serum sodium elevated, urine output elevated, hypokalemia, arterial pH low

30. A patient with chronic alcohol abuse is admitted with a serum phosphorus of 1.8 mEq/L. The nurse will need to observe this patient closely for:

    (A) massive diarrhea.
    (B) hypoventilation.
    (C) tetany.
    (D) ventricular arrhythmias.

31. Which of the following nursing behaviors is usually most helpful to patients and families regarding end-of-life decisions?

    (A) avoiding the use of words such as "death," "dying," and "suffering"
    (B) consulting the clergy for support
    (C) acting as an arbitrator between family members
    (D) requesting that only 1 person be the spokesperson

32. A patient is receiving patient-controlled analgesia, an IV infusion of morphine at 1 mg per hour, and 2 mg of morphine every 15 minutes as PRN bolus doses. The patient is having episodes of sleep apnea and is arousable only by touch. Priority interventions include:

    (A) stopping the continuous infusion and giving a slow IV push of naloxone until the patient awakens.
    (B) decreasing the morphine continuous infusion rate to 0.5 mg per hour and continuing to monitor that rate.
    (C) discontinuing the PRN bolus doses and giving a 2 mg IV bolus of naloxone.
    (D) discontinuing PCA, checking the SpO$_2$, and giving naloxone.

33. Which of the following is contraindicated when providing enteral feeding?

    (A) checking for gastric residuals every 4 hours
    (B) using a small-bore duodenal feeding tube
    (C) keeping the head of the bed flat
    (D) ensuring that free water is provided

34. A patient presented with sepsis secondary to a urinary tract infection. After the initial administration of 30 mL/kg of isotonic crystalloid, the B/P is 88/46 (the MAP is 60 mmHg), the heart rate is 102 beats/minute, the respiratory rate is 22 breaths/minute, and the lungs are clear. What intervention is indicated at this time?

    (A) Decrease the rate of fluid administration.
    (B) Start a dobutamine (Dobutrex) infusion.
    (C) Start a norepinephrine (Levophed) infusion.
    (D) Start a vasopressin infusion.

35. A patient who was admitted status post gunshot wound to the chest 2 days ago is now exhibiting signs of restlessness, hypertension, tachycardia, yawning, lacrimation, and rhinorrhea. Which of the following should be included in the nurse's plan of care?

    (A) Assess the patient further for a history of opiate abuse.
    (B) Provide scheduled pain medication.
    (C) Ensure that there is an order for sedation, and administer a sedative.
    (D) Discuss the need for an antihypertensive agent with the physician.

36. A 74-year-old female reports explosive diarrhea for several days. She is lethargic, her mucous membranes are dry and sticky, she has had dark amber urine with 40 mL output in the past hour, her urine specific gravity is 1.035, her BUN is 65, and her creatinine is 2.9. Her vital signs are a temperature of 38°C, a heart rate of 130 beats/minute, a respiratory rate of 24 breaths/minute, and a B/P of 90/40. Which of the following should the nurse anticipate administering?

   (A) antibiotics
   (B) nutrition
   (C) isotonic fluids
   (D) furosemide

37. Which of the following pathophysiological conditions will cause refractory hypoxemia that is not treatable with oxygen alone?

   (A) shunt
   (B) hyperventilation
   (C) diffusion defects
   (D) V/Q mismatch

38. A nurse is reviewing the lab results of a patient who was admitted with a stroke and a history of thyroid disease. The lab results include an Na^+ of 118 mEq/L, elevated TSH, and elevated LDH and CK. Which of the following patient signs/symptoms might the nurse anticipate?

   (A) a fever
   (B) tachycardia
   (C) elevated T3 and T4
   (D) respiratory depression, hypoxemia

39. A patient with a history of heart failure and MI presents following an episode of syncope. The assessment 2 hours later demonstrates:

   B/P 134/64 (supine); 110/70 (sitting)
   Heart rate 115 beats/minute with a weak, thready pulse (supine); 130 beats/minute (sitting)
   RR 32 breaths/minute and shallow
   U/O 30 mL over the past 2 hours
   Breath sounds: clear

   This patient most likely requires:

   (A) vasodilators.
   (B) loop diuretics.
   (C) IV fluids.
   (D) vasopressors.

40. Which of the following is an appropriate intervention when caring for a patient with a central venous catheter?

   (A) Use gauze dressing.
   (B) Provide a daily chlorhexidine bath.
   (C) Replace central lines weekly.
   (D) Disinfect access hubs prior to use by scrubbing the hubs for 5 seconds or less.

41. A patient is status post stroke and has been advanced to oral feedings after successfully completing a swallow study. The nurse knows that the patient needs to be closely monitored for signs of pulmonary aspiration. Which of the following is the earliest indication that the patient may be aspirating his oral feedings?

   (A) coughing and tachypnea
   (B) positive sputum cultures
   (C) oxygen desaturation
   (D) right middle lobe infiltrate on a chest radiograph

42. While getting a 71-year-old male patient's history, the patient tells the nurse that he has mitral valve stenosis. Based on this information, the nurse would anticipate which of the following findings?

(A) systolic murmur, sinus bradycardia
(B) systolic murmur, atrial fibrillation
(C) diastolic murmur, atrial fibrillation
(D) diastolic murmur, sinus bradycardia

43. Which of the following patients will require 0.9 NS at 1 mL/kg before and after a CT scan with an infusion of contrast media?

(A) an elderly patient who is taking NSAIDs every 6 hours for arthritis
(B) a patient with hypertension
(C) a male patient who is taking a beta-adrenergic blocker
(D) a patient with acute coronary syndrome

44. A patient was admitted status post motor vehicle crash. The patient sustained an intracranial bleed and is hypotensive and tachycardic. This patient's clinical status is most likely due to which of the following?

(A) intracranial hemorrhage
(B) neurogenic shock
(C) shock from multiple trauma
(D) brain herniation

45. A 19-year-old male patient was admitted with DKA for the third time in the past 4 months. The patient told the nurse that he is considering dropping out of college, that he cannot concentrate on his studies, that he has had insomnia, and that he is just "sick of it all." Which of the following would be the nurse's best response?

(A) Consult with the physician regarding the initiation of an antidepressant.
(B) Consult with an endocrinologist regarding the patient's symptoms.
(C) Consult with the physician regarding a psychiatric consult.
(D) Provide emotional support and encourage the patient to be positive.

46. Twelve hours after admission for a traumatic injury, a patient's arterial blood gas showed the following results:

pH	7.48
pCO_2	28 mmHg
pO_2	68 mmHg
HCO_3	25 mmol/L

Which of the following interventions is most appropriate at this time?

(A) Consider intubation and assess the blood pressure.
(B) Increase the FiO_2 and assess the electrolytes.
(C) Consider sedation and assess the blood sugar.
(D) Increase the FiO_2 and assess for pain.

47. A patient is admitted postoperatively after surgery for a crush injury of the lower left leg that was sustained in a motor vehicle crash. Which of the following is indicated for the prevention of deep vein thrombosis?

(A) compression stockings
(B) a pneumatic compression device on the right extremity
(C) daily low-molecular-weight heparin
(D) daily warfarin

48. Abdominal auscultation of a patient with early mechanical bowel obstruction would likely reveal which of the following?

    (A) normal bowel sounds
    (B) hyperactive bowel sounds
    (C) hypoactive bowel sounds
    (D) absent bowel sounds

49. A patient was admitted with an acute anterior wall myocardial infarction and suddenly develops a loud holosystolic murmur (that is loudest at the left sternal border, 5th intercostal space), tachypnea, and bibasilar crackles. Which of the following would provide the most definitive diagnosis for this problem?

    (A) decreased cardiac output
    (B) increased oxygen saturation in the pulmonary artery and the right ventricle
    (C) the central venous pressure is less than the pulmonary artery diastolic pressure
    (D) decreased arterial oxygen saturation

50. A patient who is receiving mechanical ventilation is also receiving a propofol drip at 50 mcg/kg/min in order to maintain a RASS score of –1 to –2. The patient becomes agitated with a RASS score of +3 and a behavioral pain scale (BPS) score of 10 (the range is 3–12). The SpO_2 and breath sounds are unchanged. The blood pressure and the heart rate are somewhat high. Which of the following interventions would be appropriate?

    (A) Increase the propofol infusion to 60 mcg/kg/min.
    (B) Give lorazepam 2 mg IV.
    (C) Give morphine 2 mg IV.
    (D) Order an arterial blood gas STAT.

51. Which of the following statements related to the care of a patient with a chest tube is TRUE?

    (A) Clamp the tube during patient transport.
    (B) Position the tubing in a dependent loop.
    (C) Avoid high airway pressures.
    (D) Place the collection chamber onto the cart during transport.

52. Which of the following may be the result of pulmonary hypertension?

    (A) pulmonary valve stenosis
    (B) left ventricular failure
    (C) tricuspid regurgitation
    (D) increased lung compliance

53. Which of the following interventions would a nurse anticipate for a patient with an intracerebral hemorrhage?

    (A) a STAT MRI of the brain
    (B) correction of coagulopathy
    (C) surgical evacuation of the hematoma
    (D) nitroprusside (Nipride) for an immediate correction of hypertension

54. A patient with a history of alcohol abuse sustained a traumatic injury and was admitted to the ICU. Which of the following is most likely to prevent the development of delirium tremens (DTs) for this patient?

    (A) thiamine
    (B) phenobarbital
    (C) fluids
    (D) benzodiazepines

55. A patient is receiving a heparin infusion status post pulmonary embolism. The latest lab results reveal a sudden drop in the platelet count to 80,000/mcL from 280,000/mcL the previous day. The nurse would anticipate receiving which of the following physician orders?

    (A) Begin an argatroban infusion.
    (B) Hold all anticoagulants.
    (C) Infuse platelets.
    (D) Continue heparin and order labs for heparin antibodies.

56. A patient who has a complex diabetic ulcer is receiving negative-pressure wound therapy. Which of the following is a recommended nursing intervention for this patient?

    (A) Contact the provider if suction is lost for more than 4 hours.
    (B) Change the dressing daily.
    (C) Flush the tubing daily.
    (D) Change the wound VAC canister when it is full.

57. A nurse is preparing to suction a patient who is receiving mechanical ventilation and has a history of increased ICP due to a head injury. Which of the following interventions is contraindicated for this patient?

    (A) increasing the FiO_2 to 100% during suctioning
    (B) providing sedation
    (C) limiting the procedure to 1 to 2 quick passes
    (D) stimulating coughing

58. A patient who was admitted with DKA is receiving treatment in the ICU, and he develops tachycardia, diaphoresis, and restlessness. Which of the following interventions is most likely needed?

    (A) Increase the insulin dose.
    (B) Obtain a stat 12-lead ECG.
    (C) Administer a glucose source.
    (D) Provide an increase in fluids.

59. A 70-year-old patient is admitted with a serum glucose of 850 mg/dL, a history of Type 2 diabetes, and an obtunded mental status. Which of the following laboratory findings would be expected?

    (A) pH 7.35, sodium 150 mEq/L, BUN 10 mEq/L
    (B) pH 7.25, potassium 3.2 mEq/L, serum osmolality 160 mOsm/kg
    (C) pH 7.35, potassium 5.9 mEq/L, sodium 128 mEq/L
    (D) pH 7.25, potassium 6.2 mEq/L, serum osmolality 310 mOsm/kg

60. A 28-year-old woman is in the ICU with a gunshot wound to the head. One week after admission, the physician has declared the patient brain-dead. The nurse is present when the diagnosis is shared with the patient's mother. What is one of the first issues the nurse needs to anticipate for this type of situation specifically?

    (A) the need to document this physician-family discussion
    (B) the need to initiate a discussion about organ donation
    (C) that the family may request a second opinion
    (D) that the hospital ethics committee should be contacted

61. A 55-year-old male with a history of alcohol abuse is in the ICU status post upper GI bleeding. The bleeding was controlled with an upper endoscopy and the administration of proton-pump inhibitors. Currently, the patient is complaining of extreme pain at the site of a tibial abrasion he sustained prior to admission. The abrasion has a small area of blackened tissue with an area of reddened tissue (approximately 15 cm in size) surrounding the abrasion and purplish discoloration around the borders. The priority nursing intervention for this patient is to:

(A) apply an ice pack to the abrasion.
(B) administer an analgesic.
(C) contact the provider to examine the abrasion.
(D) cover the abrasion with sterile gauze.

62. A patient develops PSVT, and synchronized cardioversion is being considered. Which of the following would be a contraindication to the cardioversion?

(A) a digoxin level of 4.0 mg/dL
(B) a potassium level of 5.1 mEq/L
(C) a magnesium level of 2.6 mg/dL
(D) a creatinine level of 3.1 mg/dL

63. An orientee asks the preceptor how IABP therapy will benefit a patient who was just admitted from the cardiac catheterization suite. The preceptor's best response would be to explain IABP therapy will increase:

(A) patient's myocardial oxygen supply.
(B) coronary artery perfusion during systole.
(C) patient's left ventricular filling volume.
(D) left ventricular diastolic pressure.

64. A shift of the oxyhemoglobin dissociation curve to the right will result in:

(A) improved SaO_2.
(B) worsening SaO_2.
(C) a decreased release of oxygen from the hemoglobin.
(D) a decreased release of 2,3-DPG in the serum.

65. A patient in septic shock received a pulmonary artery catheter. Which of the following hemodynamic profiles would this patient most likely exhibit?

(A) SVR 1,400 dynes/s/cm^{-5}, cardiac output 5 L/min, SvO_2 58%
(B) SVR 1,800 dynes/s/cm^{-5}, cardiac output 6 L/min, SvO_2 60%
(C) SVR 500 dynes/s/cm^{-5}, cardiac output 7 L/min, SvO_2 78%
(D) SVR 700 dynes/s/cm^{-5}, cardiac output 2 L/min, SvO_2 68%

66. A patient was admitted with a serum glucose of 498 mg/dL. After 2 hours of therapy with 5 units/hour of regular insulin, the patient's glucose is 478 mg/dL. Which of the following interventions is appropriate at this time?

(A) Add subcutaneous sliding scale insulin coverage, and continue to monitor the patient.
(B) Continue the insulin infusion at the current dose, and continue to monitor the patient.
(C) Increase the insulin infusion to 7 units/hour, and continue to monitor the patient.
(D) Increase the insulin infusion to 10 units/hour, and continue to monitor the patient.

67. A patient is admitted with a right cerebral hemispheric stroke. An assessment of this patient would reveal:

(A) a dilated left pupil and left-sided paresis or plegia.

(B) a dilated left pupil and right-sided paresis or plegia.

(C) a dilated right pupil and left-sided paresis or plegia.

(D) a dilated right pupil and right-sided paresis or plegia.

68. When there is a drop in the cardiac output, which of the following is a normal compensatory response?

(A) increased myocardial oxygen extraction

(B) decreased myocardial oxygen consumption

(C) decreased heart rate

(D) increased myocardial oxygen delivery

69. A 19-year-old female is admitted to the critical care unit with Type 1 diabetes. Her family reported that she was home with a "chest cold" today and became very lethargic after dinner. Her blood glucose is 490 mEq/dL, and her serum is positive for ketones. What is the most likely cause of this patient's current symptoms?

(A) dietary noncompliance

(B) an insulin omission

(C) an infection

(D) dehydration

70. Upon arrival at the ICU from the cardiac catheterization lab, where the patient had a diagnostic right heart catheterization and a percutaneous coronary intervention, the cardiologist informed the nurse that the patient had an elevated left ventricular filling pressure and a low cardiac output. Which of the following therapies would be beneficial for this patient?

(A) left ventricular afterload reduction

(B) heart rate reduction

(C) left ventricular preload elevation

(D) negative inotropic therapy

71. Which of the following assessment findings would indicate the presence of a massive hemothorax?

(A) absent breath sounds on the affected side; hyperresonance to percussion; tracheal deviation toward the affected side

(B) decreased excursion on the affected side; dullness to percussion; tracheal deviation toward the affected side

(C) absent breath sounds on the affected side; dullness to percussion; tracheal deviation toward the unaffected side

(D) decreased excursion on the unaffected side; hyperresonance to percussion; tracheal deviation toward the unaffected side

72. A patient has acute renal failure secondary to septic shock, had prolonged hypotension, and now requires hemodialysis (since his BUN is 90 mg/dL and his creatinine is 9.2 mg/dL). Which of the following findings would the nurse expect this patient to have?

(A) low urine osmolality, high urine sodium

(B) high urine osmolality, high urine sodium

(C) low urine osmolality, low urine sodium

(D) high urine osmolality, low urine sodium

73. A patient had an episode of chest pain at rest with ST elevation on the ECG. The chest pain was relieved, and the ST segments were normalized after the administration of nitroglycerin sublingual. This patient most likely had:

(A) stable angina.
(B) an ST-elevation myocardial infarction.
(C) Prinzmetal's, or variant, angina.
(D) Wellens syndrome.

74. A patient develops abdominal pain, shortness of breath, and a fever during the administration of a blood transfusion. What is the priority nursing intervention?

(A) Administer oxygen.
(B) Contact the physician.
(C) Administer acetaminophen.
(D) Stop the transfusion.

75. During initial shift rounds, the nurse notices that the patient has edema on her left hand (about 2 inches in diameter) above the insertion site of an IV that is infusing 0.9 normal saline. The patient also has blanched skin, and she denies having any pain. Which of the following is the appropriate assessment and intervention in addition to stopping the infusion?

(A) The patient has a stage 2 infiltration. Restart the IV in her right extremity.
(B) The patient has a stage 0 infiltration. Elevate the left extremity, and apply warm compresses.
(C) The patient has a stage 1 infiltration. Check for blood return.
(D) The patient has an extravasation. Contact the pharmacist for an antidote.

76. A patient has an esophageal balloon tube (Sengstaken-Blakemore) for the treatment of bleeding esophageal varices. What nursing assessment/intervention is specific to the care of a patient with this type of tube?

(A) Ensure that suction is maintained.
(B) Monitor for recurrent bleeding.
(C) Initiate fluid resuscitation as needed.
(D) Keep scissors at the bedside.

77. A 28-year-old male patient with muscular dystrophy is admitted with acute respiratory failure secondary to heart failure. He tells the nurse that he is tired of frequent hospitalizations related to his disease and does not want invasive or noninvasive ventilation since he is tired of living. Which of the following would be the nurse's best response?

(A) "You will need to sign a 'No CPR' form as soon as possible."
(B) "You are very uncomfortable right now, but you will feel differently when you are feeling better."
(C) "This is an acute problem that can be resolved with treatment, allowing you to return home to your family."
(D) "Have you discussed this decision with your family and your physician?"

78. Which of the following patients has delirium?

(A) The patient has become lethargic and is inattentive.
(B) The patient is unresponsive.
(C) The patient is acutely agitated and attentive.
(D) The patient's baseline mental status has not changed.

79. A patient received 10 units of packed red blood cells for a traumatic injury. Which of the following therapies should the nurse anticipate?

    (A) platelets and fresh frozen plasma
    (B) protamine zinc
    (C) albumin
    (D) calcium and hetastarch

80. A patient has been receiving intravenous morphine PRN for postoperative pain. When entering the room to administer an antibiotic, the nurse notices that the patient's respiratory rate has decreased to 8 breaths/minute and that the patient requires shaking to arouse. What is a priority intervention at this time?

    (A) Administer naloxone (Narcan) 0.4 mg IV.
    (B) Call the cardiac arrest team.
    (C) Administer flumazenil (Romazicon) 0.2 mg IV.
    (D) Contact the physician for a change in the analgesic orders.

81. A patient who was admitted for community-acquired pneumonia has a history of Parkinson's disease, and the nurse administers a screen for dysphagia prior to giving the patient anything by mouth. Which of the following is NOT a sign of a positive screen for dysphagia?

    (A) frequent throat clearing after the administration of water
    (B) weight loss
    (C) facial asymmetry
    (D) coughing after the administration of water

82. An infection prevention nurse reported 5 new cases of *Clostridium difficile* over the past 2 weeks in the ICU. Which of the following is an effective strategy for preventing future infections in this unit?

    (A) Test all patients and staff for *C. difficile* colonization.
    (B) Initiate the implementation of prophylactic antibiotic administration to all patients in the unit.
    (C) Place patients with documented *C. difficile* in airborne isolation.
    (D) Ensure that all staff understand the need for using soap and water for hand hygiene after contact with a patient.

83. A 59-year-old male is admitted with ST elevation in V2, V3, and V4. IV thrombolytic therapy was started in the Emergency Department. Indications of successful reperfusion would include all of the following EXCEPT:

    (A) the cessation of pain.
    (B) the absence of troponin elevation.
    (C) the reversal of ST segment elevation with a return to baseline.
    (D) short runs of ventricular tachycardia.

84. A patient with lung cancer is status post a right-sided thoracotomy with removal of the middle and lower right lung lobes. What is the main purpose of the patient's 2 chest tubes?

    (A) to provide normal ventilation
    (B) to restore negative pleural pressure
    (C) to improve lung compliance
    (D) to drain pleural fluid

85. The critical care leadership of a medical center with several ICUs has assembled a committee to decide how to implement the use of a new patient transfer device (that was recently purchased) in the critical care units. Which of the following would be an important initial action for this committee?

   (A) Benchmark area hospitals that have already implemented the use of the new device.
   (B) Consult with the manufacturer to see if printed user guides are available.
   (C) Check for any national safety warnings related to the new piece of equipment.
   (D) Include nurses from all units that will use the new patient transfer device on the committee.

86. PEEP is beneficial for the treatment of patients with pneumonia, ALI, or ARDS due to which of the following effects?

   (A) a decrease in pulmonary shunt
   (B) an increase in dead space ventilation
   (C) an increase in alveolar recruitment
   (D) a decrease in capillary leak

87. A 79-year-old male comes to the critical care unit with left-sided paralysis and paresthesia, eye deviation to the right, and a dilated right pupil. He cannot remember falling and has no signs of physical trauma. His family states that he has been "acting differently" for approximately 1 month. The patient denies having a headache. Based on this information, he probably has which of the following?

   (A) a left-hemispheric epidural hematoma
   (B) a right-hemispheric subdural hematoma
   (C) a basilar skull fracture
   (D) central herniation

88. It is suspected that a patient has appendicitis with intestinal perforation. Which of the following descriptions of abdominal pain is most specific to peritoneal irritation?

   (A) The pain is lessened while lying still with knees flexed.
   (B) There is generalized pain of the abdominal area.
   (C) The pain lasts longer than 6 hours.
   (D) The pain is becoming increasingly severe.

89. Which of the following best characterizes acute respiratory distress syndrome (ARDS)?

   (A) tachypnea, unilateral pulmonary edema on a chest X-ray
   (B) decreased lung compliance, hypercapnia, an infection
   (C) elevated PAOP, bilateral infiltrates on a chest X-ray, pO_2 is less than 60 mmHg
   (D) refractory hypoxemia, decreased functional residual capacity (FRC), an acute physiological problem

90. A 23-year-old patient with head trauma begins to have polyuria with a urine output of 900 mL in 1 hour, a urine specific gravity of 1.001, and an elevated serum osmolality. Which of the following interventions would be expected for this patient?

   (A) Administer 3% saline.
   (B) Administer phenytoin.
   (C) Administer Pitressin.
   (D) Administer dextrose 5% in water.

91. A patient complains of chest tightness and shortness of breath shortly after an IV antibiotic is initiated. Hives have appeared across her face and chest. Her vital signs include a B/P of 84/34, a heart rate of 130 beats/minute, sinus tachycardia, a respiratory rate of 28 breaths/minute with wheezing, and SpO_2 94% on room air. Which of the following interventions is most appropriate for this patient?

    (A) stat ECG, aspirin, oxygen, pressor
    (B) albuterol, steroids, oxygen, fluids
    (C) fluids, oxygen, a CT scan of the chest, heparin
    (D) epinephrine IM, steroids IV, an antihistamine, fluids

92. A patient presents with a mental status change and a history of headaches. His carboxyhemoglobin level is 45%, and the pulse oximeter is reading 98%. What is the priority treatment for this patient?

    (A) Provide 100% FiO_2.
    (B) Provide mechanical ventilation.
    (C) Provide 40% FiO_2.
    (D) Administer naloxone (Narcan).

93. A patient is admitted with chest pain and ST elevation in II, III, and aVF. He is receiving dobutamine at 10 mcg/kg/min and nitroglycerin at 20 mcg/min. His blood pressure is 90/60, and there is sinus tachycardia at 110 beats/minute. A pulmonary artery catheter is inserted, and the following values are obtained:

    RAP = 16 mmHg, PAOP = 5 mmHg, PAP = 26/10 mmHg, cardiac index = 1.9 L/min/m^2

    The patient has jugular venous distention in a Semi-Fowler's position; tall, peaked P-waves are seen in lead II. Which of the following therapies is indicated for this patient?

    (A) Increase the dobutamine infusion to 20 mcg/kg/min, and infuse 50 mL of saline.
    (B) Begin a milrinone infusion at 0.5 mcg/kg/min after a loading dose of 50 mcg/kg.
    (C) Discontinue the nitroglycerin, and infuse 500 mL of normal saline.
    (D) Discontinue dobutamine, and start a dopamine infusion at 10 mcg/kg/min.

94. Which of the following is true about an epidural hematoma?

    (A) The patient's level of consciousness will change before pupillary changes occur.
    (B) It may occur up to a month after the injury.
    (C) There is a risk of uncal herniation of the brain.
    (D) Muscle weakness will occur on the side of the injury.

95. An 81-year-old male patient was admitted with sinus arrest. The cardiologist has recommended to the patient that he receive a permanent pacemaker. The patient, who has a history of hypertension and Type 2 diabetes, told the physician that he does not want a pacemaker and that he would rather "let nature take its course." What would be the best approach for the nurse to take regarding this patient's decision?

(A) Explain to the patient that he might die without the pacemaker.

(B) Explain the consequences of the patient's decision to his family, and advise them to persuade the patient to agree to the procedure.

(C) Explore the reason for the patient's decision, and provide information on what is involved during the procedure and the usual recovery period.

(D) Advise the patient that a "No CPR" order will be needed in order to limit treatment that will prevent his heart from stopping.

96. A nurse who is caring for a patient after coronary artery bypass graft (CABG) surgery should:

(A) anticipate a possible drop in blood pressure during rewarming.

(B) strip the chest tubes hourly to maintain patency.

(C) maintain a blood sugar of 150–200 mg/dL with an insulin infusion.

(D) maintain a serum potassium of 3.0–4.0 mEq/L to prevent arrhythmias.

97. Unlike a patient with systolic dysfunction, a patient with diastolic heart failure may benefit from:

(A) digoxin.

(B) a calcium channel blocker.

(C) an ACE inhibitor.

(D) dobutamine.

98. A patient is admitted with bleeding esophageal varices. Which of the following is a sign of compensation for hypovolemic shock?

(A) a decrease in renin secretion

(B) an increase in the reabsorption of sodium and water

(C) vasodilation

(D) a capillary fluid shift to the interstitial space

99. A patient with status asthmaticus requires mechanical ventilation. Which of the following needs to be utilized?

(A) increased inspiratory phase

(B) increased PEEP

(C) increased expiratory phase

(D) increased breath rate

100. A patient has a right middle and lower lobe bacterial pneumonia and is expectorating rust-colored sputum. Which of the following interventions is most appropriate for this patient?

(A) Provide antibiotic therapy to cover MRSA.

(B) Turn the patient to the left to prevent hypoxemia.

(C) Withhold the enoxaparin that is prescribed for DVT prophylaxis.

(D) Maintain the head of the bed at less than 30°.

101. A patient had a pulmonary artery catheter, and the following values were obtained on the initial shift assessment:

Blood pressure 82/48, heart rate 126 beats/minute, pulmonary artery pressure 22/10, central venous pressure (CVP) 1 mmHg, pulmonary artery occlusion pressure 4 mmHg, cardiac output 3 L/minute, and systemic vascular resistance 1,600 dynes/s/cm^{-5}

This patient requires the administration of:

(A) a fluid bolus of 500 mL of 0.9 normal saline.
(B) dopamine at 5 mcg/kg/min.
(C) dobutamine (Dobutrex) at 10 mcg/kg/min.
(D) nitroprusside (Nipride) at 1 mcg/kg/min.

102. A patient has been admitted to the ICU with a diagnosis of esophageal varices and upper GI bleeding, the third such admission in the last year. She is hemodynamically stable, and there is no evidence of active bleeding at this time. Which of the following questions will provide the nurse with the information needed to ensure that her patient understands her diagnosis?

(A) Why do you think you are sick?
(B) When did you experience your first symptoms?
(C) Does anyone else in your family have this bleeding problem?
(D) Do you consume alcohol on a regular basis?

103. A patient is demonstrating agitated behavior with a RASS score of +3. What is a priority assessment for this patient?

(A) CAM-ICU
(B) SpO$_2$
(C) BPS
(D) blood pressure

104. It is day 3 in the ICU for a 63-year-old female patient who presented with multiple trauma. She is receiving mechanical ventilation, status post repair of a lacerated liver, and she has had a chest tube insertion for a pneumothorax. Which of the following is appropriate for the patient at this time?

(A) a chaplain consult
(B) palliative care
(C) a "No CPR" order
(D) a hospice consult

105. It is important to create a unit culture that is dedicated to patient safety, with a goal of zero patient falls. Which of the following strategies is the responsibility of the individual nurse who is caring for the patient rather than the unit manager?

(A) ensuring adequate staffing
(B) sharing data related to unit falls with and without injuries
(C) performing root cause analyses of unit falls
(D) documenting a patient's high fall risk status on the room whiteboard

106. A patient's abdominal assessment reveals a complaint of dull abdominal pain, abdominal distension, low-pitched bowel sounds, and a report of a change in bowel habits. This patient most likely has which of the following problems?

(A) large bowel obstruction
(B) acute pancreatitis
(C) small bowel obstruction
(D) acute appendicitis

107. A patient who was admitted with a traumatic injury and multiple fractures has become increasingly tachypneic, with a decrease in SpO_2 that requires an increase in the FiO_2 to 1.00 using a high-flow nasal cannula. An ABG is obtained with the following results: pH 7.52, pCO_2 29, pO_2 48, and HCO_3 25. The lungs, which were clear previously, now have bibasilar crackles, and the chest X-ray demonstrates a ground-glass appearance. This patient most likely has developed which of the following?

(A) pneumothorax
(B) acute respiratory distress syndrome
(C) pulmonary embolus
(D) pneumonia

108. Which of the following may prevent vasospasm following a subarachnoid hemorrhage secondary to a ruptured aneurysm?

(A) nimodipine (Nimotop)
(B) a loop diuretic, such as furosemide (Lasix)
(C) aminocaproic acid (Amicar)
(D) an osmotic diuretic, such as mannitol

109. A patient is admitted with a diagnosis of acute tubular necrosis (ATN). Which of the following findings would this patient be expected to manifest?

(A) hypermagnesemia, acidosis, hyperkalemia
(B) azotemia, hypocalcemia, alkalosis
(C) hypokalemia, acidosis, hypertension
(D) hyperkalemia, hypomagnesemia, acidosis

110. The preceptor for a new nurse notices that the orientee is using the printed waveform strip of the CVP to determine the reading rather than using the digital readout on the monitor. When questioned about this practice, the orientee states that he had heard that assessing the printed waveform is more accurate than using the digital display on the monitor. The preceptor has never heard of this practice. What should the preceptor do?

(A) Instruct the new nurse on the usual unit practice of using the digital display of this pressure on the monitor.
(B) Use the printed waveform strip to get the pressure and look at the digital readout on the monitor, and then compare the readings.
(C) Design a research study to compare the relationship between obtaining CVP measurements using the printed waveform vs. the digital display.
(D) Review the current literature to identify evidence and recommendations related to this practice.

111. Which of the following strategies might be used to prevent a patient from developing nosocomial anemia?

(A) Draw daily labs at a standardized time.
(B) Use small volume blood draw tubes.
(C) Obtain blood samples via stopcocks.
(D) Train unit nursing assistants to draw blood.

112. A patient is admitted with a serum sodium of 118 mEq/L and a serum osmolality of 249 mOsm/kg. Which of the following intravenous fluids is contraindicated in this situation?

(A) normal saline solution (0.9% NaCl)
(B) 3% saline solution
(C) lactated Ringer's solution
(D) dextrose in water (D_5W)

113. A patient is admitted status post motor vehicle crash with a left linear temporal skull fracture and a stable mental status upon admission. One hour after admission, he developed a right arm motor drift, a dilated left pupil, and a decreased level of consciousness. Which of the following interventions would the nurse anticipate?

    (A) cerebral arteriography and arterial stenting
    (B) emergent burr hole and clot evacuation
    (C) lower the head of the bed and administer an osmotic diuretic
    (D) intubation and a ventriculostomy

114. A nurse is initiating a vasopressin drip for a patient with GI bleeding. What is a priority assessment that is specific to a patient who is receiving this medication?

    (A) Monitor for hypertension.
    (B) Monitor the ECG for ST changes.
    (C) Monitor for a cardiac arrhythmia.
    (D) Monitor for a bowel obstruction.

115. Which of the following is associated with adrenal insufficiency?

    (A) hypocalcemia
    (B) hypernatremia
    (C) hypoglycemia
    (D) hypokalemia

116. Preload and afterload are affected by various interventions. Which of the following statements is accurate?

    (A) Afterload is increased by nitroglycerin (Tridil).
    (B) Afterload is decreased by enalapril (Vasotec).
    (C) Preload is increased by furosemide (Lasix).
    (D) Preload is decreased with the administration of fluids.

117. Which of the following patients (all of whom are receiving mechanical ventilation for pneumonia) has the greatest complexity?

    (A) the woman with 3 school-age children whose husband died 6 months ago and who just lost her job
    (B) the man who just retired, is married, has a company pension, and owns his home
    (C) the woman with 2 school-age children who is going through a contentious divorce and who works for a law firm
    (D) the man who is the caregiver for his wife, who has dementia, and whose eldest daughter is caring for his wife while he is hospitalized

118. A patient is admitted with COPD exacerbation and worsening dyspnea. The admitting vital signs are as follows: temperature 38.1°C, heart rate 120 beats/minute, B/P 180/80, SpO_2 90% on 2 L/min per a nasal cannula, and respiratory rate 35 breaths/minute and slightly labored. The initial ABG is as follows: pH 7.33, $PaCO_2$ 49, PaO_2 61, SaO_2 87%, and HCO_3 35. What intervention should the nurse anticipate based on this information?

    (A) intubation related to the hypercarbia
    (B) aggressive diuresis
    (C) sedation
    (D) increasing the O_2 to 4 L/min per a nasal cannula

119. A patient who was admitted with pneumonia and subsequent alcohol withdrawal is receiving a lorazepam (Ativan) drip at 4 mg/hour in order to maintain a RASS score of –1 to –2. The patient suddenly becomes agitated, with a RASS score of +2, and all physiological and environmental causes have been ruled out as the cause of the agitation. The most appropriate lorazepam (Ativan) adjustment would be to:

(A) increase the infusion to 5 mg/hour.
(B) give a 2 mg IV bolus dose, and then increase the infusion to 5 mg/hour.
(C) give a 5 mg IV bolus dose, and then increase the infusion to 5 mg/hour.
(D) increase the infusion to 6 mg/hour.

120. A patient was admitted with diabetic ketoacidosis, a serum glucose of 450 mg/dL, and a pH of 7.12. An IV insulin infusion was initiated. The latest serum glucose is 160 mg/dL (it was 275 mg/dL 1 hour previously), the anion gap is 22 mEq/dL, and the venous CO_2 is 14 mmol/kg. Which of the following interventions is most appropriate at this time?

(A) Discontinue the insulin infusion.
(B) Lower the insulin infusion dose.
(C) Administer sodium bicarbonate.
(D) Increase the insulin infusion dose.

121. A patient is admitted to the ICU after a motor vehicle crash related to excessive consumption of alcohol. The patient has had several previous traffic violations related to alcohol consumption, and the driver of another car in the crash had critical injuries. During the nurse's initial assessment, the patient is awake, oriented, and lying quietly. What would be the optimal approach for the nurse to use at this time?

(A) Enter the room but avoid talking about the most recent incident.
(B) Discuss nonthreatening topics such as the weather to engage in conversation.
(C) Provide nonjudgmental encouragement aimed at reducing or ceasing alcohol consumption.
(D) Ask the patient if he would like to talk about what happened.

122. A nurse evaluates the results of a patient's lumbar puncture and anticipates that the physician will order antibiotics. Which of the following results explains the nurse's evaluation of the CSF report?

(A) elevated protein
(B) clear CSF
(C) glucose 30 mg/dL
(D) elevated WBC

123. The cardiac monitor shows a pacer spike before the P-wave and a spike before the QRS, and the heart rate increases with activity. This patient has which type of pacemaker?

(A) abnormally functioning AAI pacemaker
(B) abnormally functioning VVD pacemaker
(C) normally functioning VVI pacemaker
(D) normally functioning DDD pacemaker

124. A patient is admitted with ripping upper back pain, a blood pressure of 198/106, a heart rate of 102 beats/minute, and a respiratory rate of 22 breaths/minute. A 7 cm thoracic aneurysm is identified on the CT scan. Which of the following is contraindicated in this situation?

(A) morphine for the pain
(B) a labetalol infusion
(C) immediate surgery
(D) surgery the next morning

125. Which of the following is a sign of early sepsis, especially in elderly patients?

(A) anemia
(B) heart failure
(C) fever
(D) confusion

126. A patient was admitted 2 days ago with ST elevation in II, III, and aVF. Two days later, the patient developed hypotension, tachypnea, hypoxemia, and a new loud holosystolic murmur at the apex. The definitive treatment for this patient will be:

(A) percutaneous coronary intervention.
(B) intra-aortic balloon pump therapy.
(C) surgery.
(D) intubation and mechanical ventilation.

127. Which of the following patients has the least resiliency?

(A) the 80-year-old male with STEMI but no comorbidities
(B) the 48-year-old female with multiple fractures and hypertension
(C) the 78-year-old female with lung cancer and sepsis
(D) the 59-year-old male with DKA and drug abuse

128. A patient with chronic kidney disease is admitted to the critical care unit with an acute MI. Which of the following is known to result in the highest incidences of death for patients with chronic kidney disease?

(A) wound infection
(B) dehydration
(C) fluid overload
(D) hyperkalemia

129. Despite emergent PCI and a dobutamine infusion, a patient with an acute anterior wall myocardial infarction remained hypotensive. An intra-aortic balloon (IAB) is inserted via the left femoral artery, and counterpulsation is started. The immediate effect of IABP therapy is:

(A) decreased preload and myocardial oxygen consumption.
(B) decreased preload and afterload.
(C) decreased afterload and increased coronary artery perfusion.
(D) decreased afterload and increased myocardial contractility.

130. A patient is receiving amiodarone. Which of the following assessments is important for this patient?

(A) PR interval, renal function, blood pressure
(B) QRS interval, liver function, lung sounds
(C) QT interval, thyroid function, heart rate
(D) ST segment, pulmonary function, urine output

131. A patient is 1 day post open heart surgery. The patient's spouse inquires if she might bring in the patient's favorite CD of classical music to help control the pain. Which of the following is the nurse's best response?

(A) "The use of music may reduce pain and tension."

(B) "We will give your spouse as much pain medication as needed. Music will not be necessary."

(C) "There are no studies to suggest that music will help manage postoperative pain."

(D) "We can try it, but the portable CD player will require approval by the biomedical department before it can be used."

132. Which of the following is an abnormal reflex response in an adult?

(A) The toes flare up toward the patient's head in response to plantar stimulation.

(B) The eyes turn toward the right when cold water is injected into the right ear.

(C) The eye blinks when the cornea is touched.

(D) Gagging occurs when the endotracheal tube is suctioned.

133. A patient has an ankle-brachial index of 0.8. Which of the following is important in the care of this patient?

(A) Place the bed in reverse Trendelenburg.

(B) Provide an antihypertensive.

(C) Elevate the lower extremities.

(D) Elevate the affected arm.

134. A patient is 2 days status post open reduction and internal fixation of a left tibia and fibula fracture following a fall from a ladder; additional injuries included rib and clavicle fractures. The patient is now complaining of severe left leg pain. The leg is very taut and firm, but pulses are present. The priority intervention for this patient is to:

(A) provide morphine for the pain.

(B) contact the surgeon.

(C) continue to monitor the pedal pulses.

(D) elevate the left leg.

135. A preceptor heard an orientee give an update on the patient's status, post full cardiac arrest, to the patient's family when they arrived. Although there was return of circulation, the patient was not responsive, she was receiving mechanical ventilation, and the clinical hypothermia protocol was ordered. The preceptor felt that the orientee's update was more positive than it should have been. What would be the best approach for the preceptor to take at this time?

(A) While the orientee is still in the room, tell the family that it will be best to wait for the attending physician to come in and provide an update to the family.

(B) While the orientee is still in the room, introduce herself to the family, explain the preceptor/orientee relationship, and provide a more accurate update.

(C) Ask the orientee to go get something from the storeroom. After the orientee leaves the room, introduce herself to the family, explain the preceptor/orientee relationship, and provide a more accurate update.

(D) Ask the orientee to go get something from the storeroom, tell the family that the attending physician is on the way to provide them with an update, and coach the orientee after leaving the room.

136. A patient presents with an overdose of an unknown substance. The patient is hypertensive and tachycardic and has a normal temperature. The skin is warm, the patient is flushed, and his pupils are equal and reactive with his eyes flickering up and down. The patient experienced a seizure shortly after arrival. Which of the following agents has the patient most likely taken?

    (A) PCP
    (B) heroin
    (C) LSD
    (D) amphetamines

137. A patient with dilated cardiomyopathy is most likely to have which of the following?

    (A) diastolic murmur (loudest at the right sternal border); left ventricular hypertrophy on the ECG
    (B) systolic murmur (loudest at the apex); an enlarged cardiac silhouette on the chest radiograph
    (C) diastolic murmur (loudest at the apex); normal ejection fraction
    (D) systolic murmur (loudest at the left sternal border); S4 heart sound

138. Which of the following would warrant an immediate call to the neurosurgeon postoperatively?

    (A) ICP 15 mmHg, cerebral perfusion pressure 100 mmHg
    (B) a temperature increase to 39.8°C from 37.2°C
    (C) a urine output of 100 mL in the past hour and a urine specific gravity of 1.010
    (D) the patient arouses with voice and was previously aroused with shaking

139. A patient with abdominal trauma is experiencing acute left shoulder pain. Which of the following might cause this symptom?

    (A) diaphragmatic irritation
    (B) ruptured bladder
    (C) liver contusion
    (D) ruptured kidney

140. A nursing measure designed to optimize the cerebral perfusion pressure (CPP) involves:

    (A) turning the patient every hour.
    (B) preventing the MAP from becoming greater than 65 mmHg.
    (C) maintaining the $PaCO_2$ at less than 30 mmHg.
    (D) maintaining a neutral head position.

141. The physician orders intubation and mechanical ventilation for a patient with asthma. The patient's respiratory rate is 28 breaths/minute, and she is currently receiving 3 L/nasal cannula oxygen. Which of the following arterial blood gases best supports the decision to place an endotracheal tube?

    (A) pH 7.41; $PaCO_2$ 39 mmHg; PaO_2 83 mmHg
    (B) pH 7.50; $PaCO_2$ 29 mmHg; PaO_2 72 mmHg
    (C) pH 7.46; $PaCO_2$ 33 mmHg; PaO_2 62 mmHg
    (D) pH 7.36; $PaCO_2$ 41 mmHg; PaO_2 62 mmHg

142. A 22-year-old male patient, with a known history of Wolff-Parkinson-White (WPW) syndrome, developed preexcited atrial fibrillation (AF) at a rate of 170 beats/minute. The nurse should anticipate the administration of which of the following medications?

    (A) adenosine (Adenocard)
    (B) diltiazem (Cardizem)
    (C) esmolol (Brevibloc)
    (D) digoxin (Lanoxin)

143. Which of the following patients will most likely need hemodialysis?

    (A) the patient with a BUN of 88 mg/dL and a creatinine of 3.8 mg/dL

    (B) the patient with metabolic alkalosis and hypokalemia

    (C) the patient with an aspirin overdose, a BUN of 15 mg/dL, and a creatinine of 1.5 mg/dL

    (D) the patient with a serum potassium of 5.8 mEq/L and a normal ECG

144. A Type 2 diabetic patient presents with a serum glucose of 1,050 mg/dL and negative ketones. Which of the following is the priority intervention for this patient?

    (A) insulin

    (B) bicarbonate

    (C) potassium

    (D) fluid replacement

145. A patient with acute pancreatitis has the following assessment:

Vital signs: Temperature 37°C, B/P 98/65, heart rate 110 beats/minute, respiratory rate 28 breaths/minute, SpO$_2$ 89%, FiO$_2$ of 2 L/nasal cannula

Labs: WBC count 19,000, hemoglobin 9.0 g/dL, hematocrit 40%, Na$^+$ 145 mEq/L, K$^+$ 3.0 mEq/L, Ca^{++} 7.8 mEq/L, glucose 220 mg/dL

Assessment: Lungs with left lower lobe crackles, abdomen with Cullen's sign

Which of the following additional conditions (along with pancreatitis) does this patient most likely have, and what intervention is needed?

    (A) hemorrhagic shock, stress hyperglycemia, hypoxemia; the patient needs blood

    (B) hypovolemic shock, diabetes, sepsis; the patient needs antibiotics

    (C) SIRS, hemorrhagic pancreatitis, MODS; the patient needs fluids

    (D) dehydration, ARDS, stress hyperglycemia; the patient needs intubation

146. A patient who is receiving intracranial pressure monitoring has sustained A-waves on the intracranial pressure (ICP) monitor. Which of the following interventions is contraindicated for this patient?

    (A) Discontinue opiate and sedating drugs.

    (B) Administer mannitol.

    (C) Infuse isotonic solutions.

    (D) Drain CSF from the ventricular catheter.

147. A patient arrives in the critical care unit 4 hours postpartum with bleeding that is thought to be secondary to severe uterine atony. Her blood pressure is 78/40, her heart rate is 140 beats/minute, and her respiratory rate is 30 breaths/minute. Her hemoglobin is 11.2 g/dL. Which of the following interventions is appropriate?

    (A) This patient has lost 1,500–2,000 mL of blood and is at a high risk for DIC. Initiate fluid resuscitation, transfuse blood, and check the coagulation profile.

    (B) The patient has lost 500–1,000 mL of blood and is at a high risk for septic shock. Initiate fluid resuscitation, give pressors, and obtain blood cultures.

    (C) The patient has lost 250–500 mL of blood and is at a high risk for a pulmonary embolism. Initiate fluid resuscitation, get a chest CT scan, and obtain a D-dimer.

    (D) The patient has lost over 2,000 mL of blood and is at a high risk for uterine rupture. Initiate fluid resuscitation, transfuse blood, and obtain an ultrasound of the abdomen.

148. The decision has been made to wean a patient from the ventilator. Which of the following would be an indication to stop the weaning trial?

(A) the development of a paradoxical breathing pattern with accessory muscle use

(B) the patient remains disoriented with demonstrations of mild anxiety and agitation

(C) a productive cough with activation of the ventilator alarm within the first 5 minutes of the weaning trial

(D) an increase in heart rate from 82 beats/minute to 96 beats/minute within the first 5 minutes of the weaning trial

149. A patient presents with a blood pressure of 232/129 and acute chest pain. Which of the following would be the agent of choice to use for this patient?

(A) nicardipine (Cardene)

(B) labetalol (Normodyne)

(C) nitroprusside (Nipride)

(D) diltiazem (Cardizem)

150. Which of the following findings would be expected during chest auscultation of a patient with systolic heart failure?

(A) an S4 heart sound at the apex of the heart

(B) a systolic murmur at the apex of the heart

(C) a diastolic murmur at the left sternal border

(D) an S3 heart sound at the apex of the heart

1. **B**	39. **C**	77. **D**	115. **C**
2. **D**	40. **B**	78. **A**	116. **B**
3. **B**	41. **A**	79. **A**	117. **A**
4. **D**	42. **C**	80. **A**	118. **D**
5. **C**	43. **A**	81. **B**	119. **B**
6. **B**	44. **C**	82. **D**	120. **B**
7. **C**	45. **C**	83. **B**	121. **D**
8. **A**	46. **D**	84. **B**	122. **C**
9. **C**	47. **C**	85. **D**	123. **D**
10. **C**	48. **B**	86. **C**	124. **D**
11. **A**	49. **B**	87. **B**	125. **D**
12. **C**	50. **C**	88. **A**	126. **C**
13. **D**	51. **C**	89. **D**	127. **C**
14. **C**	52. **C**	90. **C**	128. **A**
15. **B**	53. **B**	91. **D**	129. **C**
16. **A**	54. **D**	92. **A**	130. **C**
17. **B**	55. **A**	93. **C**	131. **A**
18. **B**	56. **D**	94. **C**	132. **A**
19. **D**	57. **D**	95. **C**	133. **A**
20. **A**	58. **C**	96. **A**	134. **B**
21. **B**	59. **C**	97. **B**	135. **B**
22. **A**	60. **C**	98. **B**	136. **A**
23. **B**	61. **C**	99. **C**	137. **B**
24. **C**	62. **A**	100. **B**	138. **B**
25. **D**	63. **A**	101. **A**	139. **A**
26. **D**	64. **B**	102. **A**	140. **D**
27. **C**	65. **C**	103. **B**	141. **D**
28. **B**	66. **D**	104. **B**	142. **C**
29. **A**	67. **C**	105. **D**	143. **C**
30. **B**	68. **A**	106. **A**	144. **D**
31. **C**	69. **C**	107. **B**	145. **C**
32. **A**	70. **A**	108. **A**	146. **A**
33. **C**	71. **C**	109. **A**	147. **A**
34. **C**	72. **A**	110. **D**	148. **A**
35. **A**	73. **C**	111. **B**	149. **B**
36. **C**	74. **D**	112. **D**	150. **D**
37. **A**	75. **A**	113. **B**	
38. **D**	76. **D**	114. **B**	

ANSWERS AND EXPLANATIONS

1. **(B)** An experienced nurse realizes that, to be effective, an organizational change will require input from the key stakeholders and their acceptance of the proposed change. Changing one's own practice, although admirable, will not effect broad-based change and may even cause confusion. Although getting a physician's thoughts is interesting, that response alone will not effect organizational change. Discussing the educational session with nurse colleagues provides information on possible resistance, but it is not the optimal broad-based approach that is required to be effective.

2. **(D)** Correcting the hypotension (with isotonic fluid resuscitation in order to maintain organ perfusion) is the priority at this time. Antibiotics (choice (A)) will need to be started after blood cultures are obtained. A vasopressor (choice (B)) may not be needed if the MAP is restored with fluids. Although a sputum culture (choice (C)) may be indicated, blood cultures need to be drawn first so that antibiotics can be given (within the first hour, if possible).

3. **(B)** This patient has sepsis as evidenced by an infection, organ dysfunction (hypotension), and elevated lactate upon arrival. With the administration of fluids, the hypotension was corrected, and the lactate decreased. Therefore, at this point, the patient does NOT have septic shock, which means that choice (D) is incorrect. There were signs of organ dysfunction. Therefore, the patient has more than just SIRS, which means that choice (C) is incorrect. This scenario does not describe bacteremia, so choice (A) is also incorrect.

4. **(D)** Clot formation on the valve is a major complication of valve replacement, especially for a mechanical valve. Therefore, anticoagulation will be needed. Fluid overload, a labile B/P, and infection are all possible complications. However, they are not as likely as the formation of a thrombus and a resultant stroke (if the thrombus is related to the aortic valve).

5. **(C)** This patient exhibits signs of increased ICP, and each intervention in choice (C) will decrease the ICP. Steroids, vasopressin, thiazide diuretics, and a lumbar puncture are not interventions for increased ICP.

6. **(B)** Social support is very important for a young adult to cope. A request to call friends is evidence of that need. Choices (A) and (C) do not provide the patient with the opportunity to utilize social support. This scenario does not indicate that the patient is anxious, so choice (D) is incorrect.

7. **(C)** Ensuring the competency of the staff (who insert indwelling urinary catheters) using a simulated environment is a strategy to reduce infections. Another strategy would be providing coaching related to breaks in technique. Urinary catheters should be removed on day 1 post-op, not on day 3 post-op, so choice (A) is incorrect. The drainage system of the catheter should be kept below the level of the patient's bladder at all times, not on the patient's abdomen. Thus, choice (B) is incorrect. Intermittent straight catheterization programs have been shown to help reduce catheter days, so they should not be avoided as choice (D) suggests.

8. **(A)** Mechanical devices, such as an IABP or a VAD, will increase coronary artery perfusion, which is a positive hemodynamic effect in the presence of cardiogenic shock. Beta blockers decrease myocardial contractility. Alpha-adrenergic drugs, such as

phenylephrine or norepinephrine, constrict arteries, decrease perfusion, and increase the work of the heart. Afterload reduction will decrease the work of the heart, but it will not increase coronary artery perfusion.

9. **(C)** Hospice referrals are considered for patients with a terminal illness or a chronic illness in the terminal stage. The remaining 3 choices are interventions that are included in palliative care, which all critically ill patients have a right to receive.

10. **(C)** The patient did not respond to noninvasive ventilation since the $PaCO_2$ increased, respiratory acidosis is worse, and severe hypoxemia was not corrected. BiPAP should not be continued. The issue is not metabolic acidosis. The pH is not acceptable.

11. **(A)** The plateau pressure reflects lung pressure and is needed to calculate static (lung) compliance. It is not used to calculate vital capacity, dynamic compliance, or tidal volume. Peak inspiratory pressure is used to calculate dynamic compliance.

12. **(C)** A salicylate overdose will cause renal failure. Activated charcoal will help neutralize the salicylates. Alkalinization of urine, by the administration of sodium bicarbonate in the intravenous fluids, will protect the kidneys. Emergent dialysis will ensure the clearance of the salicylates. The remaining choices will not protect the kidneys from the effects of salicylic acid.

13. **(D)** The homeless man has the fewest resources available of those listed. This lack of resiliency needs to be taken into consideration when planning care.

14. **(C)** If the patient is pulling at his central venous catheter, he is exhibiting behavior that may cause harm to himself. Assuming that alternatives to restraints were already attempted, the application of restraints to address this patient's nonviolent behavior would be appropriate. Screaming (choice (A)) and spitting (choice (B)) are not behaviors that can be controlled with restraints. The presence of an endotracheal tube alone (choice (D)) is not a reason to restrain a patient.

15. **(B)** The RA pressure is elevated in RV failure secondary to RV infarct, and a decrease in that pressure is evidence that the treatment is effective. The PAOP is a left heart pressure. It is often already low in the setting of RV infarct/failure since the preload to the left heart drops. A further decrease is not warranted. An increase in the RV pressure is a sign of worsening RV failure. The PAD pressure is already low with RV infarct, and a further decrease is not desirable.

16. **(A)** During an AAA repair, there may be prolonged decreased perfusion to the renal artery and resulting damage to the renal tubules. This population is at a high risk for acute renal failure. The remaining 3 choices are less common than renal failure.

17. **(B)** This patient has pericarditis, and the expected ECG change is global ST elevation. Choice (A) is seen in anterior wall ischemia or NSTEMI. Choice (C) is associated with RV ischemia/infarct. Choice (D) is seen with acute inferior wall STEMI.

18. **(B)** This patient has DIC, a problem that causes excessive clotting, resulting in the consumption of clotting factors, the eventual inability to clot, and bleeding. The lab profile reveals a coagulopathy. However, the key parameter is the elevated fibrin split products (also known as fibrin degradation products) of 45 mcg/dL (normal is less than 10 mcg/dL), which is evidence of excessive clot breakdown. The remaining 3 choices would not elevate the fibrin split products.

19. **(D)** Capture threshold is assessed by decreasing (not increasing) the mA output until pacer spikes are seen without a QRS. This is the point at which the capture is lost. The output is then set at about double the capture threshold. This may prevent a loss of capture even if fibrinous crust overgrows on the surface of the electrode. The pacing (or sensing) threshold is assessed by adjusting the sensitivity.

20. **(A)** This patient tolerated the current activity with head of bed elevation in high Fowler's position and is now ready to progress to sitting without back support with his legs dangling. This patient does not have contraindications to mobility progression; therefore, reducing the patient's mobility (choice (B)) or maintaining the patient's urrent level of mobility (choice (C)) would not provide progress. Although the patient might be able to progress to weight-bearing and sitting in a chair, it is best to go step-by-step and then reassess, not to proceed directly to weight-bearing (as choice (D) suggests).

21. **(B)** The primary problem is hypotension, and it should be treated with fluids. Although a reduction of PEEP would most likely increase the B/P, it would result in derecruitment of alveoli and hypoxemia. A norepinephrine drip should be initiated only if fluids alone do not correct the hypotension. An increase in the tidal volume would not increase the B/P and would cause volutrauma in a patient with ARDS.

22. **(A)** The absence of gag and corneal reflexes in a patient who recently had these reflexes needs to be further investigated. The RN should not need a physician order to call the organ procurement agency. If brain death has been diagnosed, the family should be prepared for what that diagnosis entails. However, requesting permission to remove the ventilator is not a family decision. Confirmatory tests, such as those described in choice (D), may be hospital policy. However, they are not needed to make the diagnosis of brain death.

23. **(B)** This patient with ARDS needs to receive 4–5 mL/kg tidal volume in order to prevent volutrauma. This patient is receiving 10 mL/kg tidal volume, and this level needs to be reduced. The mode of ventilation and both the PEEP and the FiO_2 settings are acceptable.

24. **(C)** A patient with asthma requires a longer expiratory time in order to decrease air trapping. A lower respiratory rate will help provide this. A short expiratory time, PEEP, and larger tidal volume will all promote air trapping or auto-PEEP. This will increase the intrathoracic pressure, decrease the venous return, and reduce the cardiac output.

25. **(D)** Large V-waves are produced by regurgitant flow backward into the left atrium during left ventricular systole. The other 3 choices do not cause this backflow of blood and the resultant large V-waves.

26. **(D)** Hypercalcemia may be associated with hypokalemia. Therefore, hypokalemia must be ruled out prior to initiating diuretic therapy (a treatment for hypercalcemia) in order to prevent life-threatening arrhythmias.

27. **(C)** The aortic, tricuspid, and mitral valves are anatomically located near conduction pathways. Therefore, a patient who has undergone mitral valve repair may develop heart block post-procedure, which is thought to be due to a local effect on the conduction pathways.

28. **(B)** The systolic pressure increases in order to try to perfuse the brain better as the pressure in the cranial vault increases. This widens the pulse pressure. Heart rate slowing and respiratory depression are the other 2 signs of the triad. Battle's sign is a sign of a basilar skull fracture. The halo sign is seen when CSF is put on sterile white gauze and results in a red center color surrounded by yellow. Chvostek sign is a cheek/facial spasm that is caused by low serum calcium.

29. **(A)** SIADH causes excessive production of antidiuretic hormone, which results in fluid retention, dilutional hyponatremia, low serum osmolality, and elevated urine specific gravity. Dilantin will decrease the production of ADH. The serum sodium would NOT be elevated, the urine output would NOT be elevated, and the urine specific gravity would NOT be low. SIADH does not cause hypokalemia or acidosis.

30. **(B)** Hypophosphatemia results in muscle weakness that may affect the diaphragm and result in hypoventilation. Low serum phosphorus causes constipation, not diarrhea. It results in depressed deep tendon reflexes, not tetany. Low serum phosphorus does not cause ventricular arrhythmias.

31. **(C)** When end-of-life decisions are required, a certain amount of family conflict usually occurs. An experienced nurse knows how to arbitrate in these matters. Choice (A) is not an effective strategy. The clergy may be consulted but only if this is the family's wish. A request that only 1 person be the spokesperson is an effective strategy for routine communication with a large family. However, when end-of-life decisions are necessary, all stakeholders need to have a voice.

32. **(A)** This patient has signs of sedation that precede hypoventilation, plus signs of sleep apnea that increase the risk of hypoventilation. The continuous infusion needs to be discontinued, not reduced. Sedation needs to be gradually (not suddenly) reversed. The patient will still need analgesia with PRN doses. A drop in SpO_2 is a late sign of hypoventilation. Although it is not a choice in this scenario, ideally the patient should have continuous waveform capnography.

33. **(C)** The head of the bed should be kept at least > 30° elevated when providing enteral feeding in order to prevent aspiration. Choices (A), (B), and (D) are correct interventions for a patient who is receiving enteral nutrition.

34. **(C)** This patient's MAP is still not > 65 mmHg. Therefore, a vasopressor needs to be initiated, and norepinephrine is the vasopressor of choice. Fluids will need to be continued at a rapid rate as long as there are no signs of fluid overload. Since fluids need to be continued, not decreased, choice (A) is incorrect. A positive inotrope (such as the one mentioned in choice (B)) is not indicated at this time. Vasopressin (choice (D)) is also not indicated and would only be started if norepinephrine at a higher dose was not increasing the blood pressure.

35. **(A)** Although restlessness, hypertension, and tachycardia may be signs of other problems, including delirium, the additional signs of yawning, lacrimation, and rhinorrhea are classic signs of opiate withdrawal. The patient will need higher doses of opiates to manage the pain due to the injury and surgical procedure. Then, the opiate dose will need to be gradually tapered. The remaining 3 choices will not address the withdrawal from opiates.

36. **(C)** This patient is dehydrated and shows signs of acute prerenal failure. Administering isotonic fluids will restore the vascular volume, increase the urine output, and correct the tachycardia, hypotension, BUN, and creatinine. The etiology of the diarrhea needs to be addressed as this is the primary problem. The remaining 3 choices will not correct the immediate acute symptoms.

37. **(A)** A shunt requires more than oxygen to correct hypoxemia; for example, PEEP therapy is needed. Hyperventilation reduces the pCO_2, not the pO_2. Diffusion defects may produce hypoxemia, but that condition responds to oxygen therapy alone. A V/Q mismatch that results in hypoxemia will respond to oxygen administration alone.

38. **(D)** This clinical picture is one of severe hypothyroidism (myxedema coma), and the patient is at risk for developing hypoventilation and hypoxemia. Since this is a case of a hypothyroid emergency, the patient will most likely have hypothermia, not a fever, so choice (A) is incorrect. Bradycardia, not tachycardia, is likely, so choice (B) is incorrect. T3 and T4 are likely to be decreased, not elevated, so choice (C) is incorrect as well.

39. **(C)** The decrease in blood pressure and increase in heart rate with a position change (orthostatic hypotension), clear lungs, and a low urine output are signs of hypovolemia. Vasodilators or diuretics will exacerbate the problem. Vasopressors will only further elevate the SVR, increasing the work of the heart.

40. **(B)** Providing a daily chlorhexidine bath (unless the patient is allergic to it) has been shown to decrease bacterial colonization and CLABSIs. A gauze dressing requires more frequent changing and does not allow the area to be readily assessed (the use of transparent dressing is preferred). Therefore, choice (A) is incorrect. Central lines should not be routinely replaced unless it is known that they were inserted emergently with breaks in technique. Thus, choice (C) is incorrect. Access hubs should be cleansed for a minimum of 5 seconds or more before using them.

41. **(A)** Coughing and tachypnea are early signs of aspiration, although not all patients will cough if their cough reflex is depressed. Positive sputum cultures are a later sign and are not always present. Oxygen desaturation and an infiltrate on a chest radiograph are also later signs of aspiration.

42. **(C)** Murmurs of stenosis occur when the valve is open, and the mitral valve is open during filling of the left ventricle (which is diastole). Chronic resistance produced by stenosis of the mitral valve will result in an enlarged left atrium, which in turn may lead to atrial fibrillation, not sinus bradycardia. During systole the mitral valve is closed. Therefore, mitral regurgitation would cause a systolic murmur. Since this patient scenario does not describe a systolic murmur or sinus bradycardia, choices (A), (B), and (D) are all incorrect.

43. **(A)** Age and the use of NSAIDs are risks for contrast-induced nephropathy. The remaining choices do not pose risks for this problem.

44. **(C)** Tachycardia and hypotension are signs of hypovolemic shock, not an intracranial hemorrhage (in which the amount of blood loss is small). Neurogenic shock and brain herniation result in bradycardia. Brain herniation also results in a widening pulse pressure.

45. **(C)** This patient is exhibiting signs of depression and perhaps suicidal tendencies, and he needs to be evaluated by a psychiatric expert in order to determine the treatment options. Initiating an antidepressant without an expert evaluation would not be the best strategy. Although he or she is able to manage the DKA, the endocrinologist is not the best person to assess the patient's signs of depression. Although it is helpful, emotional support will not necessarily focus on the cause of the patient's depression.

46. **(D)** The ABG demonstrates an uncompensated respiratory alkalosis. Common causes of this problem include hypoxemia (which the patient has) and pain (which the patient is at risk for considering the diagnosis). The patient does not require intubation since there is hyperventilation, not hypoventilation. Blood pressure abnormalities will not cause uncompensated respiratory alkalosis. Electrolyte abnormalities and blood sugar abnormalities do not cause respiratory alkalosis.

47. **(C)** Pharmacological prophylaxis is superior to mechanical prophylaxis for DVT. Daily low-molecular-weight heparin or unfractionated heparin every 8 or 12 hours are the agents of choice. Compression stockings alone are only effective for select patients with a lower risk for developing DVT. Pneumatic compression devices need to be used bilaterally on the lower extremities at all times (except when walking); they should not only be used on 1 extremity. Warfarin is used for the treatment of DVT and PE, not for prophylaxis.

48. **(B)** Early in the obstruction, bowel sounds are increased. Later, the bowel sounds become diminished. A small bowel obstruction generally causes high-pitched sounds. A large bowel obstruction typically has low-pitched sounds.

49. **(B)** This clinical picture is one of ventricular septal defect (based on the location of the murmur and the patient's chief presenting problem). It would be expected that the O_2 saturation on the right side of the heart would be higher than normal if arterial blood from the left ventricle is shunting into the right ventricle.

50. **(C)** This patient is demonstrating agitation (a RASS score of +3), and it is due to pain a (BPS score of 10). Therefore, an analgesic is indicated for the patient's agitation. An increase in the propofol dose or the administration of lorazepam would not address the pain. There is no indication that the agitation is due to a gas exchange problem. Therefore, a stat ABG is not indicated.

51. **(C)** High airway pressures may lead to an air leak. Choices (A), (B), and (D) are all contraindicated in the care of a patient with a chest tube.

52. **(C)** The pulmonary pressure gets increasingly high with pulmonary hypertension, which causes right ventricular strain and dilatation, which in turn may result in the tricuspid valve's inability to close fully. Pulmonary hypertension does not cause pulmonary valve stenosis, left ventricular failure, or increased lung compliance. Right ventricular failure and decreased lung compliance are more likely.

53. **(B)** Any sign of coagulopathy needs to be rapidly corrected in order to prevent a larger hematoma. A brain MRI is not indicated; a CT scan is done. Surgical evacuation of the hematoma may be done only in select cases if it might decrease the neurological injury. Nitroprusside is not the agent of choice to decrease the B/P of a patient with a cerebral hematoma; labetalol is the drug of choice.

54. **(D)** The "adrenergic storm" of DTs is best addressed with benzodiazepines. They enhance the effect of the neurotransmitter gamma-aminobutyric acid (GABA) at the GABA receptors, resulting in sedative, hypnotic (sleep-inducing), anxiolytic (anti-anxiety), anticonvulsant, and muscle relaxant properties. Thiamine will be needed to prevent Wernicke encephalopathy. Phenobarbital has been used for extreme cases of DTs. However, benzodiazepines are the treatment of choice for the prevention and treatment of DTs. Fluids will be needed to prevent dehydration.

55. **(A)** This patient has most likely developed heparin-induced thrombocytopenia (HIT). A direct thrombin inhibitor (DTI) needs to be started, and heparin must be immediately discontinued. The patient will still require an anticoagulant (that is not heparin). Platelets are not indicated for HIT unless the patient has life-threatening bleeding, or they may be considered if the platelet count drops to less than 10,000/mcL.

56. **(D)** A wound VAC canister needs to be changed if it is full or damaged or as recommended by the manufacturer (generally once a week). The provider needs to be contacted if suction is lost for more than 2 hours, not 4 hours as choice (A) incorrectly suggests. The dressing is not changed daily; rather, it is changed if it is no longer occlusive or if it is leaking. Therefore, choice (B) is incorrect. The tubing is not flushed daily, as choice (C) mistakenly suggests; rather, it may be flushed if it is clogged.

57. **(D)** Stimulation of the cough reflex will increase the ICP. Occasionally, lidocaine is ordered to be given prior to suctioning this patient population. The remaining choices are appropriate for this patient with increased ICP.

58. **(C)** This patient has early signs of hypoglycemia, which needs to be verified with a stat blood glucose test and treated with complex carbohydrates by mouth or a 50% dextrose IV if the patient is unable to take oral carbohydrates. An increase in the insulin dose would be given for hyperglycemia, but this patient is not manifesting signs of hyperglycemia (warm, dry skin, weakness, thirst). Thus, choice (A) is incorrect. The clinical signs described in the question do not indicate the need for an ECG or an increase in fluids. Therefore, choices (B) and (D) are also incorrect.

59. **(C)** This patient most likely has HHS. Although the patient may still produce some insulin, this problem develops less rapidly than does DKA, and the serum glucose is greater than that of DKA. Additionally, acidosis is not present, the serum osmolality is high due to fluid loss, the serum potassium may be elevated due to insufficient insulin production (not due to acidosis as in DKA), and the sodium is often low due to a loss of urine.

60. **(C)** A nurse who has experience in these situations will realize that, when faced with the diagnosis of a family member's brain death, many families may request another opinion. Documentation of physician-family discussions is done in all circumstances. A discussion about organ donation will need to happen after the family has processed the information or prior to making the diagnosis. Not every brain death diagnosis requires an ethics consult.

61. **(C)** This clinical picture is indicative of necrotizing fasciitis, which requires immediate treatment. The application of an ice pack or sterile gauze should not be done until the provider examines the abrasion. Thus, choices (A) and (D) are incorrect. This patient will need analgesia, which can be given after the provider is alerted of the change in the patient's clinical status. Thus, choice (B) is also incorrect.

62. **(A)** If synchronized cardioversion is attempted in the presence of digoxin toxicity, ventricular tachycardia or fibrillation may result. The remaining 3 options would not be contraindications to synchronized cardioversion.

63. **(A)** When the balloon inflates during diastole, coronary artery perfusion is increased, which increases the myocardial oxygen supply. This occurs during diastole, not systole. It does not increase the LV filling volume. It will not increase the LV diastolic pressure. IABP therapy will actually help to decrease the LV diastolic pressure after several hours of therapy.

64. **(B)** A shift of the oxyhemoglobin dissociation curve to the right allows hemoglobin to more easily release oxygen to the tissues, which can decrease the SaO_2 of the hemoglobin. A shift of the oxyhemoglobin dissociation curve to the right does **not** improve the SaO_2. It does **not** decrease the release of oxygen from the hemoglobin. It increases the oxygen release. A shift to the right does **not** decrease the release of 2,3-DPG. It increases the 2,3-DPG release, which results in hemoglobin more readily releasing oxygen.

65. **(C)** The endotoxins that are present in sepsis may cause massive vasodilation and the loss of vascular tone, which will decrease the SVR. The decreased SVR results in an increase in the cardiac output (although there is shunting of blood at the capillary level that can result in uneven tissue perfusion at the capillary level). The SvO_2 is elevated due to poor oxygen consumption and utilization at the cellular level. The other 3 profiles are not representative of septic shock.

66. **(D)** The dose of insulin should be doubled in order to achieve a decrease in serum glucose of 50–75 mg/dL per hour. This patient has only had a decrease in serum glucose of 20 mg/dL in 2 hours. The remaining choices would not achieve the desired goal.

67. **(C)** If the injury is on the right side, pupil changes (if present) will be ipsilateral and motor changes will be contralateral. The remaining 3 choices do not meet these criteria.

68. **(A)** Oxygen utilization is about 300 mL/min, whereas oxygen delivery is ~ 1,000 mL/min. If the cardiac output decreases, myocardial oxygen extraction will increase. (The heart rate will also increase.) A drop in oxygen consumption and a decrease in heart rate do **not** occur with a drop in the cardiac output. If the cardiac output drops, oxygen delivery will decrease, not increase.

69. **(C)** Infections are the most common cause of DKA. In this case, the patient had evidence of an infection. Even when symptoms of an infection are not reported in the patient history, all patients with DKA need to be assessed for an infection. Although the other choices may cause DKA, there is no evidence of these causes in this scenario.

70. **(A)** An elevated LV filling pressure (PAOP) and a decrease in cardiac output would benefit from decreased SVR (LV afterload). A vasodilating drug, such as an ACE inhibitor or mechanical therapy with an intra-aortic balloon pump, would provide this effect. A heart rate reduction might benefit diastolic filling, but it will not necessarily help an elevated LV filling pressure. Elevation of the LV preload or negative inotropic therapy would make the problem worse.

71. **(C)** A massive hemothorax will push the mediastinum toward the unaffected side, which will push the trachea toward the unaffected side. A simple pneumothorax (without massive pleural fluid collection or tension due to air that cannot escape) will pull the trachea toward the affected side.

72. **(A)** This patient has intrarenal failure, as evidenced by the 10:1 BUN to creatinine ratio. In intrarenal failure, the tubular basement membrane is damaged, and the tubules are no longer able to concentrate urine or hold onto sodium. The remaining choices do not meet both of these criteria.

73. **(C)** ST segment elevation that normalizes and chest pain that is relieved after the administration of nitroglycerin are indicative of Prinzmetal's, or variant, angina. Stable angina occurs with activity; it is predictable. STEMI does not respond to NTG with the normalization of ST segments and complete pain relief. Wellens syndrome does not present with ST elevation; rather, it presents with a biphasic T-wave that is specific to leads V1 and V2.

74. **(D)** This patient has signs and symptoms of a blood transfusion reaction. No further blood should be infused when a reaction is suspected. The remaining interventions will be required. However, the priority nursing intervention is to address the source of the problem (the blood transfusion), which may be life-threatening.

75. **(A)** Since this patient has blanched skin and edema that is greater than 1 inch but is less than 6 inches, this is a stage 2 infiltration, and the IV should be restarted in the opposite extremity, if possible. This is not a stage 0 infiltration, so choice (B) is incorrect. This is not a stage 1 infiltration, and if it were, there would be no need to check for blood return; it's obviously not in the vein. Thus, choice (C) is incorrect. This is not an extravasation since it was plain 0.9 normal saline that was used, not an irritant or a vesicant. Therefore, choice (D) is also incorrect.

76. **(D)** In the event that the tube becomes displaced and moves up, the esophageal balloon may obstruct the airway and result in an acute airway emergency. The scissors would be needed to cut the esophageal balloon immediately. The remaining interventions may be needed, but they are not specific to the care of a patient with an esophageal balloon tube.

77. **(D)** Gathering information is more important at this point than giving information. Telling the patient how he will feel is not advisable.

78. **(A)** There is an acute change in the level of consciousness (altered mental status) and inattention in the patient described in choice (A), both of which are required in order to make the diagnosis of delirium. Unresponsiveness alone does not meet the criteria for delirium. If the patient is attentive, delirium cannot be present. If the baseline mental status is unchanged, delirium is not present.

79. **(A)** Packed RBCs have had platelets and plasma removed. Therefore, these components will need to be replaced following the transfusion of multiple units of packed RBCs. As a result of the citrate that is present in banked blood and binds with calcium and magnesium, the patient will also need to be closely monitored for hypocalcemia and hypomagnesemia. Protamine zinc is used to reverse heparin. Albumin is not needed following the transfusion of multiple units of PRBCs. Hetastarch is not needed.

80. **(A)** This patient has signs of opioid-induced respiratory depression, and the priority is to reverse the effects of the morphine with naloxone. This patient does not require the cardiac arrest team at this time, so choice (B) is incorrect. Flumazenil reverses the effects of benzodiazepine agents, not opioids, so choice (C) is incorrect. Contacting the physician for a change in orders is not the priority intervention at this time, so choice (D) is also incorrect.

81. **(B)** Weight assessment is not included in the dysphagia screening tools. The remaining choices are signs of possible dysphagia and are indicative of the need to keep the patient NPO until the patient is further evaluated by a speech pathologist.

82. **(D)** Hand washing with soap and running water is more effective for removing *C. difficile* spores than using hand gel. The remaining 3 choices are not effective strategies for controlling *C. difficile* infections.

83. **(B)** This patient is having an anterior wall myocardial infarction. Even with reperfusion that is achieved in a timely manner, the cardiac biomarkers (troponin) will be elevated. When the artery opens, choices (A), (C), and (D) **will** occur.

84. **(B)** Chest tubes do not affect ventilation or lung compliance. Although there may be a small amount of pleural fluid drainage S/P a thoracotomy, pleural fluid drainage is not the main purpose of the chest tubes.

85. **(D)** The inclusion of all key stakeholders is necessary for the successful implementation of a change. Choices (A), (B), and (C) should have been done prior to making the decision to purchase and implement the device.

86. **(C)** Although PEEP is the therapy used for ALI/ARDS that results in a shunt, PEEP does not necessarily decrease the shunt itself. Rather, PEEP improves the severe hypoxemia by increasing alveolar recruitment. PEEP does not increase dead space ventilation or decrease capillary leak.

87. **(B)** The problem seems to be right-hemispheric in that the paralysis is on the left (contralateral), his eyes look to the right (the problem side), and his pupil changes are ipsilateral (right pupil). Additionally, a subdural hematoma develops slower and may even be chronic. An epidural hematoma usually develops with trauma and acutely; plus, the signs do not support a left-sided problem. A basilar skull fracture would present with raccoon eyes, Battle's sign, and perhaps otorrhea or rhinorrhea. Central herniation would present with bilateral pupil changes, a bilateral positive Babinski reflex, and Cushing's triad.

88. **(A)** The abdominal pain of peritonitis secondary to a perforated appendix is exacerbated by movement of the peritoneum. Therefore, lying still with knees flexed would lessen the pain. Coughing, flexing one's hips up, and positive rebound maneuver will increase the pain. Peritonitis may be generalized or localized, is not related to duration, and does not necessarily become increasingly severe.

89. **(D)** Pulmonary edema is not unilateral; it is always bilateral. ARDS is not always associated with an infection. By definition, the PAOP in the presence of ARDS is normal or low, not elevated. Elevated PAOP with pulmonary edema is due to left ventricular failure.

90. **(C)** This patient is exhibiting signs of diabetes insipidus (DI), in which there is insufficient production of antidiuretic hormone (ADH), most likely due to the head trauma. Pitressin is a form of ADH and is the treatment of choice. The massive diuresis will result in elevated serum sodium; therefore, 3% saline is not appropriate. Phenytoin may cause DI and is **not** a treatment. The main complication of DI is hypovolemic shock. Therefore, a hypotonic solution such as D_5W would not be indicated for DI.

91. **(D)** The clinical signs and symptoms indicate an allergic reaction and anaphylactic shock. The epinephrine, steroids, and antihistamine will counteract the effects of the massive histamine release. Fluids will address the hypotension and relative hypovolemia that is caused by the massive dilatation. The remaining choices include options that are not indicated or helpful for anaphylaxis.

92. **(A)** The delivery of the highest FiO_2 possible will help replace the carbon monoxide that is binding to the hemoglobin. If a hyperbaric oxygen chamber is accessible within approximately 30 minutes, the patient should be transferred there for treatment. Mechanical ventilation will provide 100% FiO_2; however, the patient does not need assistance with ventilation. In addition, 40% FiO_2 is not enough, and naloxone is indicated for an opiate overdose.

93. **(C)** This patient is having an acute inferior wall myocardial infarction. The elevated RAP, JVD, and tall, peaked P-waves are clinical indications of RV failure, most likely secondary to RV infarct. Preload reduction (nitroglycerin) will further decrease LV filling and the cardiac output. Therefore, it should be discontinued, and fluid boluses will help to increase the LV preload. Dobutamine has a mild dilating effect, and it may further decrease the blood pressure. Therefore, an increase in that dose would not be advisable. Starting milrinone would provide no benefits at this time. A dopamine infusion at 10 mcg/kg/min is a high dose. If dopamine (a pressor) is needed, it would be started at 5 mcg/kg/min, not at 10 mcg/kg/min.

94. **(C)** An epidural hematoma is caused by an injury to the meningeal artery. The meningeal artery runs along the temporal lobe (the uncal area of the brain). An epidural hematoma is one brain injury in which pupillary changes (on the side of the injury) will occur **before** a change in the LOC. Thus, choice (A) is incorrect. Choice (B) is incorrect because an epidural hematoma is an acute arterial bleed, not a chronic form. Muscle weakness that is caused by an epidural hematoma will be contralateral. Therefore, choice (D) is incorrect.

95. **(C)** An assessment of why the patient made his decision will help the nurse better intervene, and providing information will help the patient make an informed decision. Attempting to motivate the patient with fear or using family influence may cause problems in the future, even if the patient agrees to the procedure.

96. **(A)** As the patient's temperature rises, vasoconstriction that was present at lower temperatures decreases, with a possible drop in blood pressure. The chest tubes should not be stripped. A blood sugar of 150–200 mg/dL is too high for a post CABG surgery patient. The serum potassium needs to be close to 4.0 mEq/L, and 3.0–4.0 mEq/L is too low.

97. **(B)** Calcium channel blockers help to decrease pressure/stiffness and help LV filling in the presence of diastolic heart failure. Calcium channel blockers are not helpful for systolic dysfunction. Digoxin and dobutamine are positive inotropic drugs. They will increase LV wall tension and may exacerbate symptoms. ACE inhibitors are not harmful to a patient with diastolic heart failure, but they are not a first-line agent for diastolic heart failure.

98. **(B)** Volume depletion will activate the renin-angiotensin-aldosterone system (RAAS). This results in the release of aldosterone, causing sodium and water retention in an effort to increase the vascular volume. Renin secretion is increased, not decreased. The vasculature constricts. It does not dilate. A capillary fluid shift to the interstitial space would worsen the hypovolemia.

99. **(C)** Air trapping and auto-PEEP are the most lethal results of status asthmaticus, and a longer exhalation time will address these issues. The remaining 3 choices may increase air trapping and auto-PEEP.

100. **(B)** Gravity affects pulmonary perfusion, and it is best to have the "good lung down." For this patient, that would be the left side. There is not enough information available to indicate that MRSA coverage is needed. No contraindications are indicated in this scenario that would lead to the decision to withhold DVT prophylaxis. The rust-colored sputum may be due to *Streptococcus pneumoniae* bacterial pneumonia. The head of the bed should be kept at, at least, 30°, not less than that.

101. **(A)** This hemodynamic profile is one of hypovolemia. A fluid bolus should be given until the blood pressure, CVP, and PAOP increase and the heart rate and SVR decrease. A vasopressor (dopamine) would constrict an already constricted vasculature and decrease tissue perfusion. Administering a positive inotrope (dobutamine) will not correct the main problem of hypovolemia and will further increase the heart rate. Administering a potent dilator (nitroprusside) will further decrease perfusion.

102. **(A)** This question relates to assessing the patient's knowledge of the diagnosis of esophageal varices. Therefore, asking why she thinks she is sick is the most open-ended approach. Inquiring about her symptoms or her family history will not provide the information the nurse needs. Although the question posed in choice (D) is related to the diagnosis, an inquiry related to alcohol consumption does not assess the patient's understanding of the diagnosis.

103. **(B)** Ensuring adequate oxygenation and ruling out hypoxemia should be the first nursing assessment for any patient who is exhibiting agitation. Pain and hemodynamic instability also need to be ruled out and addressed, if they are present, but only after adequate oxygenation has been ensured. Delirium is also a cause of agitation and should be assessed for, but it is not as important as oxygenation, pain, or hemodynamic instability, each of which has interventions that are specific to the etiology.

104. **(B)** It is still early in the patient's ICU stay, and aggressive care for the underlying problem with symptom management (palliative care) is likely to improve the outcome. This scenario does not indicate an immediate need for a chaplain (choice (A)) or a "No CPR" order (choice (C)), although code status should be discussed with all patients and their families. This patient does not have a terminal condition; therefore, hospice care (choice (D)) is not indicated.

105. **(D)** Each nurse—not the unit manager—who is assigned to a patient is responsible for assessing the patient's fall risk. The nurse is responsible for communicating with anyone who enters the room during that particular shift, including the patient's family, that the patient is at a high risk for falling. The remaining 3 choices are interventions that are performed by the manager of the unit.

106. **(A)** Pain is boring with acute pancreatitis, and bowel habits are not remarkable. Bowel sounds are more likely to be high-pitched with small bowel obstruction, and projectile vomiting is more common than a change in bowel habits. Abdominal distension is not generally seen with appendicitis.

107. **(B)** This patient's clinical findings are typical of those seen with ARDS. The development of bibasilar crackles, the ground-glass appearance on the chest X-ray, and refractory hypoxemia are not typical of the other 3 choices.

108. **(A)** Nimodipine (Nimotop) is a calcium channel blocker that targets cerebral vessels and prevents constriction. Loop diuretics and osmotic diuretics may result in hypovolemia and increase the vessel spasm. Amicar prevents bleeding.

109. **(A)** A patient with ATN is unable to eliminate magnesium and potassium. Bicarbonate regulation is lost, resulting in a metabolic acidosis. Choices (B), (C), and (D) contain 1 or more incorrect findings.

110. **(D)** With an open mind, the preceptor will need to review the literature on this topic before forming an opinion on a practice that she is not familiar with. Choice (A) refuses to acknowledge that perhaps there is a better way to obtain the CVP value. Choice (B) may sound reasonable, but the literature on this topic needs to be consulted. Choice (C) may be decided upon only **after** the preceptor becomes more familiar with the present research on this topic.

111. **(B)** Stocking the unit with small volume blood draw tubes has been shown to prevent excessive volumes of blood from being drawn for each test. Drawing "daily" labs without a limit to the number of days, regardless of the time of day the labs are drawn (choice (A)), and obtaining blood samples via stopcocks (choice (C)) may lead to nosocomial anemia. Rather than drawing directly from stopcocks, blood conservation systems (with the ability to return blood used for waste) prevent nosocomial anemia. Training nursing assistants to draw blood (choice (D)) will not prevent nosocomial anemia.

112. **(D)** D_5W is contraindicated because it is a hypotonic solution that would exacerbate this patient's low serum osmolality. The remaining 3 types of fluid may be chosen depending upon other factors and would not harm the patient.

113. **(B)** The nature of this injury and the subsequent clinical signs indicate an epidural hematoma. An arteriogram would not be needed. A CT scan of the head would be less invasive and would confirm the diagnosis. The head of the bed should be kept at 30° at least, not lowered, in order to facilitate venous drainage from the head. Although the patient is exhibiting signs of increased ICP, emergent surgery would be the definitive treatment rather than intubation and a ventriculostomy.

114. **(B)** Vasopressin may cause myocardial ischemia that would result in chest pain and/or ST changes on the ECG. The doses used do not generally cause hypertension. Although coronary artery ischemia might result in a cardiac arrhythmia, the signs of ischemia would occur first and more reliably. Vasopressin does not result in a bowel obstruction.

115. **(C)** Adrenal insufficiency should be expected for a patient with unexplained hypoglycemia (who has no history of receiving hypoglycemic agents). Hypercalcemia (not hypocalcemia), hyponatremia (not hypernatremia), and hyperkalemia (not hypokalemia) are associated with adrenal insufficiency.

116. **(B)** Enalapril (Vasotec) is an angiotensin-converting enzyme inhibitor drug that prevents the conversion of angiotensin I to angiotensin II (a potent vasoconstrictor) and thereby causes vasodilation and a decrease in SVR. The other 3 choices are incorrect because afterload is **decreased** by nitroglycerin (high-dose NTG), while preload is **decreased** by furosemide and is **increased** with fluids.

117. **(A)** This patient has additional life stressors that add to the complexity of her care. This complexity needs to be considered when planning her care.

118. **(D)** The ABG demonstrates partially compensated respiratory acidosis and hypoxemia. The FiO_2 should be increased, and the patient response should be assessed. Intubation is not indicated since the hypercapnia is mild. This clinical picture does not support cardiogenic pulmonary edema as the source of the patient's problem. Therefore, diuresis is not indicated. Sedation will worsen the hypoventilation.

119. **(B)** This patient requires a higher dose of lorazepam. An increase in the infusion rate needs to be preceded by a 2 mg IV bolus dose. An increase in the infusion drip rate alone will not be effective since it will take an hour for the increased dose to get infused. An IV bolus dose of 5 mg is not indicated. An increase in the rate to 6 mg/hour alone will not be effective.

120. **(B)** The serum glucose should be decreased by about 50–75 mg/dL per hour for this patient with DKA. Therefore, in this situation, the insulin infusion needs to be decreased. The insulin infusion should be continued, not stopped, until the acidosis is resolved. In this case, acidosis is still present as evidenced by the anion gap and the venous CO_2. The administration of sodium bicarbonate is not indicated in this situation. The insulin infusion should not be increased.

121. **(D)** Choices (A) and (B) are passive strategies and do not provide the patient with the opportunity to share his feelings. At this point, encouragement is not an effective strategy. Being nonjudgmental is important, but the patient requires more than encouragement.

122. **(C)** CSF with glucose that is less than 60% of the serum glucose is an indication of bacterial meningitis rather than viral meningitis. Elevated protein is present in both viral and bacterial meningitis. Clear CSF is a sign of viral meningitis. Elevated WBC is present in both viral and bacterial meningitis.

123. **(D)** The spike before the P-wave is evidence of atrial pacing. The spike before the QRS is evidence of ventricular pacing. An increase in the heart rate with activity demonstrates the ability to respond to a need for a higher heart rate. Choices (A), (B), and (C) do not illustrate the pacer spikes and the increase in heart rate that is described.

124. **(D)** This clinical picture is one of a dissection of the aneurysm, which is a surgical emergency. This patient requires immediate surgery in order to have the best outcome. Therefore, waiting until the next day is contraindicated. The other 3 choices **are** indicated.

125. **(D)** Confusion is often seen with the onset of sepsis in elderly patients. Sometimes, confusion secondary to sepsis is mistaken for a stroke. The remaining 3 choices are not signs of sepsis that especially pertain to elderly patients.

126. **(C)** This patient had an acute inferior wall MI. The sudden change in condition is most likely due to acute mitral valve regurgitation secondary to papillary muscle dysfunction. With hypotension, the MV regurgitation is massive and is most likely a surgical emergency. PCI is not indicated since there is not a recurrence of ST elevation. Although IABP therapy and mechanical ventilation might help, they are not definitive treatments for this life-threatening problem.

127. **(C)** All factors, including age, acute illnesses, chronic illnesses, and support system, need to be assessed when looking at patient resiliency.

128. **(A)** Infections are the leading cause of death for patients with both acute and chronic kidney disease. The remaining choices are complications of chronic kidney disease but do not cause the greatest number of deaths.

129. **(C)** When the intra-aortic balloon closes right before systole begins, the LV afterload is decreased. When the balloon inflates during diastole, coronary artery perfusion is increased. Preload may eventually decrease as coronary artery perfusion increases and afterload decreases. However, this is an indirect effect of IABP therapy. The balloon does not directly increase myocardial contractility.

130. **(C)** Amiodarone may prolong the QT interval, and a 200 mg tablet is estimated to contain about 75 mg of organic iodide. This may result in amiodarone-induced thyrotoxicosis (AIT) or amiodarone-induced hypothyroidism (AIH), both of which can develop in apparently normal thyroid glands or in glands with preexisting abnormalities. Amiodarone does not affect the PR interval or renal function. It does not affect the QRS interval, liver function, or lung sounds. It also does not affect the ST segment or urine output. Amiodarone might decrease the B/P if a large dose (300 mg) is given in a rapid IV to a patient with a pulse, and it could affect pulmonary function (fibrosis) when used orally for long periods of time.

131. **(A)** An experienced nurse will know that there have been studies done on the effects of music on critically ill patients and would advise the spouse that this is a good idea. Choices (B) and (C) are not evidence-based. The nurse should ensure that processes are in place to provide non-pharmacological therapy that is evidence-based and know how to make that therapy happen without going into details with the spouse.

132. **(A)** Flaring of the toes up toward the patient's head is a positive Babinski reflex, which is not normal in an adult. The remaining choices describe normal reflex responses. Choice (B) is a normal oculovestibular reflex in an unconscious patient. Choice (C) is a normal corneal reflex. Choice (D) describes a normal gag reflex.

133. **(A)** An ankle-brachial index (ABI) that is < 1 is a sign of peripheral arterial disease (PAD). A patient with PAD needs to have his or her feet kept lower than the heart level in order to allow gravity to increase perfusion to the lower extremities. An ABI that is < 1 is not an indication of hypertension. Elevation of the lower extremities may worsen perfusion. The ABI has nothing to do with arm perfusion.

134. **(B)** This patient has signs and symptoms of compartment syndrome and should be examined by the surgeon since the patient may need his compartment pressure to be measured. He may also need emergent decompressive fasciotomy. The pain needs to be addressed, but only after the surgeon is notified. Thus, choice (A) is incorrect. The pedal pulses need to be monitored, but a loss of pulses is a late sign of compartment syndrome, with the possibility of permanent nerve and/or vascular damage. Thus, choice (C) is incorrect. The left leg should not be elevated because this will decrease arterial blood flow to the tissue. Thus, choice (D) is also incorrect.

135. **(B)** This strategy is the most transparent approach to use with the family, and it is also a role-modeling opportunity for the orientee. Choice (A) abdicates nursing involvement in the plan of care. Choice (C) may spare the orientee some embarrassment, but it may send the wrong message to the family and decrease trust. Choice (D) again abdicates nursing engagement with the family.

136. **(A)** Eye flickering and a seizure are most typical of a PCP overdose.

137. **(B)** As the left ventricle dilates, complete closure of the mitral valve is impeded, which prevents normal closing of the mitral valve leaflets and causes mitral regurgitation. The resultant murmur is a systolic murmur that is heard loudest at the apex of the heart, and the LV is enlarged.

138. **(B)** Temperature elevation increases the cerebral oxygen requirements and may increase the mortality of patients with neurological problems. The pressures described in choice (A) are normal. The urine assessments described in choice (C) are normal. A patient who is now arousable with voice (who had previously required shaking), as described in choice (D), shows a sign of improvement in arousability.

139. **(A)** An injury that results in diaphragmatic irritation (e.g., a splenic rupture) will result in referred pain to the left shoulder, also known as Kehr's sign. The remaining 3 choices do not cause left shoulder pain.

140. **(D)** The CPP (the MAP minus the ICP) would be lowered due to an increase of ICP that might result if the head is bent or flexed. A neutral head position facilitates venous drainage from the brain and prevents elevated ICP. Although the patient still needs to be repositioned, it does not necessarily need to be done hourly. The MAP needs to be kept > 65 mmHg, not lower than that. A $PaCO_2 < 30$ mmHg will lower the ICP by causing vasoconstriction of the brain vessels. However, this will decrease blood flow to the brain and cause hypoxemia.

141. **(D)** Normalization of the $PaCO_2$ and hypoxemia for a tachypneic patient with an asthma exacerbation is a sign that the patient is tiring and may need mechanical support. Choice (A) shows $PaCO_2$ normalization; however, the PaO_2 is acceptable. Choice (B) shows respiratory alkalosis, an early finding in an asthma exacerbation. Choice (C) shows hypoxemia, which is a worrisome sign, but hyperventilation is still present, a sign that this patient is still able to maintain ventilation.

142. **(C)** Beta blockers are able to decrease acceleration through the accessory pathway (AP). The remaining agents in choices (A), (B), and (D) should not be administered to a patient with WPW syndrome who is experiencing preexcited AF because they may enhance antegrade conduction through the AP and result in ventricular fibrillation.

143. **(C)** A patient with a confirmed aspirin overdose will require immediate dialysis in order to prevent renal tubular damage. The patient described in choice (A) has an approximately 20:1 BUN to creatinine ratio and most likely needs fluids, not dialysis. The patient described in choice (B) needs potassium replacement. The patient described in choice (D) has hyperkalemia but no ECG changes. Therefore, strategies other than dialysis are indicated.

144. **(D)** This patient most likely has HHS, and the most serious complication is hypovolemic shock. Therefore, fluid replacement is paramount. The administration of insulin is needed, but that is secondary to the administration of fluids. Bicarbonate is not needed since serious acidosis is not present. Potassium replacement will most likely not be needed.

145. **(C)** This patient has SIRS, as evidenced by the increased heart rate, respiratory rate, and WBCs. There is evidence of hemorrhagic pancreatitis, as evidenced by Cullen's sign (discoloration around the umbilicus). There is evidence of multiple organ dysfunction syndrome (MODS), as evidenced by the low SpO_2 and hypotension. Fluids are indicated since there are massive fluid shifts with acute pancreatitis with resultant hypovolemia. This patient does not have hemorrhagic shock, does not have diabetes, and does not need antibiotics. This patient is at a high risk for ARDS but does not yet have refractory hypoxemia and bilateral infiltrates.

146. **(A)** Sustained A-waves on the ICP tracing are "awful," a sign of very elevated ICP. B-waves are "bad." C-waves are OK. Discontinuing opiate and sedating drugs would **not** be indicated in the presence of A-waves/elevated ICP. The remaining 3 choices **would** be indicated in the presence of A-waves/increased ICP.

147. **(A)** This patient has hypovolemic shock secondary to a hemorrhage. A blood loss of 1,500 mL is generally required in order for compensatory responses to fail and for the patient to be hypotensive. Aggressive fluid administration is needed, and blood needs to be given. Since the sudden massive blood loss will use up coagulation factors, the patient needs to be monitored closely for the development of DIC. Choices (B) and (C) are not correct since the estimated blood loss is not accurate and there are no signs of septic shock or a pulmonary embolism. Uterine rupture, choice (D), is not likely.

148. **(A)** A paradoxical breathing pattern is evidence that the main muscle of ventilation, the diaphragm, is tiring. The remaining 3 choices are not criteria that support discontinuing the weaning trial.

149. **(B)** This patient has a hypertensive crisis, as evidenced by high blood pressure and signs of end organ damage (chest pain). The labetalol (which is a beta blocker) will help lower the blood pressure and provide some anti-ischemic effect, which this patient most likely needs in the presence of chest pain. Although nicardipine is an antihypertensive and can prevent chest pain, it is not recommended for a hypertensive crisis and active chest pain. Nitroprusside is indicated for a hypertensive crisis but is not recommended for cardiac ischemia. Diltiazem may be used for hypertension but not for a hypertensive crisis.

150. **(D)** An S3 heart sound at the apex is thought to be due to high pressure within the LV that is present in heart failure. An S4 heart sound is usually the result of hypertension or an acute MI. A systolic murmur at the apex is usually due to mitral valve regurgitation. A diastolic murmur at the left sternal border is usually due to tricuspid valve disease.

ANSWER SHEET
Practice Test 2

1. Ⓐ Ⓑ Ⓒ Ⓓ
2. Ⓐ Ⓑ Ⓒ Ⓓ
3. Ⓐ Ⓑ Ⓒ Ⓓ
4. Ⓐ Ⓑ Ⓒ Ⓓ
5. Ⓐ Ⓑ Ⓒ Ⓓ
6. Ⓐ Ⓑ Ⓒ Ⓓ
7. Ⓐ Ⓑ Ⓒ Ⓓ
8. Ⓐ Ⓑ Ⓒ Ⓓ
9. Ⓐ Ⓑ Ⓒ Ⓓ
10. Ⓐ Ⓑ Ⓒ Ⓓ
11. Ⓐ Ⓑ Ⓒ Ⓓ
12. Ⓐ Ⓑ Ⓒ Ⓓ
13. Ⓐ Ⓑ Ⓒ Ⓓ
14. Ⓐ Ⓑ Ⓒ Ⓓ
15. Ⓐ Ⓑ Ⓒ Ⓓ
16. Ⓐ Ⓑ Ⓒ Ⓓ
17. Ⓐ Ⓑ Ⓒ Ⓓ
18. Ⓐ Ⓑ Ⓒ Ⓓ
19. Ⓐ Ⓑ Ⓒ Ⓓ
20. Ⓐ Ⓑ Ⓒ Ⓓ
21. Ⓐ Ⓑ Ⓒ Ⓓ
22. Ⓐ Ⓑ Ⓒ Ⓓ
23. Ⓐ Ⓑ Ⓒ Ⓓ
24. Ⓐ Ⓑ Ⓒ Ⓓ
25. Ⓐ Ⓑ Ⓒ Ⓓ
26. Ⓐ Ⓑ Ⓒ Ⓓ
27. Ⓐ Ⓑ Ⓒ Ⓓ
28. Ⓐ Ⓑ Ⓒ Ⓓ
29. Ⓐ Ⓑ Ⓒ Ⓓ
30. Ⓐ Ⓑ Ⓒ Ⓓ
31. Ⓐ Ⓑ Ⓒ Ⓓ
32. Ⓐ Ⓑ Ⓒ Ⓓ
33. Ⓐ Ⓑ Ⓒ Ⓓ
34. Ⓐ Ⓑ Ⓒ Ⓓ
35. Ⓐ Ⓑ Ⓒ Ⓓ
36. Ⓐ Ⓑ Ⓒ Ⓓ
37. Ⓐ Ⓑ Ⓒ Ⓓ
38. Ⓐ Ⓑ Ⓒ Ⓓ

39. Ⓐ Ⓑ Ⓒ Ⓓ
40. Ⓐ Ⓑ Ⓒ Ⓓ
41. Ⓐ Ⓑ Ⓒ Ⓓ
42. Ⓐ Ⓑ Ⓒ Ⓓ
43. Ⓐ Ⓑ Ⓒ Ⓓ
44. Ⓐ Ⓑ Ⓒ Ⓓ
45. Ⓐ Ⓑ Ⓒ Ⓓ
46. Ⓐ Ⓑ Ⓒ Ⓓ
47. Ⓐ Ⓑ Ⓒ Ⓓ
48. Ⓐ Ⓑ Ⓒ Ⓓ
49. Ⓐ Ⓑ Ⓒ Ⓓ
50. Ⓐ Ⓑ Ⓒ Ⓓ
51. Ⓐ Ⓑ Ⓒ Ⓓ
52. Ⓐ Ⓑ Ⓒ Ⓓ
53. Ⓐ Ⓑ Ⓒ Ⓓ
54. Ⓐ Ⓑ Ⓒ Ⓓ
55. Ⓐ Ⓑ Ⓒ Ⓓ
56. Ⓐ Ⓑ Ⓒ Ⓓ
57. Ⓐ Ⓑ Ⓒ Ⓓ
58. Ⓐ Ⓑ Ⓒ Ⓓ
59. Ⓐ Ⓑ Ⓒ Ⓓ
60. Ⓐ Ⓑ Ⓒ Ⓓ
61. Ⓐ Ⓑ Ⓒ Ⓓ
62. Ⓐ Ⓑ Ⓒ Ⓓ
63. Ⓐ Ⓑ Ⓒ Ⓓ
64. Ⓐ Ⓑ Ⓒ Ⓓ
65. Ⓐ Ⓑ Ⓒ Ⓓ
66. Ⓐ Ⓑ Ⓒ Ⓓ
67. Ⓐ Ⓑ Ⓒ Ⓓ
68. Ⓐ Ⓑ Ⓒ Ⓓ
69. Ⓐ Ⓑ Ⓒ Ⓓ
70. Ⓐ Ⓑ Ⓒ Ⓓ
71. Ⓐ Ⓑ Ⓒ Ⓓ
72. Ⓐ Ⓑ Ⓒ Ⓓ
73. Ⓐ Ⓑ Ⓒ Ⓓ
74. Ⓐ Ⓑ Ⓒ Ⓓ
75. Ⓐ Ⓑ Ⓒ Ⓓ
76. Ⓐ Ⓑ Ⓒ Ⓓ

77. Ⓐ Ⓑ Ⓒ Ⓓ
78. Ⓐ Ⓑ Ⓒ Ⓓ
79. Ⓐ Ⓑ Ⓒ Ⓓ
80. Ⓐ Ⓑ Ⓒ Ⓓ
81. Ⓐ Ⓑ Ⓒ Ⓓ
82. Ⓐ Ⓑ Ⓒ Ⓓ
83. Ⓐ Ⓑ Ⓒ Ⓓ
84. Ⓐ Ⓑ Ⓒ Ⓓ
85. Ⓐ Ⓑ Ⓒ Ⓓ
86. Ⓐ Ⓑ Ⓒ Ⓓ
87. Ⓐ Ⓑ Ⓒ Ⓓ
88. Ⓐ Ⓑ Ⓒ Ⓓ
89. Ⓐ Ⓑ Ⓒ Ⓓ
90. Ⓐ Ⓑ Ⓒ Ⓓ
91. Ⓐ Ⓑ Ⓒ Ⓓ
92. Ⓐ Ⓑ Ⓒ Ⓓ
93. Ⓐ Ⓑ Ⓒ Ⓓ
94. Ⓐ Ⓑ Ⓒ Ⓓ
95. Ⓐ Ⓑ Ⓒ Ⓓ
96. Ⓐ Ⓑ Ⓒ Ⓓ
97. Ⓐ Ⓑ Ⓒ Ⓓ
98. Ⓐ Ⓑ Ⓒ Ⓓ
99. Ⓐ Ⓑ Ⓒ Ⓓ
100. Ⓐ Ⓑ Ⓒ Ⓓ
101. Ⓐ Ⓑ Ⓒ Ⓓ
102. Ⓐ Ⓑ Ⓒ Ⓓ
103. Ⓐ Ⓑ Ⓒ Ⓓ
104. Ⓐ Ⓑ Ⓒ Ⓓ
105. Ⓐ Ⓑ Ⓒ Ⓓ
106. Ⓐ Ⓑ Ⓒ Ⓓ
107. Ⓐ Ⓑ Ⓒ Ⓓ
108. Ⓐ Ⓑ Ⓒ Ⓓ
109. Ⓐ Ⓑ Ⓒ Ⓓ
110. Ⓐ Ⓑ Ⓒ Ⓓ
111. Ⓐ Ⓑ Ⓒ Ⓓ
112. Ⓐ Ⓑ Ⓒ Ⓓ
113. Ⓐ Ⓑ Ⓒ Ⓓ
114. Ⓐ Ⓑ Ⓒ Ⓓ

115. Ⓐ Ⓑ Ⓒ Ⓓ
116. Ⓐ Ⓑ Ⓒ Ⓓ
117. Ⓐ Ⓑ Ⓒ Ⓓ
118. Ⓐ Ⓑ Ⓒ Ⓓ
119. Ⓐ Ⓑ Ⓒ Ⓓ
120. Ⓐ Ⓑ Ⓒ Ⓓ
121. Ⓐ Ⓑ Ⓒ Ⓓ
122. Ⓐ Ⓑ Ⓒ Ⓓ
123. Ⓐ Ⓑ Ⓒ Ⓓ
124. Ⓐ Ⓑ Ⓒ Ⓓ
125. Ⓐ Ⓑ Ⓒ Ⓓ
126. Ⓐ Ⓑ Ⓒ Ⓓ
127. Ⓐ Ⓑ Ⓒ Ⓓ
128. Ⓐ Ⓑ Ⓒ Ⓓ
129. Ⓐ Ⓑ Ⓒ Ⓓ
130. Ⓐ Ⓑ Ⓒ Ⓓ
131. Ⓐ Ⓑ Ⓒ Ⓓ
132. Ⓐ Ⓑ Ⓒ Ⓓ
133. Ⓐ Ⓑ Ⓒ Ⓓ
134. Ⓐ Ⓑ Ⓒ Ⓓ
135. Ⓐ Ⓑ Ⓒ Ⓓ
136. Ⓐ Ⓑ Ⓒ Ⓓ
137. Ⓐ Ⓑ Ⓒ Ⓓ
138. Ⓐ Ⓑ Ⓒ Ⓓ
139. Ⓐ Ⓑ Ⓒ Ⓓ
140. Ⓐ Ⓑ Ⓒ Ⓓ
141. Ⓐ Ⓑ Ⓒ Ⓓ
142. Ⓐ Ⓑ Ⓒ Ⓓ
143. Ⓐ Ⓑ Ⓒ Ⓓ
144. Ⓐ Ⓑ Ⓒ Ⓓ
145. Ⓐ Ⓑ Ⓒ Ⓓ
146. Ⓐ Ⓑ Ⓒ Ⓓ
147. Ⓐ Ⓑ Ⓒ Ⓓ
148. Ⓐ Ⓑ Ⓒ Ⓓ
149. Ⓐ Ⓑ Ⓒ Ⓓ
150. Ⓐ Ⓑ Ⓒ Ⓓ

18

Practice Test 2

1. A patient's blood pressure is 82/48 after an infusion of 30 mL/kg of 0.9 NS over the past hour. The heart rate is 126 beats/minute, the temperature is 35°C, the hemoglobin is 8.9 g/dL, the WBC count is 4,000, and the bands are 22%. A pulmonary artery catheter was inserted, and the following measurements were obtained: pulmonary artery pressure 22/8 mmHg, central venous pressure 1 mmHg, pulmonary artery occlusion pressure 4 mmHg, cardiac output 7.0 L/minute, and systemic vascular resistance 600 dynes/s/cm^{-5}.

   This patient needs:

   (A) continued fluids, a blood transfusion, and pressors.
   (B) discontinuation of fluids, a blood transfusion, and warming.
   (C) reduction in the fluid rate, positive inotropes, and preload reducers.
   (D) continued fluids, vasopressors, and antibiotics.

2. A nurse notices that patients who are receiving PCA therapy have had more adverse effects and have generated a lot of safety reports over the past month. She asks the clinical nurse specialist whether anyone else has noticed these increases, and the CNS says "No." What would be the ideal strategy for the nurse to follow at this point?

   (A) Poll the unit nurses and 2 noncritical care units about whether an increase in adverse effects has been noticed.
   (B) Discuss the finding with the author of the hospital PCA Standing Orders.
   (C) Undertake a chart audit of all patients who have received PCA therapy in the previous 6 months.
   (D) List all future adverse effects for the next 30 days.

3. The physician asks the nurse to call if there are any signs of increased intracranial pressure. Clinical changes that are indicative of an increase in the ICP for the majority of neurological problems are seen in which order of progression (early to late) of those listed below?

(A) pupillary inequality, change in the level of consciousness, vital sign changes

(B) change in the level of consciousness, vital sign changes, pupillary inequality

(C) vital sign changes, pupillary inequality, pupils fixed and dilated

(D) change in the level of consciousness, pupillary inequality, vital sign changes

4. Which of the following sets of assessments indicates organ dysfunction according to the qSOFA score?

(A) B/P 96/48, respiratory rate 28 breaths/minute, Glasgow Coma Scale (GCS) 12

(B) temperature 39°C, heart rate 104 beats/minute, respiratory rate 24 breaths/minute

(C) B/P 104/48, heart rate 106 beats/minute, WBC count 18,000

(D) temperature 34°C, respiratory rate 24 breaths/minute, bands 12%

5. Which of the following would a nurse anticipate with the initiation of a nitroprusside (Nipride) infusion?

(A) decreased contractility

(B) increased pulmonary vascular resistance

(C) decreased afterload

(D) increased preload

6. A patient was admitted 12 hours ago with an acute inferior wall MI. Which of the following would be expected on the 12-lead ECG?

(A) ST elevation and deep Q-waves in I, II, and aVL

(B) ST depression in I and aVL

(C) ST elevation and deep Q-waves in V2, V3, and V4

(D) ST depression in II, III, and aVF

7. Which of the following is NOT a negative outcome of immobility?

(A) increased resting heart rate

(B) dementia

(C) pain

(D) urinary retention

8. A patient was admitted status post fall from a third-story roof. A chest X-ray reveals a fracture of left ribs 4 through 6, and chest excursion on the left side is diminished. The patient's vital signs include: B/P 84/54, heart rate 130 beats/minute, and respiratory rate 32 breaths/minute. Which of the following immediate interventions is indicated?

(A) oxygen, a fluid bolus, left-sided chest tube insertion

(B) intubation, pressors, left-sided chest tube insertion

(C) oxygen, a fluid bolus, pericardiocentesis

(D) intubation, fluids, emergency surgery

9. Which of the following is an evidence-based indication of the need for an indwelling urinary catheter?

(A) the presence of an infection

(B) an acute pelvic fracture

(C) the presence of a stage 1 pressure injury

(D) a provider order for shift intake and output

10. A Type 1 diabetic is training for a 10K run and develops tachycardia, slurred speech, and confusion. Which of the following does this patient most likely need?

    (A) an immediate glucose source
    (B) insulin
    (C) a CT scan of the head
    (D) fluids

11. Fluid and electrolyte balance require close monitoring for a patient with acute pancreatitis due to which of the following?

    (A) increased diuresis secondary to pancreatic enzyme release
    (B) increased incidences of hypercalcemia
    (C) increased capillary permeability, resulting in fluid loss from the vascular space
    (D) hypoglycemia due to pancreatic cell destruction

12. A patient is status post percutaneous coronary intervention, and labs reveal a PTT of 210 seconds. Which of the following is indicated?

    (A) heparin
    (B) vitamin K
    (C) protamine sulfate
    (D) fresh frozen plasma

13. A nurse notices that a patient who was admitted with acute pancreatitis demonstrates a left hand spasm when she inflates the B/P cuff on the patient's left arm. Which of the following is the most likely assessment?

    (A) positive Chvostek sign, hypophosphatemia
    (B) positive Trousseau sign, hypocalcemia
    (C) positive Kernig's sign, hypermagnesemia
    (D) positive Cullen's sign, hypercalcemia

14. A nurse is interested in getting approval for a protocol that he learned from a nationally known expert at a nursing conference he recently attended. Which of the following strategies would be most effective in convincing hospital leadership that the new protocol is financially worthwhile?

    (A) Send copies of the protocol and the conference presentation to the nursing leadership.
    (B) Present a summary of research (that relates the protocol to a decreased length of patient stay) to the nursing leadership.
    (C) Outline favorable patient outcomes that have been demonstrated at other hospitals that adopted the protocol.
    (D) Ask for a meeting with the unit medical director to request adoption of the protocol.

15. A patient develops an acute onset of inspiratory and expiratory wheezing throughout the lung fields. Which of the following statements about this patient is correct?

    (A) The patient has acute heart failure and requires morphine.
    (B) The patient has an asthma exacerbation and immediately requires bronchodilators.
    (C) The patient has an asthma exacerbation and immediately requires corticosteroids.
    (D) The patient has acute heart failure and requires a diuretic.

16. Which of the following ventilator settings or patient assessments is most likely to predict success with ventilator liberation or weaning?

    (A) FiO_2 70% or less
    (B) negative inspiratory force of < -25 cm H_2O
    (C) minute ventilation 15 L/min
    (D) vital capacity 3–5 L/min

17. Pressure support ventilation has which of the following positive effects?

    (A) It decreases the oxygen requirements.
    (B) It decreases the work of breathing.
    (C) It decreases the work of all muscles.
    (D) It decreases the tidal volume requirements.

18. A patient had a prolonged period of hypotension status post surgical repair of a leaking AAA. The patient developed ATN. Which of the following are likely to develop?

    (A) acidosis, azotemia, hyperkalemia
    (B) anemia, alkalosis, hypercalcemia
    (C) acidosis, hypertension, hypomagnesemia
    (D) hypertension, azotemia, hypokalemia

19. A patient who is receiving mechanical ventilation and tube feeding is suspected of having aspiration. Which of the following is most likely to develop if the patient has aspiration?

    (A) a decrease in the minute ventilation and a drop in the SaO_2
    (B) a decrease in the respiratory rate and a low-pressure alarm
    (C) an increase in the negative inspiratory force and bilateral infiltrates on the chest film
    (D) an increase in the peak inspiratory pressure and a right-sided infiltrate on the chest film

20. A patient presents with a methamphetamine overdose. Which of the following initial interventions should the nurse anticipate?

    (A) Monitor the renal function and protect the patient from self-harm.
    (B) Monitor for rhabdomyolysis and prepare for intubation.
    (C) Initiate cooling and fluid replacement.
    (D) Initiate naloxone (Narcan) and monitor the renal function.

21. Which of the following is CORRECT regarding continuous venovenous hemofiltration (CVVH) therapy?

    (A) It directly prevents a life-threatening electrolyte imbalance.
    (B) It removes immunoglobulins for those with an autoimmune disease.
    (C) It corrects a fluid imbalance.
    (D) It increases the colloid oncotic pressure.

22. A man is admitted with a gunshot wound to the head. His right pupil is dilated and nonreactive. This indicates damage to cranial nerve:

    (A) II.
    (B) III.
    (C) V.
    (D) IX.

23. A patient is admitted with a fever and nuchal rigidity. A lumbar puncture is performed. Which of the following findings most likely indicates bacterial meningitis rather than viral meningitis?

    (A) a CSF glucose of 30 mg/dL
    (B) CSF with elevated WBCs and protein
    (C) a fever greater than 40°C
    (D) a decreased level of consciousness

24. Which of the following assessment findings indicates possible ARDS?

    (A) PaO_2 95 mmHg on FiO_2 1.00
    (B) SvO_2 0.65
    (C) PaO_2 65 mmHg on room air
    (D) A-a gradient 8 mmHg

25. A 78-year-old female patient with a history of Class IV heart failure was admitted with septic shock secondary to bowel perforation. On day 13 of her hospital stay, after an extremely complicated course without significant improvement, she expressed that she no longer wanted aggressive therapy and wanted to be kept comfortable. Which of the following consults is appropriate to discuss with the patient at this time?

    (A) home health care
    (B) palliative care
    (C) ethics
    (D) hospice care

26. A patient is admitted with intestinal obstruction. Which of the following assessments would the nurse anticipate for this patient?

    (A) rigid, boardlike abdomen; absent bowel sounds; rebound tenderness; pain worse with movement
    (B) dull, right upper quadrant pain; rebound tenderness
    (C) tympanic percussion note; cramping pain; abdominal distension; high-pitched tinkling sounds
    (D) boring, epigastric pain; abdominal tenderness; normal bowel sounds

27. The sepsis protocol was started at 10:00 A.M., when it was first determined that the patient has sepsis. At 10:20 A.M., the serum lactate was drawn. Why is it important for the nurse to assess the results of the serum lactate?

    (A) If it is > 4 mmol/L, vasopressors will need to be initiated.
    (B) If it is > 2 mmol/L, another level needs to be drawn within 2–4 hours.
    (C) If it is elevated, that is a sign of aerobic metabolism.
    (D) If it is < 4 mmol/L, fluids can be decreased.

28. A patient who was admitted with systolic heart failure developed hypotension, tachycardia, a decreasing urine output, cool and clammy skin, a decreasing level of consciousness, and tachypnea. Which of the following medical orders should the nurse anticipate?

    (A) negative inotropes, antiarrhythmics, cardiac glycoside
    (B) a positive inotrope, a diuretic, a vasodilator
    (C) beta blockers, ACE inhibitors, diuretics
    (D) calcium channel blockers, positive inotropes, amiodarone

29. A patient with status asthmaticus will most likely have which of the following?

    (A) wheezing, atrial fibrillation
    (B) silent chest, diastolic murmur
    (C) wheezing, giant V-waves
    (D) silent chest, pulsus paradoxus

30. Which of the following would be contraindicated in the treatment of SIADH?

    (A) hypertonic saline and diuretics
    (B) vasopressin
    (C) fluid restriction
    (D) phenytoin (Dilantin)

31. A patient was admitted with signs of an acute embolic stroke, and fibrinolytic therapy is being considered. Which of the following is a priority determination?

    (A) home medications the patient has been taking
    (B) when the symptoms began
    (C) the patient's allergy history
    (D) whether the patient has a history of hypertension

32. A patient is admitted with community-acquired pneumonia, and she only speaks Spanish. Which of the following strategies is effective in this situation?

(A) Get a hospital translator; stand next to the translator while speaking and as close to the patient as possible.

(B) Allow extra time for the hospital translator to decode medical terms when providing the translation.

(C) Speak slowly in English, using hands and pictures when indicated.

(D) Ask the patient's wife to translate, provide all of the information, and then take patient questions through the translator.

33. A patient was admitted with ST elevation and deep Q-waves in V1, V2, and V3. The patient suddenly complains of shortness of breath and develops a loud holosystolic murmur that is loudest at the left sternal border, 5th intercostal space. Which of the following has this patient most likely developed?

(A) ventricular septal defect
(B) acute ischemia
(C) cardiac tamponade
(D) papillary muscle dysfunction

34. A patient was admitted with confusion, agitation, a fever, sinus tachycardia, and dyspnea. She has a history of hyperthyroidism and was found to have hypertension 2 weeks prior to admission, for which she was prescribed hydrochlorothiazide (HCTZ). Her lungs are clear, and her blood pressure is 138/88. Which of the following therapies is indicated for this patient?

(A) aspirin, cooling measures
(B) a beta blocker, discontinue hydrochlorothiazide
(C) levothyroxine (Synthroid), IV fluids
(D) glucocorticoids, 3% saline

35. A patient is experiencing alcohol withdrawal, and he reports that bugs are crawling on his arms and on the walls. Which of the following nursing interventions is most appropriate for this patient?

(A) Whisper to colleagues to control the noise.
(B) Explain the actual circumstances to the patient.
(C) Provide a therapeutic touch to calm the patient.
(D) Explain to the patient that the hallucinations are not real.

36. Which of the following is most indicative of cardiogenic shock?

(A) cardiac index 1.9 L/min/m^2
(B) PAOP 9 mmHg
(C) SvO$_2$ 70%
(D) SVR 1,000 dynes/s/cm^{-5}

37. A patient is admitted with upper GI bleeding, hypotension, and tachycardia. Which of the following lab results would be expected?

(A) elevated BUN, elevated serum sodium
(B) metabolic acidosis, decreased PT
(C) elevated PTT, decreased sodium
(D) decreased WBC, elevated platelets

38. A 90 kg male patient with ARDS is receiving mechanical ventilation with the following settings: assist-control mode, breath rate of 18 breaths/minute; FiO$_2$ 70%; Vt 450 mL; PEEP 5 cm H$_2$O. An ABG is obtained that reveals the following: pH 7.36, pCO$_2$ 50, pO$_2$ 49, HCO$_3$ 25. Which of the following interventions should the nurse anticipate?

(A) Increase the FiO$_2$.
(B) Increase the breath rate.
(C) Increase the Vt.
(D) Increase the PEEP.

39. Which of the following is most indicative of distributive shock?

    (A) SVR 490 dynes/s/cm^{-5}
    (B) CVP 1 mmHg
    (C) heart rate 130 beats/minute
    (D) PAOP 7 mmHg

40. Which of the following is TRUE about surfactant?

    (A) It is produced by the Type I alveolar cells.
    (B) It prevents atelectasis.
    (C) It increases the work of breathing.
    (D) It decreases lung compliance.

41. Which of the following are related to hypokalemia?

    (A) ACE inhibitors and crush injuries
    (B) diarrhea and hemolysis
    (C) alkalosis and thiazide diuretics
    (D) acidosis and vomiting

42. A research study is being conducted to look at the effectiveness of a newer drug designed to manage patient agitation. A patient is too ill to make his own decisions. While the nurse is in the patient's room, a family member is approached by one of the research staff members and is asked to consent to letting the patient participate in the study. When the family member asks if there are any risks, she is told not to worry about risks, and the research staff member says, "Here is the form. Sign here." How should the patient's nurse immediately respond?

    (A) Report what was overheard to the ethics committee.
    (B) Contact the primary investigator on the study.
    (C) Review the protocol for this research study with the patient's surrogate decision maker.
    (D) Smile at the family member, and leave the room.

43. An 81-year-old patient who was admitted 4 days ago is experiencing periods of agitation alternating with withdrawal. Which of the following is the most appropriate initial nursing intervention?

    (A) Keep the lights on, and put the television on the music station.
    (B) Provide a private room, and restrict visiting to family.
    (C) Review the medication list, and ensure periods of uninterrupted sleep.
    (D) Contact the physician for an order for benzodiazepines.

44. A patient has been in the ICU with respiratory failure and hepatic failure secondary to metastatic cancer for 6 days without improvement. The family seems to understand the patient's condition and refuses to agree to a do-not-resuscitate order and requests that full therapy be continued at a family meeting with the multidisciplinary team. The patient's SpO_2 acutely drops to 74%, and the physician orders the FiO_2 to be maintained at 40%. Which of the following should the nurse do at this time?

    (A) Ask the physician to provide a rationale for the order.
    (B) Continue the FiO_2 at 40%.
    (C) Request that the family speak with the physician.
    (D) Administer analgesia and sedating medication to avoid discomfort.

45. A 22-year-old patient presented to the Emergency Department with weakness and a history of aching and fever for 2 days. The patient was hypotensive, was not responsive to fluids, and was admitted to the critical care unit with a blood pressure of 80/60. A pulmonary artery catheter was inserted, and the following values were obtained: right atrial pressure 14 mmHg; PAOP 16 mmHg; cardiac output 2.0 L/min; SVR 1800 dynes/s/cm^{-5}. Which of the following treatments would the nurse anticipate?

(A) emergent pericardiocentesis
(B) antibiotics
(C) pressors
(D) aggressive fluids

46. A patient is in cardiogenic shock and is not responsive to positive inotropic drug therapy. The nurse asked the cardiologist if preparation should begin for an intra-aortic balloon insertion, but the physician said that the patient has a contraindication to this therapy. This patient most likely has which of the following?

(A) ventricular septal defect
(B) aortic valve regurgitation
(C) mitral valve regurgitation
(D) aortic valve stenosis

47. Which of the following is most likely a pressure injury?

(A) a diabetic venous ulcer on the left leg
(B) a knee abrasion following a fall
(C) a lip ulcer post-extubation
(D) a skin tear following IV dressing removal

48. Heart failure is most often associated with which of the following arrhythmias?

(A) third-degree AV block
(B) atrial fibrillation
(C) ventricular bigeminy
(D) atrial tachycardia

49. While preparing a patient for transfer from the critical care unit, the patient states to the nurse, "I will probably end up back here tomorrow since they don't know what to do for me on the other unit." Which of the following is the most appropriate response for the nurse?

(A) "You seem concerned about going to the other unit."
(B) "The nurses are very well-trained on that unit."
(C) "The doctors all feel you don't need us anymore."
(D) "We need your bed for an extremely ill lady in the emergency room."

50. After admitting a 19-year-old trauma patient who is in critical condition, the nurse enters the family waiting room and is approached by 8 family members with questions. Which of the following INITIAL responses is appropriate?

(A) Tell the family that the trauma surgeon will come and speak with them.
(B) Explain to the family that all questions will be answered when the chaplain arrives.
(C) Request that the family identify a spokesperson.
(D) Inform the family that the patient's condition is critical.

51. An obstetrical patient who is 1 hour status post abruptio placental delivery has pink urine and oozing from the IV insertion site. Which of the following laboratory tests would most likely be ordered at this time?

(A) D-dimer and PT
(B) fibrin split products and creatinine
(C) Pitocin level and magnesium
(D) BUN and factor X

52. A patient was admitted with a history of several syncopal episodes at home. Upon arrival, the patient was in normal sinus rhythm with a QTc of 0.50 seconds. The patient suddenly developed a non-sustained episode of polymorphic ventricular tachycardia. Which of the following interventions would be most appropriate at this time?

(A) defibrillation
(B) an amiodarone IV
(C) a magnesium IV
(D) synchronized cardioversion

53. A patient with DKA would most likely present with which of the following?

(A) decreased anion gap
(B) volume overload
(C) hypokalemia
(D) low serum osmolality

54. Which of the following will worsen hepatic encephalopathy?

(A) normal saline
(B) carbohydrates
(C) Aldactone
(D) GI bleeding

55. A patient has a temporary transvenous pacemaker set at 70 beats/minute on demand. The nurse notices that the patient's heart rate is 78 beats/minute, and pacer spikes are noted in the patient's native beats. Which of the following interventions is indicated at this time?

(A) Check the pacing connection to the generator.
(B) Decrease the pacing rate.
(C) Increase the sensitivity.
(D) Increase the mA output.

56. A 21-year-old female patient is being treated for necrotizing fasciitis of the left forearm at the site of an insect bite. Which of the following is TRUE regarding the treatment for this problem?

(A) Vancomycin is the antibiotic of choice.
(B) Hyperbaric oxygen therapy must be initiated immediately.
(C) The administration of a vasopressor should be avoided.
(D) Treatment may include the loss of the limb.

57. A patient with which of the following signs most likely has a tension pneumothorax?

(A) absent breath sounds on the affected side, hypotension, distended neck veins
(B) dull to percussion on the affected side, hypertension, flat neck veins
(C) diminished breath sounds on the affected side, tracheal deviation to the affected side, hypotension
(D) absent breath sounds on the affected side, tracheal deviation to the opposite side, flat neck veins

58. A patient who is 2 days status post a head injury keeps asking for water and has a urine output of 300 mL/hour. Which of the following lab findings and treatment should the nurse expect?

(A) serum sodium decreased, serum osmolality increased; administer phenytoin
(B) serum sodium decreased, serum osmolality decreased; administer phenytoin
(C) serum sodium increased, serum osmolality decreased; administer vasopressin
(D) serum sodium increased, serum osmolality increased; administer vasopressin

59. A patient is status post a craniotomy. Which of the following positions is optimal for this patient?

(A) a position that prevents postoperative pain

(B) a position that increases the intracranial pressure

(C) on the side opposite of the surgery

(D) upright to maximize cerebral venous outflow

60. A patient was admitted with a history of sustaining sudden cardiac death (SCD) at home and required insertion of an implantable cardioverter-defibrillator (ICD). The patient's wife is anxious that the patient's ICD will not work and that the patient will have another cardiac arrest after being discharged. Which of the following would be the most appropriate response of the nurse?

(A) "Now that he has the ICD, you do not need to worry."

(B) "Would you be less anxious if you learned how to do CPR?"

(C) "Your town has an excellent EMS system."

(D) "I will ask the cardiologist to speak with you and give you more information."

61. A measurement of hemodynamic data is most accurate when obtained:

(A) at the end of the T-wave.

(B) every hour.

(C) at the end of the respiratory cycle, end expiration.

(D) from the digital readout on the monitor.

62. A patient has acute respiratory failure secondary to a pulmonary embolism. The patient has a respiratory rate of 28 breaths/minute, the lungs are clear, the SpO_2 is 88% on 4 L/minute per a nasal cannula, and the blood pressure is 88/58. Which of the following is accurate regarding this patient?

(A) The embolism is massive, and alveolar dead space is increased.

(B) The patient's D-dimer is negative, and fibrinolytic therapy is indicated.

(C) The patient requires mechanical ventilation and a norepinephrine infusion.

(D) The shunting is massive, and PEEP therapy is indicated.

63. A patient was ordered prophylactic antibiotics for a neutropenic fever. Which of the following assessments does this patient have?

(A) an absolute neutrophil count (ANC) of 1,550 cells/mcL and a temperature of 38.2°C (100.8°F) for the past 60 minutes

(B) an absolute neutrophil count (ANC) of 450 cells/mcL and a temperature of 37.3°C (99.1°F) for the past 180 minutes

(C) an absolute neutrophil count (ANC) of 1,530 cells/mcL and a temperature of 38.3°C (101.0°F) for the past 60 minutes

(D) an absolute neutrophil count (ANC) of 480 cells/mcL and a temperature of 38.2°C (100.8°F) for the past 90 minutes

64. Which of the following is least likely to be linked with adrenal insufficiency?

(A) head trauma

(B) diabetes

(C) phenytoin

(D) Addison's disease

65. Which of the following hemodynamic profiles is indicative of hypovolemic shock?

(A) SvO_2 55, PAOP 16, SVR 1,600
(B) SvO_2 65, PAOP 8, SVR 1,200
(C) SvO_2 55, PAOP 3, SVR 1,500
(D) SvO_2 85, PAOP 3, SVR 500

66. Which of the following unit strategies is likely to result in the lowest rate of CLABSIs?

(A) The nurse manager evaluates central line necessity for each patient during daily rounds.
(B) Unit house staff insert femoral central venous lines.
(C) Unit leadership provides adequate staffing for day shifts.
(D) The hospital Infection Control Department provides data related to unit CLABSIs every 3 months.

67. A patient has acute respiratory distress syndrome (ARDS) and septic shock. Which of the following assessments of oxygenation would be most likely for this patient?

(A) pO_2 50, SvO_2 50
(B) pO_2 80, SvO_2 80
(C) pO_2 50, SvO_2 85
(D) pO_2 55, SvO_2 50

68. A patient was admitted with a carboxyhemoglobin level of 55%. Which of the following is appropriate treatment for this patient?

(A) Provide FiO_2 of 100% until the SpO_2 is > 95%.
(B) Provide positive-pressure ventilation until the patient's level of consciousness is normal.
(C) Provide FiO_2 of 100% until the carboxyhemoglobin level is < 10%.
(D) Provide treatment in a hyperbaric oxygen chamber until the patient's level of consciousness is normal.

69. Which of the following would be expected for a patient with renal hypoperfusion?

(A) urine sodium greater than 20 and serum osmolality greater than urine osmolality
(B) urine sodium less than 20 and serum osmolality greater than urine osmolality
(C) urine sodium greater than 20 and urine osmolality greater than serum osmolality
(D) urine sodium less than 20 and urine osmolality greater than serum osmolality

70. A patient is admitted with a middle meningeal artery bleed. Which of the following problems does this patient most likely have?

(A) subdural hematoma
(B) subarachnoid hemorrhage
(C) epidural hematoma
(D) AV malformation

71. A patient developed confusion and combativeness 2 days post-op. Which of the following would support that this patient has delirium?

(A) The patient's mental status has fluctuated over the past 24 hours.
(B) The patient's family reports that this is the patient's usual behavior.
(C) The patient is attentive when spoken to.
(D) The patient has a history of word-finding difficulty.

72. A 55-year-old female is admitted with subarachnoid hemorrhage (SAH). Which of the following interventions is indicated for this patient?

(A) Provide hypotonic intravenous fluids.
(B) Secure her airway in the event of respiratory arrest.
(C) Prevent hypoventilation.
(D) Administer antibiotics to prevent an infection.

73. A patient has ST elevation in V1, V2, and V3. Which of the following is this patient at risk for developing?

(A) sinus exit block or sinus arrest
(B) second-degree AV block, Type I
(C) second-degree AV block, Type II
(D) third-degree AV block, complete

74. A newly admitted patient has had a STEMI, is hypotensive, and has a heart rate of 42 beats/minute, with more P-waves than QRS complexes, a wide QRS, and constant PR intervals. Which of the following arteries is most likely blocked?

(A) left anterior descending
(B) left main coronary
(C) left circumflex coronary
(D) right coronary

75. A patient presents 1 month status post gastric bypass bariatric surgery with vomiting, a headache, diplopia, and memory loss. This patient most likely needs which of the following?

(A) vitamins
(B) antibiotics
(C) potassium
(D) emergent surgery

76. Which of the following would be the goals of therapy for a patient with dilated (congestive) cardiomyopathy?

(A) Decrease the preload, and decrease the afterload.
(B) Increase the preload, and increase the afterload.
(C) Decrease the preload, and increase the afterload.
(D) Increase the preload, and decrease the afterload.

77. A patient was admitted with chest pain and ST elevation in leads II, III, and aVF. Several hours after PCI, the patient developed a drop in blood pressure to 82/52, bibasilar crackles, and a urine output of 25 mL in the past hour. Which of the following hemodynamic profiles would this patient be expected to have?

(A) CO 5.8; SVR 500; PAP 19/6
(B) CO 2.8; SVR 725; PAP 25/14
(C) CO 3.5; SVR 1800; PAP 42/22
(D) CO 4.8; SVR 950; PAP 32/11

78. A patient was admitted with an anterior MI 2 days ago with no pertinent past medical history. He needs to use the commode to have a bowel movement. Since metoprolol and lisinopril were recently prescribed, the nurse checked his blood pressure while the patient was lying down and again while he was standing. His blood pressure was 101/52 with a heart rate of 76 beats/minute after standing, compared to a blood pressure of 134/70 with a heart rate of 68 beats/minute when lying in bed in Semi-Fowler's position. The patient denied dizziness when standing. Which of the following is the preferred intervention at this time?

(A) Advise the patient that the physician will be called immediately.
(B) Order a stat ECG.
(C) Explain the reason for the difference in B/P and heart rate to the patient.
(D) Accompany the patient to the commode, and instruct him to call when he's done.

79. A patient is admitted with hepatic failure. Which of the following treatments should the nurse anticipate?

(A) Provide higher doses of insulin to treat hyperglycemia.
(B) Provide sedation with benzodiazepines.
(C) Treat dehydration with lactated Ringer's.
(D) Treat ascites with spironolactone (Aldactone).

80. A patient was admitted status post full cardiac arrest on the Step Down Unit and died prior to his wife's arrival at the hospital. Which of the following should the nurse do in order to prepare for the wife's arrival?

(A) Plan to provide the wife with information about the care that was provided to the patient prior to his death.
(B) Arrange to allow the wife to view the patient in the morgue after she arrives.
(C) Ensure that the physician is available when the wife arrives.
(D) Have the chaplain available to escort the wife to the waiting room when she arrives.

81. A patient has a right-sided chest tube. The nurse notices that during inspiration and expiration, the water in the water seal chamber rises and falls. What does this assessment indicate?

(A) a pleural leak
(B) a tension pneumothorax
(C) normal fluctuation in the pleural pressure
(D) an intact connection to suction

82. A patient with acute respiratory distress syndrome (ARDS) is receiving mechanical ventilation with the following settings: FiO_2 60%; assist-control mode, breath rate of 12 breaths/minute; Vt 4 mL/kg; and PEEP 15 cm H_2O pressure. Which of the following is an important nursing intervention for this patient?

(A) Avoid disconnecting the ventilator circuit from the ETT.
(B) Increase the Vt.
(C) Ensure that suction passes are greater than 15 seconds.
(D) Decrease the PEEP and then decrease the FiO_2.

83. A pulmonary assessment reveals bronchial breath sounds and whispered pectoriloquy. Which of the following should the nurse expect?

(A) a partial pneumothorax
(B) air trapping
(C) pulmonary consolidation
(D) pulmonary edema

84. A patient sustained a crush injury at a construction site. The patient's urine is tea-colored, and the urine output is 20 mL/hour. The creatine kinase (CK) is 15,000 U/L. The nurse knows that this patient is at risk for which of the following?

(A) heart failure
(B) hyperkalemia
(C) alkalosis
(D) acute liver failure

85. A patient is receiving assist-control ventilation and is not assisting the ventilator with spontaneous breaths. The ABG reveals the following results: pH 7.29; pCO_2 52; pO_2 69; HCO_3 29. Based on this information, which of the following statements is correct?

(A) The patient has partially compensated respiratory acidosis; increase the breath rate.
(B) The patient has uncompensated metabolic acidosis; increase the FiO_2.
(C) The patient has uncompensated respiratory acidosis; decrease the tidal volume (Vt).
(D) The patient has partially compensated metabolic acidosis; decrease the peak flow rate.

86. A patient presented with a lower leg wound with purulent drainage, and generalized weakness. The patient's temperature was 39°C, the B/P was 82/38 mmHg (MAP 53), the heart rate was 140 beats/minute, the hemoglobin was 9.1 gm/dL, the WBC count was 3,000, the bands were 25%, and the lactate was 3.9 mmol/L. A total of 30 mL/kg of isotonic solution was infused. After fluids, the B/P was 80/40 mmHg (MAP 53), the heart rate was 132 beats/minute, the repeat lactate was 3.7 mmol/L, and the lungs were clear. Which of the following interventions is appropriate?

(A) Resume the fluids at 50 mL/hour, start a dopamine infusion, and titrate to a urine output of 30 mL/hour.
(B) Continue the fluid boluses, start a norepinephrine infusion, and titrate to a mean arterial pressure (MAP) ≥ 65 mmHg.
(C) Continue the fluid boluses, infuse PRBCs, and titrate to a CVP of 8 mmHg.
(D) Discontinue the isotonic fluids, begin 0.45 normal saline at 50 mL/hour, and begin a phenylephrine infusion.

87. A patient is receiving an angiotensin-converting enzyme (ACE) inhibitor. Which of the following signs/symptoms should be assessed for in this situation?

(A) heart failure symptoms and hypokalemia
(B) proteinuria and hyperkalemia
(C) thrombocytopenia and hepatotoxicity
(D) dysrhythmias and hyponatremia

88. A 19-year-old presents with raccoon eyes and bruising behind his right ear after falling from a 1-story roof. The nurse notices clear fluid draining from his nose. The most appropriate intervention would be to:

(A) insert a nasogastric tube to prevent vomiting.
(B) suction the nasopharynx as needed.
(C) insert nasal packing until the physician arrives.
(D) tape rolled sterile gauze under his nose.

89. Which of the following may trigger a vasospasm post-aneurysm repair for subarachnoid hemorrhage?

(A) hypokalemia
(B) dehydration
(C) nimodipine
(D) hypertension

90. A patient who is receiving mechanical ventilation for acute respiratory failure developed agitation, with a RASS score of +2 and a BPS score of 6. Propofol is infusing at 25 mcg/kg/min. The patient's vital signs are stable, and the SpO_2 is 0.94. Which of the following interventions is indicated?

(A) Increase the propofol infusion.
(B) Order a chest X-ray.
(C) Administer morphine 2 mg IV.
(D) Obtain an ABG.

91. A patient presents with eye deviation to the left, right homonymous hemianopsia, right-sided weakness, and left pupil dilation. This patient most likely has which of the following?

(A) a left-sided stroke
(B) a right-sided temporal lobe tumor
(C) central herniation
(D) meningitis

92. A patient with chronic hepatic failure with acute GI bleeding is likely to receive which of the following agents?

   (A) octreotide (Sandostatin)
   (B) lactulose
   (C) lactated Ringer's
   (D) beta blockers

93. A patient is admitted with acute-onset chest pain at rest, ST elevation, and deep Q-waves in leads V5, V6, I, and aVL. Which of the following statements is the most accurate?

   (A) The patient is having an acute posterior wall MI; emergent PCI is indicated.
   (B) The patient is having an acute anterior wall MI; fibrinolytic therapy is indicated.
   (C) The patient is having an acute inferior wall MI; emergent PCI is indicated.
   (D) The patient is having an acute lateral wall MI; fibrinolytic therapy is indicated.

94. The purpose for and management of a mediastinal chest tube include which of the following?

   (A) promote lung reexpansion; keep the drainage system lower than the chest, clamp when transporting the patient
   (B) improve gas exchange postoperatively; report bubbling in the negative pressure chamber, monitor the SpO_2
   (C) remove serosanguinous fluid from the operative site; gently milk visible clots to keep patent, report an output of greater than 100 mL/hour for 2 consecutive hours
   (D) prevent cardiac tamponade postoperatively; prepare to transfuse PRBCs if the output is greater than 100 mL for the hour, report bubbling in the suction chamber

95. Which of the following is indicative of cor pulmonale?

   (A) right ventricular failure secondary to pulmonary hypotension
   (B) right ventricular enlargement secondary to pulmonary hypertension
   (C) pulmonary edema secondary to right ventricular failure
   (D) left ventricular failure secondary to chronic hypoxemia

96. Differentiating between DKA and HHS is best done by examining which of the following?

   (A) serum osmolality
   (B) serum sodium
   (C) serum glucose
   (D) serum potassium

97. A patient who is 1 month status post burr hole and evacuation of a subdural hematoma presents with a positive Brudzinski's sign and a positive Kernig's sign. Which of the following is most likely the etiology of these signs?

   (A) a recurrence of the subdural hematoma
   (B) hydrocephalus
   (C) a central nervous system infection
   (D) increased intracranial pressure

98. All members of the health care team (such as nurses, physicians, dietitians, and physical and speech therapists) are responsible for documenting that discharge teaching has been provided to the patient. Which of the following is the best strategy to ensure the coordination of this teaching between all health care team members?

   (A) Discuss patient teaching at daily care conferences.
   (B) Review each discipline's flow sheet of documentation every week.
   (C) The same flow sheet should be used (to document patient teaching) by all members of the health care team.
   (D) Each team member documents on their own flow sheet that they reviewed the other team members' flow sheets.

99. Hypotension, distended neck veins, distant heart sounds, a widening mediastinum, clear lungs, a narrowing pulse pressure, and pulsus paradoxus are signs of what problem and require which interventions?

(A) hypovolemia; fluid resuscitation, identify and correct the underlying cause

(B) diastolic heart failure; control the heart rate, calcium channel blockers, avoid positive inotropes

(C) cardiac tamponade; emergent pericardiocentesis or a return to the operating room if the individual is a post-op cardiac surgical patient

(D) cardiogenic shock; positive inotropes, afterload reduction, IABP therapy

100. Which of the following is correct regarding a shift of the oxyhemoglobin dissociation curve to the left?

(A) It may be due to a decrease in the arterial pH.

(B) It will cause an easier release of oxygen from hemoglobin.

(C) It may drop the SaO_2.

(D) It may be due to hypothermia.

101. A patient is admitted with acute pancreatitis. Which of the following lab profiles will this patient most likely have?

(A) elevated serum calcium, elevated serum amylase, elevated total protein

(B) decreased serum glucose, elevated bilirubin, decreased serum lipase

(C) decreased serum calcium, elevated serum amylase, decreased total protein

(D) elevated serum glucose, decreased alkaline phosphatase, elevated calcium

102. A patient sustained multiple fractures due to a motor vehicle crash and has a left arm cast. It is now suspected that the patient has left arm compartment syndrome, and the provider is examining the patient. Which of the following is an appropriate intervention for this patient?

(A) Add additional padding to the cast.

(B) Monitor for postischemic tissue swelling after a decompression procedure.

(C) Maintain the left arm above the level of the heart.

(D) Perform an emergent fasciotomy for a compartment pressure of 18 mmHg.

103. Which of the following is a primary treatment for a patient with sepsis?

(A) vasopressors

(B) antibiotics

(C) steroids

(D) antipyretics

104. Which of the following strategies for reducing multi-drug resistant organisms (MDROs) is evidence-based?

(A) Train nurses to clean the rooms of and equipment used by patients with an MDRO.

(B) Provide universal MRSA decolonization upon admission to the ICU.

(C) Order antibiotics for a minimum of 72 hours for a VRE infection.

(D) Administer metronidazole (Flagyl) prophylactically to all patients during a *C. difficile* outbreak.

105. A patient has septic shock. Which of the following assessments would the nurse expect?

(A) SVR 1,400, ejection fraction 30%

(B) SVR 525, cardiac output 9 L/minute

(C) SVR 1,200, ejection fraction 60%

(D) SVR 600, cardiac output 3 L/minute

106. Arterial hypoxemia may occur with a pulmonary embolism due to which of the following?

    (A) anatomic shunt
    (B) diffusion defect
    (C) pulmonary hypotension
    (D) ventilation-perfusion mismatch

107. A nurse is caring for a patient with rhabdomyolysis secondary to a crush injury. Which of the following orders should the nurse question?

    (A) Administer mannitol.
    (B) Monitor the serum potassium level.
    (C) Test the patient's urine for myoglobin.
    (D) Infuse 0.45 normal saline at 100 mL/hour.

108. While orienting a new nurse to the unit, the orientee's patient experiences cardiac arrest and requires resuscitation. The preceptor sees that the orientee has not lowered the head of the bed. Which of the following represents the best initial action the preceptor could take to instruct this new nurse?

    (A) Immediately begin chest compressions.
    (B) Reposition the patient in a supine position.
    (C) Initiate the unit's code blue response.
    (D) Ask the orientee why she did not lower the head of the bed.

109. A patient is admitted with a pelvic fracture. Which member of the health care team should be consulted first in order to optimize this patient's recovery?

    (A) physical therapist
    (B) wound care consultant
    (C) social services consultant
    (D) dietitian

110. Which of the following results in death for a patient with status epilepticus?

    (A) respiratory failure
    (B) pulseless electrical activity
    (C) cerebral hypermetabolism
    (D) intracranial hemorrhage

111. Which of the following nursing interventions is appropriate regarding the care of a post-PCI patient?

    (A) Apply a pressure dressing after 5 minutes of direct pressure for acute groin bleeding.
    (B) Administer atropine and dopamine for hypotension secondary to vasovagal response.
    (C) Monitor for ST changes (in the lead that showed the greatest change) on the bedside monitor.
    (D) Adjust the head of the bed, administer an analgesic, and reposition the patient if there is acute back pain.

112. A patient presents with complaints of ripping back pain, dizziness, dyspnea, and a widening mediastinum on the chest radiograph. Which of the following should the nurse anticipate that this patient most likely has?

    (A) a dissecting thoracic aneurysm, which requires vasopressors and surgery if the aneurysm is greater than 6 cm in size
    (B) an abdominal aortic aneurysm, which requires a blood transfusion and surgery if the aneurysm is greater than 5 cm in size
    (C) a dissecting thoracic aneurysm, which requires aggressive blood pressure control and emergent surgery
    (D) cardiac tamponade, which requires fluids and emergent pericardiocentesis

113. A patient had an arteriogram. Which of the following should the nurse closely assess?

    (A) serum creatinine
    (B) mean arterial pressure
    (C) WBC count
    (D) liver enzymes

114. Which of the following assessments is most important in order to identify a complication for a patient with Guillain-Barré syndrome?

    (A) vital capacity
    (B) O₂ saturation
    (C) pupil reaction
    (D) temperature

115. A potassium chloride infusion infiltrated into a patient's left forearm. Which of the following is an appropriate intervention in this situation?

    (A) Administer phentolamine, and apply cold compresses.
    (B) Administer hyaluronidase, and apply warm compresses.
    (C) Administer hyaluronidase, and apply cold compresses.
    (D) Administer phentolamine, and apply warm compresses.

116. A patient's wife is expressing concern about the meaning of the numbers on the patient monitor. Which of the following is the most appropriate response for the nurse?

    (A) "The nurses are closely watching the numbers."
    (B) "There is no problem unless an alarm sounds."
    (C) "The trend of the numbers is more important than intermittent changes."
    (D) "What about the numbers concerns you?"

117. Two days after admission for a pulmonary embolism (PE), the patient's laboratory report reveals a 55% decrease in the platelet count and no clinical changes. Which of the following is indicated FIRST?

    (A) Infuse platelets.
    (B) Discontinue all heparin exposure.
    (C) Order an enzyme-linked immunosorbent assay (ELISA).
    (D) Start a direct thrombin inhibitor.

118. A patient who has had an acute ischemic stroke screened positive for dysphagia. After an evaluation by the speech pathologist, the patient was ordered a diet along with dysphagia precautions. Which of the following nursing interventions is essential for this patient?

    (A) Cut all meats for the patient.
    (B) Instruct the patient to track the amount of water he drinks.
    (C) Assist the patient with meals.
    (D) Deliver all meals at scheduled times.

119. Which of the following are signs of syndrome of inappropriate antidiuretic hormone (SIADH) secretion?

    (A) low urine output, elevated serum osmolality, hypernatremia, and elevated urine sodium
    (B) elevated urine output, elevated serum osmolality, hypernatremia, and low urine sodium
    (C) elevated urine output, low serum osmolality, hyponatremia, and low urine sodium
    (D) low urine output, low serum osmolality, hyponatremia, and elevated urine sodium

120. During an assessment of a patient, a nurse notices that the patient has developed Cullen's sign. Which of the following problems has most likely developed?

(A) acute hepatic failure
(B) esophageal varices
(C) small bowel obstruction
(D) hemorrhagic pancreatitis

121. A patient who was admitted with acute respiratory failure is very upset regarding his new diagnosis of lung cancer. The nurse understands that a useful strategy to use for this type of situation is to frame the new diagnosis as a new life challenge for the patient to meet. Which of the following actions would help the patient see the new diagnosis in this light?

(A) Determine how the patient has met past life challenges.
(B) Explain that the tumor is small and that the diagnosis was caught early.
(C) Assist the patient in preparing for death.
(D) Remind the patient that therapeutic options are now more successful.

122. Which of the following physiological responses may occur during the induction phase of targeted temperature management (TTM)?

(A) a decrease in blood glucose
(B) hyperkalemia
(C) increased cardiac output
(D) platelet dysfunction

123. Care for a critically ill, mechanically ventilated patient includes:

(A) routine instillation of saline down the ETT for suctioning.
(B) the use of a higher tidal volume and airway pressure if the patient has ARDS.
(C) disconnecting a patient with critical PEEP from the ventilator to ventilate with a bag valve mask during patient transport.
(D) hyperoxygenation before, during, and after the suctioning procedure.

124. A patient with Type 1 diabetes is admitted with DKA and a stuporous mental status, and she responds to shaking with moaning. Which of the following is the most likely cause of this patient's mental status?

(A) acidosis
(B) hypovolemia
(C) hyperkalemia
(D) an infection

125. A patient has a right-sided temporal lobe tumor and a history of a seizure prior to admission. Which of the following would be the most ominous sign for this patient?

(A) the right pupil is 5 mm, and the left pupil is 3 mm
(B) left-sided weakness since admission
(C) left-sided headache
(D) right-sided facial bruise

126. Acute care and critical care nurses may be required to teach patients and their families how to perform care. Which of the following principles of teaching is accurate?

(A) Teaching is best done at the beginning of the day.
(B) A complex procedure is best taught in one session.
(C) Written instruction is the most effective method for adult learners.
(D) Knowledge about the importance of learning is the first step.

127. A magnesium infusion is being administered to a patient after several non-sustained episodes of torsades de pointes ventricular tachycardia. Which of the following clinical findings would indicate that the infusion should be discontinued?

(A) hyperreflexia
(B) hypotension
(C) supraventricular tachycardia
(D) tachypnea

128. A patient who is receiving mechanical ventilation has a peak inspiratory pressure of 70 cm H_2O and a plateau pressure of 35 cm H_2O. Which of the following assessments and interventions is most likely correct?

(A) The patient has ARDS; decrease the tidal volume.
(B) The patient has a pulmonary embolus; begin anticoagulation.
(C) The patient has pneumonia; increase the FiO_2.
(D) The patient has an asthma exacerbation; administer a bronchodilator.

129. Management of acute pancreatitis includes which of the following?

(A) antibiotics for all patients
(B) a close lung assessment for all patients
(C) a nasogastric tube for all patients
(D) avoiding narcotics for all patients

130. Which of the following statements about transcatheter aortic valve replacement (TAVR) is true?

(A) All patients require daily aspirin therapy for life.
(B) Procedure access is most often achieved via the subclavian artery.
(C) The ideal candidates for TAVR are those who are at a low risk for an open procedure.
(D) Paravalvular regurgitation is a common post-procedure complication.

131. A patient presents with a salicylate overdose. Which of the following acid-base disturbances is expected?

(A) metabolic alkalosis, respiratory alkalosis
(B) metabolic acidosis, respiratory acidosis
(C) metabolic alkalosis, respiratory acidosis
(D) metabolic acidosis, respiratory alkalosis

132. Which of the following is indicative of a massive pulmonary embolism?

(A) B/P 78/58, SpO_2 88%, increased PAOP
(B) B/P 170/102, SpO_2 86%, decreased mean pulmonary artery pressure
(C) B/P 82/52, SpO_2 85%, increased alveolar dead space
(D) B/P 158/98, SpO_2 89%, decreased pulmonary vascular resistance (PVR)

133. A patient is receiving volume resuscitation. Which of the following would be indicative of successful resuscitation?

(A) cardiac index of 2.3 $L/min/m^2$
(B) CVP of 1 mmHg
(C) base deficit of 5 mmol/kg
(D) oxygen consumption of 225 $mL/min/m^2$

134. A definitive diagnosis of a pulmonary embolism is made with which of the following?

(A) a pulmonary angiogram
(B) a chest X-ray
(C) a ventilation/perfusion scan
(D) an arterial blood gas

135. A patient was admitted with multiple trauma and brief hypotension. The following day, the patient is hypertensive, tachycardic, and tachypneic with bilateral lung crackles. The BUN is 100 mg/dL, and the creatinine is 3.2 mg/dL. Which of the following should be the initial treatment?

(A) hemodialysis
(B) mannitol 25% IV
(C) hemofiltration
(D) a fluid bolus

136. What is the pathophysiology of sepsis that requires fluid resuscitation for all patients and, for many, vasopressors?

(A) impaired oxygen extraction and maldistribution of blood flow
(B) vasodilation and increased capillary permeability
(C) accelerated coagulation and microemboli formation
(D) pulmonary dysfunction and myocardial dysfunction

137. A patient has had a stormy course, with numerous complications, and she is manifesting signs of depression. Which of the following interventions is contraindicated for this patient?

(A) Force the patient to make decisions related to her care.
(B) Provide a safe environment.
(C) Encourage the patient to express her feelings.
(D) Involve family members and the patient's support system.

138. A patient sustained trauma from a fall down the basement stairs. Which of the following is the highest priority?

(A) Stabilize the cervical spine.
(B) Assess the blood pressure.
(C) Identify facial fractures.
(D) Initiate IV access.

139. A patient was admitted with an acute anterior wall MI and is now hypotensive, with sinus tachycardia, tachypnea with an SpO_2 of 0.89, lung crackles, an S3 heart sound, and restlessness. Which of the following interventions is anticipated at this time for this patient?

(A) a negative inotrope, antiarrhythmics, digoxin
(B) beta blockers, diuretics, aspirin
(C) a positive inotrope, vasodilators, diuretics
(D) adenosine, ACE inhibitors, calcium channel blockers

140. What positive hemodynamic effects do nitrates provide for chest pain secondary to coronary artery disease?

(A) They increase afterload and decrease the myocardial oxygen demand.
(B) They decrease afterload and increase myocardial contractility.
(C) They increase preload and increase myocardial contractility.
(D) They decrease preload and decrease the myocardial oxygen demand.

141. A patient with chronic alcoholism is at risk for which of the following?

(A) hyperkalemia
(B) hypomagnesemia
(C) hyperphosphatemia
(D) hyponatremia

142. A patient is admitted with chest pain. The ECG shows ST elevation in leads V1, V2, and V3. The day after admission, the patient developed a drop in blood pressure and a holosystolic murmur on the left sternal border, 5th intercostal space. The nurse suspects that this patient has developed:

(A) a ventricular septal defect.
(B) left ventricular failure.
(C) acute mitral valve regurgitation.
(D) right ventricular failure.

143. A 72-year-old patient who was admitted with pneumonia has a known history of Alzheimer's disease and is cared for by his daughter. The patient keeps trying to pull out his intravenous lines and get out of the bed. Which of the following interventions is most effective for maintaining this patient's safety?

(A) Maintain wrist restraints around the clock.

(B) Involve the family members in the patient's care for as many hours as possible.

(C) Request and order a psychotropic medication.

(D) Reorient the patient frequently, and remind him of the need for the intravenous lines.

144. A patient has a blood pressure of 150/96, a heart rate of 110 beats/minute, a respiratory rate of 32 breaths/minute, and an SpO_2 of 0.89. Auscultation reveals diminished breath sounds over the right lung fields, and tracheal deviation to the right is present. Which of the following interventions is the definitive treatment?

(A) Initiate oxygen and observe the response.

(B) Prepare for a right-sided needle thoracostomy.

(C) Call the provider for the insertion of an endotracheal tube.

(D) Prepare for a right-sided chest tube insertion.

145. Which of the following is a major effect of acute respiratory distress syndrome (ARDS)?

(A) decreased lung compliance

(B) increased alveolar surface area

(C) decreased capillary permeability

(D) increased oxygen delivery

146. A patient with a 3-year-long history of intermittent claudication is now complaining of left foot pain at rest. Which of the following assessment findings is likely, and which of the interventions is indicated?

(A) absent pulses, cool toes, edema; apply TED hose and SCDs

(B) an ankle-brachial index of 1.2, edema, pallor; elevate the left leg above the level of the heart

(C) a positive venous Doppler test, reddish color; apply warm compresses

(D) an ankle-brachial index of 0.8, minimal edema, cool toes; use reverse Trendelenburg

147. A patient is 3 hours status post percutaneous coronary intervention (PCI) with the successful deployment of a stent to the LAD coronary artery. The patient suddenly complains of low back pain, and a vital sign assessment reveals the following: a B/P of 82/58, heart sinus tachycardia of 122 beats/minute, and a respiratory rate of 28 breaths/minute. No bleeding is seen at the femoral insertion site. Which of the following has most likely occurred?

(A) retroperitoneal bleeding

(B) cardiac tamponade

(C) thoracic aneurysm dissection

(D) stent reocclusion

148. A physician ordered a propofol infusion to provide deep sedation for a patient immediately after the patient exhibited status epilepticus. What should the nurse anticipate this patient's response will be during deep sedation?

(A) The patient will respond normally to verbal commands.

(B) The patient will respond purposefully to verbal commands with light tactile stimulation.

(C) The patient will not be arousable to painful stimulation.

(D) The patient will respond purposefully to repeated or painful stimulation.

149. A patient with known alcohol abuse is admitted 2 weeks status post tendon repair due to a hand laceration. The patient is lethargic. The skin is warm and flushed. The surgical site is red, hard, and tender to touch. The patient's vital signs are as follows: a temperature of 39.2°C (102.6°F), a B/P of 78/39 (MAP 52), a heart rate of 130 beats/minute, and a respiratory rate of 24 breaths/minute. The nurse should anticipate that initial treatment will include which of the following?

(A) stat CBC, antipyretics, the rapid administration of fluids

(B) the administration of dopamine, a CT scan of the head, monitoring for alcohol withdrawal

(C) the rapid administration of isotonic fluids, antipyretics, the administration of vitamins

(D) blood cultures, antibiotics, the rapid administration of isotonic fluids

150. A patient is admitted with ST elevation in leads II, III, and aVF and an S4 heart sound at the apex. The patient developed hypotension; the lungs are clear. Which of the following is accurate regarding this patient?

(A) The patient most likely has an anterior myocardial infarction and requires pressors.

(B) The patient most likely has a right ventricular myocardial infarction and requires fluids.

(C) The patient most likely has an anterior myocardial infarction and requires positive inotropes.

(D) The patient most likely has an inferior myocardial infarction and requires afterload reduction.

ANSWER KEY
Practice Test 2

1.	D	39.	A	77.	C	115.	B
2.	C	40.	B	78.	D	116.	D
3.	D	41.	C	79.	D	117.	B
4.	A	42.	C	80.	A	118.	C
5.	C	43.	C	81.	C	119.	D
6.	D	44.	A	82.	A	120.	D
7.	B	45.	A	83.	C	121.	A
8.	A	46.	B	84.	B	122.	D
9.	B	47.	C	85.	A	123.	D
10.	A	48.	B	86.	B	124.	B
11.	C	49.	A	87.	B	125.	A
12.	C	50.	C	88.	D	126.	D
13.	B	51.	A	89.	B	127.	B
14.	B	52.	C	90.	C	128.	D
15.	B	53.	C	91.	A	129.	B
16.	D	54.	D	92.	B	130.	A
17.	B	55.	C	93.	D	131.	D
18.	A	56.	D	94.	C	132.	C
19.	D	57.	A	95.	B	133.	D
20.	C	58.	D	96.	A	134.	A
21.	C	59.	D	97.	C	135.	B
22.	B	60.	B	98.	C	136.	B
23.	A	61.	C	99.	C	137.	A
24.	A	62.	A	100.	D	138.	A
25.	D	63.	D	101.	C	139.	C
26.	C	64.	B	102.	B	140.	D
27.	B	65.	C	103.	B	141.	B
28.	B	66.	A	104.	B	142.	A
29.	D	67.	C	105.	B	143.	B
30.	B	68.	C	106.	D	144.	D
31.	B	69.	D	107.	D	145.	A
32.	A	70.	C	108.	B	146.	D
33.	A	71.	A	109.	D	147.	A
34.	B	72.	C	110.	C	148.	D
35.	B	73.	C	111.	C	149.	D
36.	A	74.	A	112.	C	150.	B
37.	A	75.	A	113.	A		
38.	D	76.	A	114.	A		

ANSWERS AND EXPLANATIONS

1. **(D)** This clinical picture is one of septic shock. The patient needs continued fluids and also vasopressors to restore vascular tone. The patient does not require a blood transfusion, since a transfusion is not indicated unless there is active bleeding or unless the hemoglobin is < 7.0 g/dL. Neither a reduction in the fluid rate nor preload reducers are indicated since the right and left ventricular preload is already low.

2. **(C)** Taking the initiative to collect accurate data will determine the scope of the problem, if there actually is one, and thus is the first step in getting additional support from key stakeholders. Choices (A) and (B) do not produce evidence of the problem. Although it is an attempt to produce data, choice (D) will not produce data that is as powerful as a 6-month retrospective analysis.

3. **(D)** Changes occur from "higher" to "lower" centers of the brain, cerebrum to brain stem. A change in the level of consciousness (LOC) is representative of higher (cerebrum) centers. Pupillary change is at the level of the transtentorial notch. Vital sign changes are the last to occur and are representative of brain stem compression.

4. **(A)** The qSOFA score is a bedside assessment that evaluates 3 criteria, assigning 1 point to each. The criteria include systolic B/P ≤ 100 mmHg, respiratory rate ≥ 22 breaths/minute, and Glasgow Coma Scale < 15 (altered mentation). A score of 2 or 3 indicates organ dysfunction. The remaining 3 choices do not meet these criteria.

5. **(C)** Nitroprusside (Nipride) is a potent dilator drug that decreases preload and afterload. This drug does not affect contractility and does not increase either PVR or preload.

6. **(D)** The leads that represent the inferior wall of the LV are II, III, and aVF. Therefore, acute changes would occur in 2 or more of these 3 leads. ST depression and positive troponin would be found in an NSTEMI of the inferior wall. Leads I and aVL represent the high lateral wall of the left ventricle. V2, V3, and V4 represent the anterior wall of the LV.

7. **(B)** Dementia is not caused by immobility during hospitalization; it is a chronic problem that develops over time. (Dementia, however, may **cause** immobility.) Immobility affects the neurological system, but it does so as delirium, which is an acute problem. The remaining choices **are** negative outcomes of immobility.

8. **(A)** If O_2, fluids, and a chest tube are rapidly initiated, intubation may not be needed, and pressors should not be used for this type of traumatic injury. There are no signs of cardiac tamponade. Although surgery may be needed later, the immediate need is not surgery based on the information provided.

9. **(B)** Trauma (such as a pelvic fracture), when stabilization of the injury is important, is an indication of the need for an indwelling urinary catheter. The remaining choices are not indications for a urinary catheter.

10. **(A)** The physical exertion increases glucose utilization and decreases insulin requirements, which results in hypoglycemia. Hypoglycemia increases adrenaline production (tachycardia) and affects brain cells, resulting in mental status changes.

11. **(C)** The massive fluid shifts may result in hypovolemic shock. Pancreatic enzyme release does not result in diuresis. Acute pancreatitis results in hypocalcemia, not hypercalcemia. Pancreatitis results in hyperglycemia, not hypoglycemia.

12. **(C)** This patient received heparin during the procedure, had inadequate heparin reversal, and needs the agent that reverses heparin. Heparin will further prolong the PTT. Vitamin K is the reversal agent for warfarin. There is no evidence that the patient's prolonged PTT is due to a deficiency of clotting factors and requires FFP.

13. **(B)** Chvostek sign causes twitching of facial muscles. Kernig's sign, due to meningeal irritation, results in hamstring pain when the leg is straightened. Cullen's sign is discoloration around the umbilicus, a sign of retroperitoneal bleeding.

14. **(B)** Information that demonstrates a decreased length of patient stay will reduce costs. Knowledge of the protocol does not demonstrate financial benefit. Although outlining favorable patient outcomes is an important selling point, it does not demonstrate financial benefit. Ensuring the support of unit key stakeholders is important, but doing so does not necessarily address the financial benefit.

15. **(B)** Although the pulmonary edema of heart failure may trigger bronchospasm, resulting in wheezing, there would also be pulmonary crackles. Although steroids are used for an asthma exacerbation, bronchodilators are a higher priority. Diuretics are not used for bronchospasm but, rather, for pulmonary edema and fluid overload.

16. **(D)** A vital capacity of at least 3 L/min indicates the strength to support independent ventilation. The remaining 3 choices are not predictive of successful weaning.

17. **(B)** Pressure support (PS) assists the inspiratory phase of spontaneous breathing (the degree of support depends upon the PS setting) and decreases the work of breathing. It does not decrease the oxygen requirements or the tidal volume requirements. Pressure support may prevent tiring of the diaphragm, but choice (C) does not specify this muscle.

18. **(A)** ATN does not result in alkalosis, and anemia is usually seen in chronic renal failure. The blood pressure may be high or low with ATN. Therefore, the B/P is not a definitive sign of ATN. ATN generally results in high electrolyte levels, not low magnesium and potassium levels.

19. **(D)** Lung aspiration will result in increased airway secretions that will cause an increase in the peak inspiratory pressure. Due to the shorter, straighter right mainstem bronchus, most aspirations occur in the right lung, not bilaterally. The minute ventilation would be expected to increase (not decrease) due to an increase (not a decrease) in the respiratory rate. The negative inspiratory force would most likely drop, not increase.

20. **(C)** Although the renal function and the potential development of rhabdomyolysis should be monitored, these are not **initial** interventions. Respiratory depression with a need for intubation is not a common effect of a methamphetamine overdose, and naloxone is not an antidote.

21. **(C)** CVVH does remove some body waste products (although it is not as efficient as hemodialysis). However, CVVH is mainly used for a critically ill, unstable patient who may not tolerate hemodialysis. CVVH provides for the replacement of fluids as needed to the vasculature. It may indirectly prevent a life-threatening electrolyte imbalance, although close electrolyte monitoring during CVVH is needed in order to prevent a severe imbalance. Choice (B) describes plasmapheresis. The purpose of CVVH is not to increase the colloid oncotic pressure.

22. **(B)** Pupillary changes are due to compression of the oculomotor nerve, cranial nerve (CN) III. CN II does not affect the pupil response. CN II is the optic nerve, which is responsible for vision. If CN II is damaged, the result may be homonymous hemianopsia. CN V is the trigeminal nerve (corneal reflex), and CN IX is the glossopharyngeal nerve (gag reflex).

23. **(A)** Viral meningitis will not lower the CSF glucose, but bacterial meningitis will. The remaining 3 choices may be seen with both bacterial meningitis and viral meningitis.

24. **(A)** The PaO_2 to FiO_2 ratio is < 200 for a patient with ARDS, as choice (A) demonstrates. (Additionally, the patient would need to meet the other criteria for ARDS.) An ARDS patient would not have normal mixed venous oxygen. The oxygen would be low. The PaO_2 to FiO_2 ratio in choice (C) is 310, which is too high for ARDS. An A-a gradient of 8 mmHg is normal and would not be seen in the presence of ARDS.

25. **(D)** This patient's history of Class IV heart failure and septic shock, along with her current wish to not pursue aggressive therapy, suggest that a hospice consult would now be appropriate. Home health alone (choice (A)) would not meet all of the patient and family needs at this time. Palliative care (choice (B)) is appropriate for patients for whom aggressive therapy is still an option. There are no ethical issues described in this scenario. Therefore, an ethics consult (choice (C)) is not needed.

26. **(C)** Choice (A) describes peritonitis. Choice (B) describes appendicitis. Choice (D) describes acute pancreatitis.

27. **(B)** If the serum lactate is > 2 mmol/L, a second serum lactate is needed in 2–4 hours. If this second serum lactate is still greater than 2 mmol/L and the MAP is 65 mmHg or less, septic shock is present, and vasopressors should be initiated. Also, if the second serum lactate is > 4 mmol/L and the MAP remains below 65 mmHg, the fluid status needs to be evaluated to see if the patient would benefit from ongoing aggressive fluid administration. The remaining choices are not accurate.

28. **(B)** This clinical picture is one of cardiogenic shock. A positive inotrope (dopamine 5 to 10 mcg/kg/min, not a high dose) will increase contractility. A diuretic (usually given after the positive inotrope) will decrease LV preload. A vasodilator will decrease LV afterload. All of these will increase the coronary artery perfusion and the cardiac output. The remaining choices include negative inotropic agents that may make the shock worse. Antiarrhythmics are not needed.

29. **(D)** Atrial fibrillation, diastolic murmur, and giant V-waves are not clinical signs of status asthmaticus.

30. **(B)** Vasopressin is ADH, and there is excessive ADH production in SIADH. Therefore, the administration of vasopressin is contraindicated in the treatment of SIADH. Hypertonic saline and diuretics may be indicated in order to treat the hyponatremia and fluid overload. Fluid restriction, especially free water, is indicated. Phenytoin may be ordered since it decreases the production of ADH.

31. **(B)** Fibrinolytic therapy is indicated if the patient presents within 4.5 hours of symptom onset. Once this is established, contraindications for fibrinolytic therapy are identified, and then a more comprehensive history is obtained.

32. **(A)** When using a translator, the patient needs to know that the information is coming from the nurse through the translator, and the nurse needs to stay physically present. Refrain from using medical jargon when communicating with patients, directly or through a translator, in order to avoid creating a misunderstanding. If the patient does not know English, there is no point in speaking English. Although using gestures may be helpful when the translator is not present, it is not adequate for providing an overview of the plan of care. It is **not** advisable to use a family member as a translator since subjectivity may enter the translation. Additionally, when using a translator, give small bits of information, stop and allow the translation, and then resume with more information in order to prevent any omissions of information.

33. **(A)** This patient has an acute anterior wall MI, which is usually caused by an LAD plaque rupture. LAD occlusion may lead to interventricular septal ischemia/necrosis and a VSD. This patient has ST elevation and deep Q-waves, signs of a myocardial infarction; acute ischemia results in ST depression or T-wave inversion, not ST elevation. An acute anterior wall MI does not cause cardiac tamponade or papillary muscle dysfunction.

34. **(B)** The history and clinical picture reflect a thyroid storm, most likely precipitated by the initiation of hydrochlorothiazide (HCTZ). This patient will need beta blocker therapy to control the effects of elevated thyroid hormone on the heart, and discontinuation of the HCTZ. While cooling measures are appropriate, the use of aspirin may inhibit T3 and T4 binding and further aggravate the hyperthyroidism. Therefore, choice (A) is incorrect. Levothyroxine will worsen the problem and is contraindicated. Therefore, choice (C) is incorrect. There is no indication of hypotension, for which glucocorticoids might be used, and there is no evidence of a need for 3% saline. Therefore, choice (D) is also incorrect.

35. **(B)** Whispering may trigger paranoia. Touch may aggravate the symptoms. Logical explanations are not especially useful for a patient with DTs.

36. **(A)** Cardiogenic shock will cause a very low cardiac index. The left heart pressure (PAOP) would be elevated, not normal as in choice (B). The SvO_2 would be low, not elevated as in choice (C). The SVR would be elevated, not normal as in choice (D).

37. **(A)** The volume depletion that is associated with a hemorrhage results in factitious dehydration (high BUN and sodium). As the volume is restored, the BUN and sodium will normalize.

38. **(D)** The PEEP setting of 5 cm H_2O is too low for the treatment of ARDS, so there is an opportunity to adjust this setting. Since PEEP is still quite low, there would not be a need to increase an already high FiO_2 setting. Permissive hypercapnia is expected and tolerated quite well for a patient with ARDS since the tidal volume needs to be kept low (permissive hypercapnia). Therefore, choices (B) and (C) would not be good interventions.

39. **(A)** The chief characteristic of distributive shock (septic, anaphylactic, neurogenic) is massive vasodilation, which results in a low SVR. Although the other choices are associated with distributive shock, they may also be seen in hypovolemic shock.

40. **(B)** Surfactant prevents alveolar collapse. Surfactant is produced by the Type II alveolar cells, not the Type I alveolar cells. Surfactant decreases, not increases, the work of breathing. Surfactant increases, not decreases, lung compliance, thereby decreasing the work of breathing.

41. **(C)** There is an increased loss of potassium with the use of thiazide diuretics. Additionally, chloride is lost. When chloride is lost, the renal tubules reabsorb bicarbonate, which may lead to metabolic alkalosis. Vomiting and diarrhea may cause hypokalemia. However, the use of ACE inhibitors, crush injuries, hemolysis, and acidosis (metabolic) may all lead to hyperkalemia.

42. **(C)** Immediate nurse engagement to correct the research staff member's omission of providing information to the patient and his family will be most effective for all sides. Involvement of the ethics committee may be needed at a later time. Eventually, a discussion with the primary investigator will need to occur. Right now, though, nurse engagement is the best strategy. Choice (D) is passive and is not best for the patient or his family.

43. **(C)** Medications and sleep deprivation may cause the signs that this patient is experiencing. Environmental stimulation, isolation, and benzodiazepines increase the incidences of delirium in elderly patients. Benzodiazepines may be used for this population if other strategies are not effective or if immediate patient safety is an issue.

44. **(A)** The family still desires full therapy, and the patient now requires an increase in the FiO_2 in order to maintain oxygenation. The nurse needs to advocate for the family's wishes, and a discussion between the nurse and the physician is the first step. Keeping the FiO_2 at 40% would not be honest because the family still wants full therapy. Advising the family to speak with the physician is a passive approach. Choice (D) is palliative care, but that is not the family's choice at this time.

45. **(A)** This patient has cardiac tamponade, as evidenced by equilibration of the right and left heart pressures and a narrowing pulse pressure. This question is more challenging in that the usual signs of cardiac tamponade (bulging neck veins, distant heart sounds, a widening mediastinum, pulsus paradoxus) are not provided. Antibiotics are not indicated since there is no indication of a bacterial infection or sepsis (since the hemodynamics are not reflective of sepsis). Pressors would increase an already high SVR (afterload) and increase the work of the heart. Fluids are not indicated for a patient with an elevated RAP and an elevated PAOP. The etiology of cardiac tamponade may be a viral infection that led to a pericardial effusion, resulting in tamponade.

46. **(B)** If the aortic valve is unable to close completely, when the IAB inflates during diastole, blood will go backward into the left ventricle, which would not provide the desired hemodynamic benefits. IABP therapy may be done with any of the other conditions.

47. **(C)** A patient with a lip ulcer post-extubation had an endotracheal tube that caused pressure to the lip; this would be classified as a pressure injury (PI). Diabetic venous ulcers (choice (A)), a knee abrasion after a fall (choice (B)), and a skin tear due to tape removal (choice (D)) are not caused by pressure. Therefore, they are not pressure injuries.

48. **(B)** Due to increased left heart pressures, the left atrium often enlarges and predisposes the patient to atrial fibrillation. Heart failure is also associated with ventricular tachycardia (but not ventricular bigeminy). However, VT is not a choice. As a result of the predisposition to VT, the patient may qualify for an ICD device. Third-degree AV block and atrial tachycardia are not specifically associated with heart failure.

49. **(A)** It is best to explore the source of the patient's point of view and then address it. The remaining choices are not as effective.

50. **(C)** Communication through one designated person is most efficient for the nursing staff, and this family decision can be passed on from shift to shift. It is not best practice for the nurse to defer family communication to other health care team members. Choice (D) does not provide the family with sufficient information and is open to many interpretations.

51. **(A)** This patient, who most likely had excessive bleeding during the complicated delivery with resultant consumption of clotting factors, has signs of early DIC. A prolonged PT and a positive D-dimer would help confirm this diagnosis. Although elevated FSP is the most definitive lab test for DIC, the creatinine level would not be helpful. The Pitocin, magnesium, BUN, and factor X levels are not definitive tests for DIC.

52. **(C)** This patient is having episodes of torsades de pointes VT, a polymorphic VT, secondary to a prolonged QT interval. Magnesium is indicated in order to decrease the QT. Defibrillation may briefly return the rhythm to normal sinus rhythm, but without the administration of magnesium, the torsades de pointes VT arrhythmia will recur. Lidocaine and amiodarone will increase the QT and exacerbate the torsades VT (as will procainamide and any other drug that prolongs the QT). Since the torsades de pointes VT arrhythmia is not sustained, synchronized cardioversion is not indicated.

53. **(C)** Although acidosis results in an elevated serum potassium, the total body potassium is low in DKA due to fluid loss. This becomes evident as the acidosis is corrected. Therefore, potassium replacement needs to begin as soon as the serum potassium reaches "normal."

54. **(D)** The blood in the intestine results in the breakdown of protein, which will raise the serum NH_3, and the NH_3 further irritates the brain. The remaining three choices do not increase the NH_3 or worsen hepatic encephalopathy.

55. **(C)** The pacemaker is not effectively sensing the patient's own beats, and an increase in the sensitivity is needed. To increase the sensitivity, the sensitivity dial on the device is **decreased** so that the pacemaker will sense "smaller size" (the patient's ECG waves). The remaining three choices would not be helpful.

56. **(D)** When aggressive debridement fails to halt the progression of the fasciitis, life-saving amputation may need to be done. The choice of antibiotic is initially decided upon empirically, based on the patient's history and an evaluation, and then it is subsequently reevaluated based on the blood culture results. Vancomycin may be chosen, but it is not the antibiotic of choice for all cases. Thus, choice (A) is incorrect. Hyperbaric oxygen therapy has shown some benefits and may be implemented if it is available, but it is not required to improve the outcome. Thus, choice (B) is incorrect. If the patient develops septic shock, then a vasopressor should be administered. Thus, choice (C) is also incorrect.

57. **(A)** Hypertension, flat neck veins, and tracheal deviation to the affected side are not signs of a tension pneumothorax.

58. **(D)** This patient has signs of diabetes insipidus (DI). There is a deficiency of antidiuretic hormone (ADH) with large volume fluid loss, resulting in dehydration and potential

hypovolemic shock. Water loss will increase the serum sodium and the serum osmolality. The treatment is to provide what the patient is not able to produce—vasopressin. Additionally, the urine specific gravity will be very low. Phenytoin (Dilantin) may cause DI.

59. **(D)** Elevation of the head of the bed will allow venous outflow and help decrease the ICP. None of the other positions listed will prevent elevated ICP.

60. **(B)** The literature has demonstrated that learning CPR has been beneficial to families of patients who have sustained sudden cardiac death (SCD). The ability to provide CPR provides a sense of empowerment, and at times has saved a patient's life. Choice (A) may not be true. Choice (C) does not provide a sense of empowerment. Even if the family knows how and when to access the EMS system, early, effective CPR improves the outcome. Choice (D) is deferring nurse accountability.

61. **(C)** During end expiration, there is no interference from the thoracic pressure changes that are seen during inspiration. There is no evidence that obtaining measurements at the end of the T-wave or obtaining measurements every hour affects the accuracy of the measurements. The digital readout on the monitor may not always be accurate, especially in the presence of respiratory artifact. The printed waveform strip or an analysis of the waveform on the monitor using the scale is the most accurate method to determine hemodynamic readings.

62. **(A)** This patient has hypotension and hypoxemia, which are evidence of a massive PE. A pulmonary embolus prevents pulmonary perfusion, which results in dead space. The larger the PE is, the greater the degree of dead space. The D-dimer would be positive, not negative, since a clot is present. There are possible options other than mechanical ventilation and a pressor infusion, such as fibrinolytic therapy if the patient does not have contraindications. A PE results in increased dead space, not shunting. PEEP therapy is not indicated.

63. **(D)** A patient with an ANC of 480 cells/mcL has severe neutropenia, and a single oral temperature of 38.3°C (101.0°F) or a temperature greater than 38.0°C (100.4°F) that is sustained for more than 1 hour in a patient with neutropenia most likely indicates a neutropenic fever, which needs to be treated accordingly. In choices (A) and (C), the patient does not have severe neutropenia (severe neutropenia is defined as an ANC < 500 cells/mcL). The assessment described in choice (B) reflects severe neutropenia, but that assessment does not meet the temperature criteria for a neutropenic fever.

64. **(B)** A diagnosis of diabetes has not been linked with adrenal insufficiency. The remaining choices are potential etiologies of adrenal insufficiency/crisis.

65. **(C)** The mixed venous O_2 will drop in hypovolemic shock due to a drop in oxygen delivery. The left heart pressure will drop due to decreased venous return (left ventricular preload). The SVR will increase due to compensatory vasoconstriction.

66. **(A)** Considering central line necessity each day and the engagement of unit leadership are known strategies to reduce CLABSIs. The remaining choices put patients with central venous lines at a greater risk for CLABSIs.

67. **(C)** The refractory hypoxemia that is seen with ARDS/ALI results in an abnormally low pO_2. Poor oxygen utilization (VO_2), which is typical of septic shock, results in an elevated SvO_2.

68. **(C)** Do not use the SpO₂ to monitor the oxygenation status for a patient with CO poisoning. Positive-pressure ventilation (PPV) will not achieve the goal of therapy (a CO level that is returned to normal), and the LOC alone is not the endpoint of therapy.

69. **(D)** Initially, renal hypoperfusion results in prerenal failure. The renal tubules are not yet destroyed. Therefore, they will hold onto sodium (resulting in decreased urine sodium) and concentrate urine in an attempt to counteract the effects of decreased perfusion. After the renal tubular basement membrane is damaged (intrarenal failure), the tubules can no longer do the above. Urine sodium will be high, and urine osmolality will be low.

70. **(C)** The middle meningeal artery lies above the dura, a tough covering of the brain right under the temporal bone, and if the middle meningeal artery is traumatized the result is an arterial epidural bleed. The remaining choices are due to problems other than middle meningeal artery disruption.

71. **(A)** A fluctuation in mental status over the past 24 hours is a sign of delirium. Delirium is an acute problem, not a chronic one. Inattentiveness, not attentiveness, is a component of delirium. A history of word-finding difficulty is a sign of dementia.

72. **(C)** Acidosis secondary to hypoventilation will result in cerebral vasodilation that, in turn, will increase the ICP. Hypotonic fluids should be avoided due to their propensity for leaving the vascular space and increasing the ICP. Respiratory arrest should be avoided. Antibiotics are not given prophylactically for SAH.

73. **(C)** This patient is having an anteroseptal myocardial infarction, which is most often due to an occlusion of the left anterior descending (LAD) artery. This problem may affect perfusion to the common bundle of His of the conduction system, which may result in a second-degree AV block, Type II. (If the patient is symptomatic, he will most likely require transcutaneous pacing since atropine is not generally effective.) The remaining three choices are more often associated with an acute inferior wall MI, which is due to a right coronary artery occlusion and decreases perfusion to the SA and AV nodes.

74. **(A)** This patient has bradycardia secondary to high-grade, second-degree AV block, Type II, which often occurs due to a conduction defect of the bundle of His (not the AV node). The bundle of His is supplied by the LAD. Occlusion of the arteries described in the remaining three choices would not usually lead to a second-degree AV block, Type II.

75. **(A)** Patients who have had bariatric surgery may have alteration in absorption, which results in vitamin deficiency. There is no indication for any of the other three choices.

76. **(A)** A patient with dilated cardiomyopathy has signs of systolic heart failure that would benefit from a reduction of LV preload (PAOP) and a decrease in afterload (decreased SVR). The other choices would either not benefit this patient or may actually cause harm.

77. **(C)** This patient seems to have developed acute heart failure that is severe enough to drop the B/P. Therefore, the cardiac output (CO) will drop. Afterload will increase in an attempt to compensate. The left heart pressure will be elevated due to the LV's inability to empty, which will result in an elevated pulmonary artery diastolic pressure.

78. **(D)** The immediate priority at this time is to prevent the patient from falling. Although the patient denies dizziness when standing and is able to get to the commode, walking assistance may be needed. The physician should be notified since she may want to adjust the medication dosage or provide other orders. However, this is not an emergency, so choice (A) is incorrect. There is no evidence of acute ischemia or a rhythm change. Therefore, a stat ECG is not required, which means that choice (B) is incorrect. The patient should be provided information about the effects of the medications, but the immediate need is to allow the patient to use the commode safely.

79. **(D)** Aldactone is a potassium-sparing diuretic that is used to prevent the hypokalemia that is associated with a thiazide diuretic. It is important to prevent hypokalemia in the presence of liver failure since a secondary acidosis may result. Patients with liver failure tend to develop hypoglycemia, not elevated blood glucose. Sedation should be avoided since it may mask encephalopathy. Lactated Ringer's may result in acidosis if the liver cannot metabolize the lactate. Therefore, 0.9 normal saline is the preferred isotonic solution.

80. **(A)** Although the wife will be grief-stricken, the knowledge that everything possible was done offers some comfort. (Do not say, "We did everything we could," without providing a few details.) Choice (B) may not meet the wife's needs (although it could be arranged if specifically requested). Although having the physician or chaplain present may provide the nurse with support, choices (C) and (D) may not be as effective as choice (A) is in terms of meeting the wife's needs.

81. **(C)** The water level in the water seal chamber should decrease during inspiration, as the pleural pressure increases, and rise back up to baseline during expiration. This fluctuation of the water level, known as "tidaling," indicates a normally functioning, patent chest tube. A pleural leak or a tension pneumothorax would result in bubbling in the water seal chamber. An intact connection to suction would be assessed by evaluating the suction chamber or suction indicator, not the negative-pressure water seal chamber.

82. **(A)** PEEP enables alveolar recruitment. Disconnecting the ventilator circuit from the ETT will result in massive derecruitment and hypoxemia. Even with an immediate reconnection, time will be needed for the hypoxemia to resolve. The remaining three choices are not beneficial strategies and may be harmful for a patient with ARDS/ALI.

83. **(C)** The remaining three choices do not typically present with bronchial breath sounds or whispered pectoriloquy.

84. **(B)** This patient has signs of rhabdomyolysis, a result of massive destruction of skeletal muscle cells. When these cells lyse, they release CK and intracellular potassium. None of the other choices is a typical result of rhabdomyolysis.

85. **(A)** An increase in the breath rate (or in the Vt) would decrease the pCO_2. The remaining choices have incorrect acid-base interpretations.

86. **(B)** This patient has septic shock. There is SIRS, organ dysfunction (hypotension), and an incomplete response to fluids, as evidenced by the B/P and the lactate after the initial administration of 30 mL/kg of isotonic fluids. The aggressive administration of fluids should be continued, and norepinephrine needs to be initiated. Dopamine is not a first-line agent for septic shock. The administration of blood is not indicated for

a patient who is not actively bleeding and has a hemoglobin of 9.1 gm/dL. A hypotonic solution, such as 0.45 normal saline, and the pressor phenylephrine are not indicated for septic shock.

87. **(B)** The ACE inhibitor may affect renal function, as evidenced by proteinuria and/or hyperkalemia (or elevated serum creatinine). The clinical signs listed in choices (A), (C), and (D) are not caused by ACE inhibitors.

88. **(D)** The clinical signs seem to be that of a basilar skull fracture. Clear drainage from the nose is most likely CSF, which should be allowed to drain. Nasogastric tube insertion may be dangerous in the presence of a skull fracture since the tube may get displaced to the brain. Suctioning or inserting nasal packing may result in an infection of the meninges.

89. **(B)** Hypovolemia needs to be avoided since it has been associated with a cerebral vasospasm post-aneurysm repair for SAH. The remaining three choices are not associated with a vasospasm.

90. **(C)** Guidelines for the treatment of agitation include "analgesia first." Pain is underappreciated in the medical population, and it is important to assess medical patients for pain, not just agitation, using a validated behavioral pain tool (e.g., BPS, CPOT). It is recommended to treat a BPS score of 5 or greater with an analgesic. Propofol (choice (A)) does not provide analgesia. There is no indication that the patient needs a chest X-ray (choice (B)) or an ABG (choice (D)).

91. **(A)** A left-sided problem will result in ipsilateral pupil change, eye deviation toward the problem, and contralateral vision and motor changes.

92. **(B)** It is important to increase the transit time of blood through the gut in order to prevent the breakdown of protein, which will increase the serum NH_3 and increase the chance of encephalopathy. Although octreotide may be used for GI bleeding, it is used for all types of GI bleeding, not only for those with hepatic failure. Lactated Ringer's may cause acidosis. Beta blockers have no special role in the treatment of GI bleeding or hepatic failure.

93. **(D)** Leads V5 and V6 represent the lower LV lateral wall, and leads I and aVL represent the higher lateral wall of the LV. PCI is generally preferred, but when that is not available, fibrinolytic therapy may be used for coronary reperfusion for a patient who meets the criteria. The remaining three choices are not correct.

94. **(C)** The mediastinal chest tube does **not** promote lung reexpansion. A mediastinal chest tube does not improve gas exchange. A transfusion would not be anticipated for a chest tube output of > 100 mL in 1 hour; rather, a transfusion would more likely be indicated for that same quantity of output for 2 consecutive hours.

95. **(B)** Pulmonary hypotension (choice (A)) and left ventricular failure (choice (D)) are not signs of cor pulmonale. There may be pulmonary edema if there is concomitant LV failure. However, the pulmonary edema would not be due to RV failure; rather, it would be due to LV failure. Thus, choice (C) is also incorrect.

96. **(A)** Although HHS generally has higher serum glucose than DKA, DKA may, at times, present with a serum glucose > 600 mg/dL. However, the serum osmolality is always elevated in HHS due to the higher fluid loss, whereas the serum osmolality in DKA may be normal or only slightly elevated. This is due to the fact that DKA develops more rapidly, and fluid loss occurs over a shorter period of time.

97. **(C)** A positive Brudzinski's sign and a positive Kernig's sign (along with nuchal rigidity) indicate meningeal irritation/infection. These signs are not typical of the remaining three choices.

98. **(C)** When all team members document on the same flow sheet, effective communication is more likely to occur. Choice (A) does not ensure that all members of the interdisciplinary team have access to the daily documentation or that they can participate in the daily care conferences. Choices (B) and (D) are less efficient and foster a "silo mentality" when planning patient care.

99. **(C)** These are signs of cardiac tamponade. Treatment for a medical patient would be emergent pericardiocentesis. Treatment for a post-op cardiac surgical patient would be an emergent return to the OR. The clinical picture described would not be seen with hypovolemia, diastolic heart failure, or cardiogenic shock.

100. **(D)** A shift of the oxyhemoglobin dissociation curve to the **left** will occur with alkalosis, a low pCO_2, a low temperature, or a low 2,3-DPG. Each of these prevents the release of O_2 from hemoglobin, which may slightly raise the SaO_2.

101. **(C)** Calcium is used in the autodigestive process in acute pancreatitis, which will decrease the serum calcium. Amylase is produced in the pancreas and increases with pancreatic inflammation. Protein may decrease due to increased capillary permeability caused by inflammation. Additionally, the serum glucose may increase due to beta 2 cell damage, the serum lipase increases, and the alkaline phosphatase rises, which make the other choices incorrect.

102. **(B)** About 3 hours after a decompression procedure, there may be tissue swelling due to altered capillary permeability. If this occurs, mannitol may be useful. Padding should not be added to the cast; the cast should be cut to loosen it. Thus, choice (A) is incorrect. The left arm should not be elevated since this will decrease arterial perfusion to the limb. Thus, choice (C) is incorrect. An emergent fasciotomy is generally not performed unless the compartment pressure is greater than 30 mmHg. Thus, choice (D) is also incorrect.

103. **(B)** The early initiation of antibiotics decreases the mortality of sepsis. Vasopressors are only indicated for sepsis that is not responsive to fluid resuscitation, which is then defined as septic shock. Steroids are not a primary intervention for sepsis. Antipyretics are provided for a fever, when present, but are not considered life-saving.

104. **(B)** Universal decolonization for MRSA and/or treating MRSA prophylactically for all ICU admissions has been shown to be effective in the prevention of MRSA in ICUs. Cleaning staff require special training, so choice (A) is incorrect. However, nurses need to be aware of the importance of environmental cleaning. Choices (C) and (D) have not been shown to prevent MDROs.

105. **(B)** A patient with septic shock has massive vasodilation (a low SVR). Due to low arterial resistance, the CO is initially high.

106. **(D)** Complete occlusion of a pulmonary vessel obstructs blood flow past the ventilated alveoli. It results in a mismatch of ventilation and perfusion. Gas exchange cannot occur. A PE is not an anatomic defect. Diffusion is not impeded. The pulmonary pressure increases, not decreases.

107. **(D)** A patient with rhabdomyolysis requires large volumes of 0.9 normal saline (an isotonic solution) and bicarbonate in some of the IV fluid in order to flush and buffer the renal tubules. The 0.45 normal saline is a hypotonic solution and will not adequately flush the renal tubules. Instead, it will rapidly leave the vascular compartment and get displaced intracellularly. The remaining three choices are appropriate interventions for this patient.

108. **(B)** The preceptor needs to do what is best for the patient in this emergency situation. Beginning chest compressions with the head of the bed elevated would not be the best intervention for the patient. Although the unit's code blue response needs to be initiated, the initial priority is to reposition the patient. Discussing the situation with the orientee at this moment is not correct. This needs to be done later, after the emergency.

109. **(D)** The most immediate need of a patient with a pelvic fracture is adequate nutrition and the prevention of malnutrition, which will delay recovery. Physical therapy and social services consults may be needed at a future time, but they are not immediate priorities. No information in the question indicates that the patient presented with a wound. Therefore, a wound care consultant is not indicated. Preventative measures should be instituted by nurses for all trauma patients.

110. **(C)** The continual firing of neurons in the brain tissue consumes a great deal of O_2. The brain does not store O_2. Therefore, hypermetabolism results in massive brain cell death. Although ventilation is not normal during a generalized tonic-clonic seizure, respiratory failure is addressed with intubation and would not be fatal. Although skeletal muscle breakdown may lead to hyperkalemia, which may in turn result in PEA, the continuous muscle activity can be controlled with clinical paralysis. Status epilepticus does not cause an intracranial hemorrhage.

111. **(C)** Monitoring the patient in his "fingerprint" lead will detect artery reocclusion. If acute groin bleeding occurs, it would require more than 5 minutes of manual pressure. Vasovagal response generally occurs during sheath removal. Acute back pain is a sign of possible retroperitoneal bleeding, which may occur post-PCI. However, interventions include a stat CT scan and fluids, not the interventions described in choice (D).

112. **(C)** These symptoms are typical of a dissecting thoracic aneurysm, which requires both B/P control and emergent surgery (regardless of the size of the aneurysm). The signs and symptoms are different for an abdominal aortic aneurysm and cardiac tamponade.

113. **(A)** Any patient who has been exposed to contrast media is at risk for nephropathy. Renal function should be closely monitored, especially for those at a high risk for contrast-induced nephropathy. The remaining three choices are not usually affected by an arteriogram.

114. **(A)** Guillain-Barré syndrome (GBS) results in ascending bilateral paralysis, and monitoring the patient's vital capacity will identify diaphragmatic involvement. An O_2 saturation decrease is a late sign of hypoventilation. Pupil monitoring is done for a change in the ICP, which is not typical of GBS. A temperature change is not typical of GBS.

115. **(B)** Potassium chloride is a vesicant, and the appropriate antidote is hyaluronidase along with warm compresses, which will facilitate diffusion and the absorption of fluids from the affected area. Cold compresses are not used with hyaluronidase, which makes choice (C) incorrect. Phentolamine (Regitine) is not indicated for a potassium chloride

extravasation, but phentolamine is used for an extravasation of pressor agents. Since phentolamine is not the appropriate antidote in this situation, choices (A) and (D) are incorrect. Choice (A) is also incorrect because when phentolamine is used warm compresses (not cold compresses) are indicated.

116. **(D)** It is best to determine what specifically is causing anxiety rather than begin an explanation that may further confuse the patient's wife and increase her anxiety. Choice (A) is too vague and will most likely not reduce the wife's anxiety. Choice (B) will be problematic since many times the alarms are false and are not a sign of patient deterioration. Although choice (C) is an attempt to reassure the wife, it might not directly relate to the wife's concerns.

117. **(B)** This patient, who would have had heparin for the PE, has signs of heparin-induced thrombocytopenia (HIT). The first intervention is to stop all heparin to prevent progression of the problem. Infusing platelets is only indicated for active bleeding or extremely low platelets (a platelet count of ∼ 10,000). Although the ELISA test may be ordered, the decision to discontinue heparin should not be delayed until the ELISA results are available. A direct thrombin inhibitor will be needed, but all heparin must be stopped first.

118. **(C)** Dysphagia precautions include assisting the patient with meals to ensure that aspiration does not occur during oral intake. It is unlikely that a patient who requires dysphagia precautions would be served meat that requires cutting. Therefore, choice (A) is incorrect. This patient would most likely not be ready to independently drink water, and he may even require thickened water. Therefore, choice (B) is incorrect. Serving meals on time is desired but not essential for a patient who is on dysphagia precautions. Therefore, choice (D) is also incorrect.

119. **(D)** There is increased production of antidiuretic hormone with SIADH, resulting in a drop in the urine output. As a result, there is a dilutional hyponatremia, a sodium loss in urine, and a drop in the serum osmolality due to fluid retention.

120. **(D)** Hemorrhagic pancreatitis may result in retroperitoneal bleeding. Cullen's sign is not typical of the other 3 problems.

121. **(A)** Exploring how the patient has met past life challenges will assist the patient in identifying coping mechanisms. Choices (B) and (D) may give the patient hope, but they may not assist the patient in identifying coping strategies. Choice (C) may not be warranted at this time.

122. **(D)** Altered coagulation may occur due to platelet dysfunction at lower body temperatures. The remaining choices are not expected during the induction phase of TTM. Rather, hyperglycemia, hypokalemia, and decreased cardiac output are the expected physiological changes due to hypothermia.

123. **(D)** Hyperoxygenation will prevent potential adverse effects of hypoxemia during the suctioning procedure. The remaining three choices are contraindicated for the situation described.

124. **(B)** The total body fluid loss results in intracellular dehydration of the brain cells, which results in mental status changes. The other three choices have little or no effect on mental status changes. They affect other organ systems.

125. **(A)** This patient has a right-sided brain abnormality. An acute increase in the ICP will cause a sudden pupil change on the side of the problem. Weakness since admission is not a sign of an acute change. A unilateral headache is not an ominous sign for a patient with a brain tumor. A facial bruise may have occurred during the seizure, but it is not as ominous as a pupil change.

126. **(D)** Adults learn best when they understand the importance of and the reason for the need to learn. Choice (A) is not a proven fact. Choice (B) is not true. A complex procedure should be broken down into several sessions in order to prevent sensory overload, which impedes learning. Adults (as well as children) have various preferred learning styles (written, auditory, kinesthetic). Therefore, the same approach cannot be used for all individuals. A combination of written, auditory, and kinesthetic (hands-on) learning styles may be best.

127. **(B)** Hypermagnesemia may result in hypotension. It may also cause depressed reflexes, not hyperreflexia, and it may cause bradyarrhythmias, not SVT. Hypermagnesemia may result in hypoventilation, not tachypnea.

128. **(D)** The extremely elevated peak inspiratory pressure reflects bronchospasm. The relatively normal plateau pressure reflects that the problem is not at the lung level.

129. **(B)** The inflamed pancreas may result in elevation of the diaphragm, left lower lobe atelectasis, bilateral crackles, and even ARDS. The patient needs a close lung assessment. Antibiotics and gastric decompression are not needed for most patients. The patient does need opiate drugs for the severe pain, even though all opiates may constrict the sphincter of Oddi. This constriction is not going to worsen the pain, as was thought in years past.

130. **(A)** Daily aspirin therapy is required for life for all patients who have had TAVR. Clopidogrel will also be prescribed, but only for a limited time of 3 to 6 months post-procedure. Access for the procedure is most often achieved via the femoral artery, not the subclavian artery. Thus, choice (B) is incorrect. Ideal candidates are those with severe aortic valve disease and those who are classified as high risk for an open procedure. Thus, choice (C) is incorrect. Paravalvular regurgitation can occur, but it is not a common complication of TAVR. Thus, choice (D) is also incorrect.

131. **(D)** Hyperventilation results from direct stimulation of the respiratory center by the salicylic acid. Increased bicarbonate excretion results in metabolic acidosis.

132. **(C)** There is increased dead space ventilation with a pulmonary embolism (PE) since there is ventilation without perfusion. Additionally, with a massive PE, hypotension and hypoxemia are present due to the severity of the pulmonary hypertension and the degree of V/Q mismatch. The PAOP is a left heart pressure, and it does not increase with a PE. The mean PA pressure increases with a massive PE. It does not decrease. The PVR increases (not decreases). Hypertension is not a clinical indicator of a massive PE.

133. **(D)** Successful volume resuscitation would result in normal oxygen consumption/ utilization. The remaining three choices would not indicate that the target has been reached during volume resuscitation.

134. **(A)** Although not often done due to its invasiveness, only an angiogram allows visualization of the occluded vessel. A PE does not alter the chest X-ray in any specific,

unique manner. A V/Q scan demonstrates a perfusion defect. However, COPD may also cause perfusion defects due to alveolar destruction. Although the ABG may be altered, there is no finding that is specific for a PE.

135. **(B)** Administering diuretics in order to "challenge" the kidneys is an initial treatment for acute renal failure (as long as obstructions and hypotension are not present). An isotonic fluid bolus may also be given initially as long as there are no signs of fluid overload. In this case, the patient does have signs of fluid overload. Hemodialysis may be needed if initial interventions are not effective. Hemofiltration (or continuous renal replacement therapy (CRRT)) may be used if the initial treatment is not effective for a patient with hypotension.

136. **(B)** The inflammatory response due to the release of mediators of endotoxins causes massive vasodilation with decreased systemic vascular resistance. The administration of fluids addresses these effects by "filling up" the larger "space" in the vasculature, and vasopressors help restore vascular tone. The increased capillary permeability results in a loss of fluid from the vascular space, and fluid resuscitation helps restore vascular volume. The remaining pathophysiological processes that are described in choices (A), (C), and (D) may be caused by the inflammatory response that is associated with sepsis, but fluids and pressors are not intended to directly address these issues.

137. **(A)** A patient with signs and symptoms of clinical depression has trouble making decisions. Forcing the patient to make decisions may increase her anxiety and anger and is not therapeutic. The remaining three choices have been shown to be effective interventions for depression and are indicated.

138. **(A)** If a patient sustained any injury at all to the cervical spine, any movement will worsen the injury and may lead to respiratory arrest secondary to paralysis. All of the other choices will need to be dealt with, but they are not as important as cervical spine stabilization.

139. **(C)** This clinical picture is one of extreme heart failure: cardiogenic shock. The patient needs an increase in contractility (a positive inotrope), a decrease in preload (diuretics), and a decrease in afterload (vasodilators). Providing a positive inotrope first (perhaps dopamine) will help increase the B/P, and then the other 2 agents can be given. Negative inotropes and antiarrhythmics are not indicated and may even be harmful. Aspirin is not an agent that is used for cardiogenic shock. Beta blockers and calcium channel blockers are negative inotropes and are not indicated.

140. **(D)** Nitrates dilate the venous bed, which decreases left ventricular preload. In turn, this decreases the myocardial workload. Nitrates do not increase afterload. They mildly decrease afterload at higher doses, but they do not directly affect contractility either positively or negatively. Nitrates do not increase preload; vasoconstriction or fluids have this effect.

141. **(B)** A chronic alcohol abuser is at risk for low magnesium due to a poor nutritional status and due to the effect of alcohol on the proximal renal tubules, which prevents the reabsorption of magnesium. There is also a risk for low potassium, phosphate, and calcium.

142. **(A)** A VSD is associated with an anteroseptal MI and hypotension due to a drop in the cardiac output and due to the murmur as described. LV failure generally results in an S3 heart sound and lung crackles. Mitral valve regurgitation results in a systolic murmur at the apex. RV failure will not result in the murmur described in the question.

143. **(B)** A patient with dementia needs familiarity to minimize agitated behavior and to feel safe. Therefore, family involvement is highly recommended. Restraints will increase anxiety and fear. Non-pharmacological solutions are always preferable to pharmacological ones. Reorientation is more effective for delirium, whereas it is not very effective for dementia.

144. **(D)** This patient has a right pneumothorax. The initiation of oxygen will resolve the hypoxemia, but it is not the definitive treatment. A needle thoracostomy is not indicated for this patient; it is indicated for a tension pneumothorax. However, this patient does not have signs of a tension pneumothorax (hypotension, tracheal deviation away from the side of the lung collapse). The insertion of an endotracheal tube will not resolve this patient's problem.

145. **(A)** In ARDS, the Type II alveolar cells no longer produce the surfactant that is needed to prevent alveolar collapse. With massive atelectasis, lung compliance and the functional residual capacity drop. The alveolar surface area decreases (not increases). Capillary permeability increases (not decreases), which results in pulmonary edema. In addition, O_2 delivery decreases due to severe hypoxemia. It does not increase.

146. **(D)** This patient's peripheral artery disease (PAD) is worsening. The ankle-brachial index is abnormal (it should be > 1), and perfusion to the foot may be aided by keeping the extremity down. Each of the remaining choices has clinical signs that are not typical of PAD or interventions that are not beneficial.

147. **(A)** The low back pain that is associated with hypotension after the PCI procedure, which involved a puncture of the femoral artery, is indicative of retroperitoneal bleeding. The remaining problems would not present with the same signs and symptoms.

148. **(D)** During deep sedation, the patient responds purposefully to repeated or painful stimulation. Choice (A) describes light sedation. Choice (B) describes a moderate level of sedation. Choice (C) describes general anesthesia.

149. **(D)** This patient has signs of sepsis. The interventions described in the other three choices are not all indicated for sepsis.

150. **(B)** The ECG changes are indicative of an acute inferior wall MI, which has a higher probability for an RV myocardial infarction than any other type of STEMI. When the RV infarct is large, it results in RV failure with decreased perfusion to the left side of the heart. This, in turn, causes hypotension with clear lungs and is treated with fluids and pressors (if fluids alone are not effective). This patient is not having an anterior MI. Afterload reduction would exacerbate this patient's symptoms and is not indicated.

References

19

AACN. "Practice Alerts: Assessing Pain in Critically Ill Adults," published December 1, 2018. *www.aacn.org/practicealerts*, accessed February 6, 2020.

AACN. "Practice Alerts: Assessment and Management of Delirium Across the Life Span," *Critical Care Nurse*, 2016: 36: e14–e19.

AACN. "Practice Alerts: Assessment and Management of Delirium Across the Life Span, Evidence Update," published October 1, 2016 (Evidence Update: October 1, 2018). *www.aacn.org/practicealerts*, accessed February 6, 2020.

AACN. "Practice Alerts: Family Presence: Visitation in the Adult ICU," published February 1, 2016. *www.aacn.org/practicealerts*, accessed February 6, 2020.

AACN. "Practice Alerts: Initial and Ongoing Verification of Feeding Tube Placement in Adults," published April 1, 2016 (Evidence Update: January 29, 2020). *www.aacn.org/practicealerts*, accessed February 6, 2020.

AACN. "Practice Alerts: Oral Care for Acutely and Critically Ill Patients," published June 1, 2017. *www.aacn.org/practicealerts*, accessed February 6, 2020.

AACN. "Practice Alerts: Prevention of Aspiration in Adults," published February 1, 2016 (Evidence Update: May 17, 2018). *www.aacn.org/practicealerts*, accessed February 6, 2020.

AACN. "Practice Alerts: Prevention of CAUTI in Adults," published July 31, 2016. *www.aacn.org/practicealerts*, accessed February 6, 2020.

AACN. "Practice Alerts: Ventilator Associated Pneumonia VAP," published June 1, 2016. *www.aacn.org/practicealerts*, accessed February 6, 2020.

Adler, L., Yi, D., Li, M., et al. "Impact of Inpatient Harms on Hospital Finances and Patient Clinical Outcomes," *Journal of Patient Safety*, 2018: 14(2): 67–73.

American Association of Blood Banks (AABB). *Standards for Blood Banks and Transfusion Services, 28th Edition,* 2012.

American Heart Association. *Advanced Cardiovascular Life Support Provider Manual, 16th Edition,* 2016.

Brewer, B.B., Wojner-Alexandrov, A.W., Triola, N., et al. "AACN Synergy Model's Characteristics of Patients: Psychometric Analyses in a Tertiary Care Health System," *American Journal of Critical Care*, 2007: 16(2): 158–167.

Burns, S.M. and Delgado, S.A. *AACN Essentials of Critical Care Nursing, 4th Edition*, 2018.

Devlin, J.W., Skrobik, Y., Gélinas, C., et al. "Executive Summary: Clinical Practice Guidelines for the Prevention and Management of Pain, Agitation/Sedation, Delirium, Immobility, and Sleep Disruption in Adult Patients in the ICU," *Critical Care Medicine*, 2018: 46(9): 1532–1548.

Duh, S.H. and Cook, J.D. "Laboratory Reference Range Values," Stedman's Online, *www.stedmansonline.com/webFiles/Dict-Stedmans28/APP17.pdf*, accessed June 17, 2014.

Frat, J.P., Coudroy, R., Marjanovic, N., et al. "High-Flow Nasal Oxygen Therapy and Noninvasive Ventilation in the Management of Acute Hypoxemic Respiratory Failure," *Annals of Translational Medicine*, 2017: 5(14): 297–305.

Gasparis Vonfrolio, L. *CCRN Certification Examination Review Cram—Audio CDs*, 2012.

Haight, K. "Caring for Patients After Transcatheter Aortic Valve Replacement," *American Nurse Today*, 2017: 12(8): 10–16.

Hartjes, T.M. (editor). *AACN Core Curriculum for High Acuity, Progressive, and Critical Care Nursing, 7th Edition*, 2017.

Jorgensen, A.L. "Nurse Influence in Meeting Compliance With the Centers for Medicare and Medicaid Services Quality Measure: Early Management Bundle, Severe Sepsis/Septic Shock (SEP-1)," *Dimensions of Critical Care Nursing*, 2019: 38(2): 70–82.

Kleinman, M.E., Brennan, E.E., Goldberger, Z.D., et al. "2015 American Heart Association Guidelines Update for Cardiopulmonary Resuscitation and Emergency Cardiovascular Care: Part 5: Adult Basic Life Support and Cardiopulmonary Resuscitation Quality," *American Heart Association*, 2015: 132: S414–S435.

Levy, M.M., Fink, M.P., Marshall, J.C., et al. "2001 SCCM/ESICM/ACCP/ATS/SIS International Sepsis Definitions Conference," *Critical Care Medicine*, 2003: 31(4): 1250–1256.

Lo, E., Nicolle, L.E., Coffin, S.E., et al. "Strategies to Prevent Catheter-Associated Urinary Tract Infections in Acute Care Hospitals: 2014 Update," *Infection Control and Hospital Epidemiology*, 2014: 35(5): 464–479.

Marschall, J., Mermel, L.A., Fakih, M., et al. "Strategies to Prevent Central Line-Associated Bloodstream Infections in Acute Care Hospitals: 2014 Update," *Infection Control and Hospital Epidemiology*, 2014: 35(7): 753–771.

McClave, S.A., Taylor, B.E., Martindale, R.G., et al. "Guidelines for the Provision and Assessment of Nutrition Support Therapy in the Adult Critically Ill Patient: Society of Critical Care Medicine (SCCM) and American Society for Parenteral and Enteral Nutrition (A.S.P.E.N.)," *Journal of Parenteral and Enteral Nutrition*, 2016: 40(2): 159–211.

Mion, L.C. "Physical Restraint in Critical Care Settings: Will They Go Away?" *Geriatric Nursing*, 2008: 29(6): 421–423.

Otto, C., Kumbhani, D., Alexander, K., et al. "2017 ACC Expert Consensus Decision Pathway for Transcatheter Aortic Valve Replacement in the Management of Adults With Aortic Stenosis," *Journal of the American College of Cardiology*, 2017: 69(10): 1313–1346.

Singer, M., Deutschman, C.S., Seymour, C.W., et al. "The Third International Consensus Definitions for Sepsis and Septic Shock (Sepsis-3)," *JAMA*, 2016: 315(8): 801–810.

Society of Thoracic Surgeons Blood Conservation Guideline Task Force, Ferraris, V.A., Brown, J.R., et al. "2011 Update to the Society of Thoracic Surgeons and the Society of Cardiovascular Anesthesiologists Blood Conservation Clinical Practice Guidelines," *The Annals of Thoracic Surgery*, 2011: 91(3): 944–982.

Vincent, J.L., de Mendonça, A., Cantraine, F., et al. "Use of the SOFA Score to Assess the Incidence of Organ Dysfunction/Failure in Intensive Care Units: Results of a Multicenter, Prospective Study. Working Group on "Sepsis-Related Problems" of the European Society of Intensive Care Medicine," *Critical Care Medicine*, 1998: 26(11): 1793–1800.

Wiegand, D.L. *AACN Procedure Manual for High Acuity, Progressive, and Critical Care, 7th Edition*, 2016.